Mental Health in Historical Perspective

Series Editors

Catharine Coleborne, School of Humanities and Social Science, University of Newcastle, Callaghan, NSW, Australia

Matthew Smith, Centre for the Social History of Health and Healthcare, University of Strathclyde, Glasgow, UK

Covering all historical periods and geographical contexts, the series explores how mental illness has been understood, experienced, diagnosed, treated and contested. It will publish works that engage actively with contemporary debates related to mental health and, as such, will be of interest not only to historians, but also mental health professionals, patients and policy makers. With its focus on mental health, rather than just psychiatry, the series will endeavour to provide more patient-centred histories. Although this has long been an aim of health historians, it has not been realised, and this series aims to change that.

The scope of the series is kept as broad as possible to attract good quality proposals about all aspects of the history of mental health from all periods. The series emphasises interdisciplinary approaches to the field of study, and encourages short titles, longer works, collections, and titles which stretch the boundaries of academic publishing in new ways.

Gordon David Lyle Bates

The Uncanny Rise of Medical Hypnotism, 1888–1914

Between Imagination and Suggestion

palgrave
macmillan

Gordon David Lyle Bates
School of Arts
Birkbeck, University of London
London, UK

ISSN 2634-6036 ISSN 2634-6044 (electronic)
Mental Health in Historical Perspective
ISBN 978-3-031-42727-5 ISBN 978-3-031-42725-1 (eBook)
https://doi.org/10.1007/978-3-031-42725-1

Cover illustration: Science History Images/Alamy Stock Photo

This Palgrave Macmillan imprint is published by the registered company Springer Nature Switzerland AG
The registered company address is: Gewerbestrasse 11, 6330 Cham, Switzerland

Paper in this product is recyclable.

For Vanessa, Gulliver and Kingsley
my support team

Preface

The genesis of this book is thirty years of clinical practice of psychiatry. When I started the Ph.D. which informs this monograph, I had little idea of my motives. But as I reflected over the time of writing and attempted to justify the subject matter, there are three moments that came to mind as formative. Firstly, my experience working with Dr. Michael Prendergast at the original Birmingham Children's Hospital. The early nineties saw an increase in severe somatising illness in young people: an epidemic of ME (myalgic encephalomyelitis). Over a 6-month training placement, I witnessed children who were stuporous, unresponsive and immobile in bed, start eating and return to home and school. It was nothing short of miraculous. This was a form of holistic treatment that did not require pharmacology skills but leadership, a clear therapeutic model based on suggestion and an excellent team. I was hooked!

The second formative incident forms the basis of an anecdote that I have often repeated. My wife is a general practitioner who confessed to one of her patients that she sometimes asked for my advice about patients because I was a psychiatrist. The lady that she told this to did not seem reassured by the source of her psychiatric treatment plan. 'I should hate that,' she said seriously, 'he must always know what you're thinking.' This was my first realisation of the unusual beliefs that the public hold about psychiatry and psychiatrists. I just thought it was an interesting job. However, it did make me consider the projections and bizarre ideas that the public have about my profession and I started to look out for them in popular culture. While it was flattering that we were thought to be able to read minds, within films and books this was portrayed as a bad thing and people with such powers inevitably abused them.

Finally, in researching my dissertation for a course in Medical Humanities, I discovered that the roots of talking therapies and dynamic psychiatry lay in mesmerism and a Victorian gentleman's club called the Society for Psychical Research. While medicine is a highly pragmatic discipline with most time spent doing the job rather than thinking about it, I wondered why I had never previously heard about this exotic heritage. I realised that the lady who thought I could read my wife's mind and the parents who wanted me to hypnotise their son to make him behave better were on to something. Somehow, the time when early doctors used hypnotism or investigated telepathy has remained in our cultural memory. It was my profession that had air-brushed away this inconvenient truth from our accepted institutional history. I was determined to find out more about the New Hypnotists and this book is the result.

London, UK Gordon David Lyle Bates

Acknowledgements

I have often wondered who reads the acknowledgements and at whom they are aimed. I like to read them, as for me, this part of any work allows a fascinating glimpse of the oily, spluttering machinery that lies under the gleaming bonnet of the highly polished creation. It is the chance to see behind the curtain of the Great Oz and observe the people who made it all possible. Therefore, it is particularly important that I mention the people that I owe.

For their practical help, I must thank Peter Henderson, the school archivist at King's school, Canterbury; Sue Young, internet historian for her vast online resource on homeopathy and the Golden Dawn, particularly her help with re-finding her original sources for me; Francis Maunze, Archivist at the Royal College of Psychiatrists; Tom Carter at Blackpool Heritage Service and Wendy Townsend and her staff, lead librarian at Coventry and Warwickshire Partnership Trust. Special mention must go to the anonymous librarians at the Wellcome collection, the National Archive at Kew, the National Library of Scotland, Aberdeen University Special Collections and Allard Pierson Museum, Amsterdam University.

This work would be much poorer without the conceptual contributions of many people. The historians, Mathew Thomson and Philip Kuhn were generous with their time and supportive of my efforts exploring their domains. Closer to home, the Birmingham Psychiatry and Philosophy group introduced me to 'looping kinds' and listened kindly and attentively to the first draft of an early chapter. Jamie Scott, Chris Adams and Didge were so enthusiastic about the topic when my confidence in its merit was low. Andrew Duffy went above and beyond the duties of a Best Man by reading both the thesis and the Ph.D. His suggestions helped me to work out the hard decision of which material to jettison.

My Ph.D. supervisors were Roger Luckhurst and Jo Winning. I met both of them during a Master's course in Medical Humanities at Birkbeck College. Despite the threats to their jobs and their department, they have remained positive and inspirational over the last seven years. Roger's love for late Victorian genre fiction and the weird and wonderful is infectious. Jo helped to convince me that my choice of topic was not only important for the whole field of medical humanities but also that writing it was possible. They both helped with my successful application for a Birkbeck Wellcome Institutional Strategic Support Fund grant which enabled me to prioritise the writing of this book over my clinical commitments for six months.

I should mention too, William Hughes and Rhodri Hayward, the two examiners of the thesis and the anonymous book reviewer. Jointly, their helpful suggestions alerted me to the gaps and weaknesses of my story and inevitably improved this book. At the publishers, Lucy Kidwell took a punt on the unusual subject matter and Eliana Rangel helped with the practical aspects.

The chapter on imaginary hypnotism contains close readings of Arthur Conan Doyle's 'John Barrington Cowles' and *The Parasite*. Some of this material has previously appeared in a different form: 'Arthur Conan Doyle in Mesmeric Edinburgh and Hypnotic London', *Victoriographies* 11, 3 (pp. 314–30) and 'The Fascinating Fictions of Arthur Conan Doyle: Hypnotism and Mesmerism in "John Barrington Cowles" and *The Parasite*' in *Re-examining Arthur Conan Doyle,* edited by Nils Clausson, 59–74, Newcastle: Cambridge Scholars Publishing.

I would also like to thank Robert Wozniak, the editor and curator of the series *Classics in Psychology: 1855–1914* (Bristol: Thoemmes) for his unknowing help. Not only did he include Lloyd Tuckey's *Psycho-Therapeutics* (1888) as one of the key psychology texts of the era but his comment that 'Biographical Information on Tuckey is not readily available', was the critical spur for this work.[1]

[1] Robert Wozniak, 'Tuckey, Psycho-Therapeutics', *Classics in Psychology, 1855-1914: Historical Essays* (London: Thoemmes Continuum, 1998) pp. 100–2 (p. 100).

Finally, a word about my wife and sons, Vanessa, Gulliver and Kingsley. They have had to put up with my mental and physical absence over the last few years. They have heard more stories about the New Hypnotists and hypnotism than anyone should have to. They have witnessed me tell the same stories to their friends and rarely complained. They have supported me throughout and I will take this opportunity to thank them.

Contents

About the Author

Gordon David Lyle Bates is a child and adolescent psychiatrist and writer. He was recently appointed as the Historian in Residence at the Royal College of Psychiatrists. He lives in a Victorian house in Birmingham which is too cold for writing. He has written many papers and several chapters on psychiatric and medical humanities topics. This is his first book.

Abbreviations

BHS	British Homeopathic Society
BJH	British Journal of Homeopathy
BMA	British Medical Association
BMJ	British Medical Journal
JMS	Journal of Mental Science
MPC	Medico-Psychological Clinic (also known as the Brunswick Square Clinic)
MSSST	Medical Society for the Study of Suggestive Therapy
MTHG	Medical Times and Hospital Gazette
PMS	Psycho-Medical Society
RLHH	Royal London Homeopathic Hospital
SPR	Society for Psychical Research
SRIA	Societas Rosicruciana in Anglia

List of Figures

CHAPTER 1

Introduction

Introduction

In May 1897, Bram Stoker published *Dracula*, his well-researched and medically informed version of the vampire myth.[1] By the end of the nineteenth century, most of the iterations of the literary vampire had powerful new gifts: unspoken communication, irresistible compulsions and the psychic connection. Using their strange mesmeric eyes and their Byronic charm, they could compel their victims to do whatever they wanted, 'speak' to them across great distances and even steal their life force and energy. This uncanny and intimate link was to be part of the enduring appeal of the modern vampire tale.

Bram Stoker's network of friends and his medical links mean that it is no coincidence that at this time British Medicine was battling another dangerous but appealing foreign invader, hypnotism. Hypnotism too, was linked to telepathy, rapport, neurasthenia (nervous tiredness) and automatic obedience. It had been scientifically sanctioned by the recent clinical experiments of the eminent French neurologist Jean-Martin Charcot of the Salpêtrière, making it a reputable subject for medical scrutiny once more. This was not just a trivial or parochial professional matter. Its mystical and disreputable predecessor mesmerism had become an integral

[1] Bram Stoker, *Dracula* (London: Archibald Constable, 1897).

G. D. L. Bates, *The Uncanny Rise of Medical Hypnotism, 1888–1914*, Mental Health in Historical Perspective,
https://doi.org/10.1007/978-3-031-42725-1_1

part of European cultural life in the form of travelling lectures, magical stage shows and spiritualist séances, even in Britain.

Mesmerism was the name given to the pseudoscience which had initially enchanted Paris nearly 120 years before. The Austrian physician Franz Anton Mesmer had brought his animal magnetism to the capital in 1778 and entertained, fascinated and apparently cured many of the nobility and peasants of pre-revolutionary France. It was characterised by close theatrical 'passes' or manual gestures over the sick body parts which required a close proximity between 'operateur' (mesmerist) and 'somnambulist' (patient). It was explained as a rebalancing of the patient's magnetic fluid by the healer.

The healing potential of mesmerism had been popularised in the UK somewhat later, by John Elliotson (1791–1868), a distinguished physician and founder of University College Hospital (UCH) in London. He had started to trial the techniques of Mesmer and his followers in the late 1820s and was most impressed by the medical conditions that he could improve. However, despite his successes and his prominence, he had been forced to resign his chair in 1838, when his consultant colleagues turned against him and banned further displays of mesmerism at UCH. Elliotson would continue to work in the capital but died in poverty.

Mesmerism had become the crucible for the new objective and scientific credentials of Victorian medicine. It's associations with magic, fraud, quackery and inappropriate intimacy between male doctors and usually female patients made it too hazardous for the precarious newly established medical profession. John Elliotson and mesmerism were direct challenges to orthodox medical practice and were brought down by the combined might of the medical institutions using the specialist medical and lay press. The new journal the *Lancet* and its editor Thomas Wakley played a prominent role in Elliotson's downfall.

Despite the orthodox medical response to mesmerism, the general public remained fascinated. Hovering between life and death, the indeterminate trance state held a pervasive influence on Victorian life. A powerful reason for the interest was the widespread rejection of the prevailing scientific materialism, the belief that the objective world available to the natural sciences was all that existed. This led to interest in esoteric new philosophies like Occultism and Theosophy which re-emerged and emerged respectively in the 1870s. Both Theosophy and ceremonial magic resonated with the Victorian drive for self-improvement and both included trance as an important technique for creativity, mental communication and astral projection.

Elliotson's clinical demonstrations were shamelessly duplicated and repeated across the country, initially as a form of education and entertainment hybrid, the mesmerism lecture. These always began by inducing a shift in the consciousness of the somnambulist, the trance state. The power of the trance would be demonstrated to the audience by imperviousness to pain. The success of travelling hypnotists and their shows had kept trance alive in the UK. By the 1890s, any self-respecting stage magician would incorporate a hypnotic or trance mind-reading act into their performance. This trivialisation of trance was one of several negative associations taken on by mesmerism.

Another important connotation was the link of the trance state to spiritualism and contact with the dead as a result of the popular growth and slow evolution of the Church of Spiritualism. Starting with the Fox sisters' experiences with 'rapping' to communicate with the dead in the United States in 1848, the Church of Spiritualism had spread across America and quickly to the UK. Both formal religious Spiritualism and its less religious variants tapped into a very real Victorian need to communicate with their deceased relatives, which was usually made possible by the entrancement of the spirit medium. Spiritualist mediums and mesmeric lecturers frequently overlapped both in terms of personnel and belief systems. By the latter half of the century, spiritualist seances were increasingly commonplace in stately homes and middle-class parlours. The spirit mediums who interceded with the afterlife became more and more likely to enter a self-induced trance or one induced by a fellow spiritualist. After the exposure of many spirit mediums as frauds, trance itself was viewed sceptically by many.

This book is about the courageous and ambitious British physicians who risked their reputations and livelihoods to fight for medical hypnotism just fifty years after Elliotson's very public disgrace. Firstly, they had to convince a sceptical medical professional that the trance state of hypnotism was safer and different to that of mesmerism. Both procedures induced a state of reduced awareness and increased suggestibility to facilitate healing. Unlike Mesmer's dramatic induction techniques, most hypnotic inductions were provoked visually through sustained focus on a bright object and verbally, through calming and positive affirmations. Some proximity between patient and physician was required but close 'passes' were not.

The physicians also needed to provide a rationale for the therapeutic benefits that did not rely upon the doctrine of the imagination, an ancient mystical concept developed by the alchemists, which had little place in modern scientific Victorian medicine. The effects of trance were theorised to be the result of suggestion, a theory proposed by Hippolyte Bernheim and Ambrose Liébeault based in Nancy, France. The usefulness and shortfalls of this theory will be reviewed.

The New Hypnotists

Throughout this book, I will use 'New Hypnotism' as the name for the British medical hypnotism movement of the time and the 'New Hypnotists' for the loose affiliation of extraordinary doctors who advocated for it. This is based upon the title of Charles Lloyd Tuckey's essay for the gentleman's periodical the *Contemporary Review*.[2] Without television or radio, the printed word played a major part in promoting scientific literacy in the general public. Tuckey, Robert Felkin, George Kingsbury and John Milne Bramwell had all visited and learned about hypnotism from Hippolyte Bernheim and Ambroise-Auguste Liébeault.

The New Hypnotists had to fight the negative perceptions of other British physicians and the general public to achieve acceptance. I will describe the ways that, against the odds, medical hypnotism managed to achieve its goal of mainstream credibility, going up against the innate conservatism and reactionary nature of British institutional medicine. The British Medical Association and Ernest Hart, editor of the *British Medical Journal* (*BMJ*), were formidable opponents and did not always fight fairly. Hart went so far as to set up a 'sting' in which some of the New Hypnotists were duped into unsuccessfully hypnotising an actor who had previously worked for stage magicians, feigning entrancement and enduring painful procedures. Hart took great glee in exposing the doctor's gullibility in the *BMJ*. His attitude can be easily discerned from the titles of his journal articles and books: *Hypnotism, Mesmerism and the New Witchcraft, Hypnotism and Humbug*, and *The Eternal Gullible*.[3] The

[2] Charles Lloyd Tuckey, 'A New Hypnotism: A Reply to Mr E Hart's "The Revival of Witchcraft"', *The Contemporary Review,* 63 (1893) (pp. 416–9).

[3] Ernest Hart, 'Hypnotism and Humbug', *Nineteenth Century,* 31 January, 1892 (pp. 24–37); Ernest Hart, 'Mesmerism and the New Witchcraft' (London: Smith and Elder, 1893). His articles on hypnotism were collected and republished in Ernest Hart,

dispute took place across both the medical and lay press. At first, the New Hypnotists had to use the gentleman's journals to promote their ideas as the medical journal editors strictly controlled access to their pages. Later they used their own medical journal the *General Practitioner* to advocate for suggestive therapy.

Throughout, the New Hypnotists used their personal connections in the London club culture to disseminate their message and were in turn influenced by those that they met there. They formed a part of an unlikely series of networks of late Victorian esoteric knowledge. Their connections with the investigations of the Society for Psychical Research (SPR), whose elite membership included Government Ministers and Nobel Prize winners, and the Hermetic Order of the Golden Dawn, an occult ceremonial magical group founded by two physicians, helped to both shape and propagate their views. It is these links to psychism and the occult which make the rise of medical hypnotism 'uncanny'. Its rise was also uncanny in the sense that it was counterintuitive. The power of the medical establishment was such that it was successful in supressing other fringe practices such as homeopathy, hydrotherapy (balneotherapy) and electrotherapy.

As well as its representation in the scientific literature and factual articles in gentleman's periodicals, imaginary or fictional hypnotism was very popular in the 1890s. *Dracula* was just one of many literary narratives concerning hypnotism. These stories were not only shaped by the information and attitudes in the public domain but also helped to shape the public's beliefs about hypnosis. In order to examine some of the persistent themes of hypnotic fiction which include automatic obedience, gender, sexuality and medical professionalism, I will offer close readings of L. T. Meade's medical mystery 'The Red Bracelet' and Arthur Conan Doyle's gothic novella *The Parasite*.[4] These stories show the complex and frequently conflicting views about hypnotism. Hypnotism was simultaneously seen as highly dangerous, needing tight regulation and as ineffective, the result of trickery and the preserve of mountebanks. Analysis of fiction is rarely used in medical histories but this untapped resource helps to illustrate the shifting cultural landscape around hypnotism.

Hypnotism, Mesmerism and the New Witchcraft, enlarged ed. (London: Smith and Elder, 1896).

[4] L. T. Meade and Clifford Halifax, 'The Red Bracelet', *Strand Magazine*, 9 May, 1895, (pp. 545–61); Arthur Conan Doyle, 'The Parasite' in *The Parasite and the Watter's Mou,* ed. by Catherine Wynne (Kansas City: Valancourt Books, 2009) (pp. 3–47).

The final chapters describe the way that suggestive therapy was eventually accommodated by orthodox medicine. In part, this was because there was a growing appetite for the insights of psychology and talking therapies in the general population. However, for suggestive therapy to be adopted by the mainstream of medicine it had to be adapted and the hypnotic induction techniques and the depth of the trance state both lost their importance. Meanwhile, the personality of the doctor, the suggestive affirmations that he used and the relationship with the patient moved to centre stage. The theory of suggestion found its way into various early psychological therapies from early Freudian analysis to mixed hypnotic catharsis and the auto-suggestions of Émile Coué: 'every day and in every way, I am getting better and better'.

The understanding of this early history of psychological therapy requires the recovery of both the cultural context and the wide-ranging therapeutic practices that were found in London between 1900 and 1914. Early British psycho-therapeutics was heterogenous and treatments were often hybrid. This early history is little known and not well told but hypnotism and suggestion were important components. The New Hypnotists played a key role in two early psychotherapeutic institutions: the Medical Society for the Study of Suggestive Therapy ((MSSST) founded in 1907) and the Medico-Psychological Clinic (MPC), established in 1914. Both groups utilised an empirical form of treatment using different psychological therapies depending on the patient's need.

By the start of the twentieth century, the medical environment and popular culture were much more conducive to talking therapies. The British Freudian myth of massive medical and public resistance to Freudian ideas at this time is just that. There were cogent criticisms of the prominence of sex and the time commitment for both analyst and analysand but these were quibbles rather than wholesale rejection. Freud's ideas were well-known to those interested in psychological therapies. In addition there was increasing public curiosity about all forms of mental work. This included practical 'mind-drills' like Pelmanism to exercise one's brain and new North American influences like the New Thought movement and self-help books both of which were strongly influenced by the idea of suggestion. Non-medical mind cure therapists started to emerge, threatening the medical monopoly. Probably the most prominent of these was Arthur Hallam's lay London Psycho-Therapeutic Society (LPS). It offered free treatment and was a centre of learning for medical and non-medical therapists. Hypnotism, magnetism and suggestive therapy were routinely used by its therapists. There was good take-up of the free service and its lecture programme.

The outbreak First World War suddenly raised the profile of psychotherapeutics. The scale of the trench-based warfare and the constant fear of death or injury led to massive numbers of psychologically damaged soldiers on both sides. When the British Army looked for help from the medical psychologists, the solutions that they offered were mostly variations on hypnotism and suggestive therapy. It was to be the highest profile for the treatment which soon fragmented into other forms of therapy after the war.

Suggestion was incorporated into more general medical practice as a mechanism for the nonphysical healing aspects of the doctor-patient relationship. It came to mean that a cheerful and optimistic physician had better outcomes. This belief and form of practice were typified by the work and writings of the charismatic Canadian-born physician William Osler, who established Johns Hopkins Medical School and became the Regius Professor of Medicine at Oxford in 1905. Curiously, the importance of this part of the clinical relationship became more actively considered and better described by the physicians when the profession's monopoly on healing was threatened from an unlikely source: the meteoric rise of faith-healing and the Church of Christian Science in the early twentieth century. This interest predated the experimental investigation of the concept of the placebo effect in the 1950s. However, the ideas of suggestion and expectancy continue to be important ways that placebo effects are understood today.

References

Doyle, Arthur Conan. 2009. 'The Parasite' in *The Parasite and the Watter's Mou*, ed. by Catherine Wynne. Kansas City: Valancourt Books. 3–47.

Hart, Ernest. 1892. 'Hypnotism and Humbug', *Nineteenth Century* (31 January, 1892): 24–37.

Hart, Ernest. 1893. 'Mesmerism and the New Witchcraft'. London: Smith and Elder.

Hart, Ernest. 1896. *Hypnotism, Mesmerism and the New Witchcraft*, enlarged ed. London: Smith and Elder.

Meade, L.T. and Halifax, Clifford. 1895. 'The Red Bracelet', *Strand Magazine* 9 (May): 545–61.

Stoker, Bram. 1897. *Dracula* (London: Archibald Constable).

Tuckey, Charles Lloyd. 1893. "A New Hypnotism: A reply to Mr E Hart's 'The Revival of Witchcraft.'" *Contemporary Review* 63: 416-9.

CHAPTER 2

The New Hypnotists

The birth of the New Hypnotism can be traced back to two events and four innovative British physicians: Charles Lloyd Tuckey, John Milne Bramwell, George Kingsbury and Robert Felkin. They were quite different men with different backgrounds, abilities and strengths. While there is evidence that they were familiar with each other, there is no evidence that they were particularly close (with the exception of Kingsbury and Tuckey) or worked in concert to promote hypnotism, despite my claim for a movement. They did share interests and clubs: Tuckey and Bramwell were senior members of the Society for Psychical Research (SPR), an elite society which examined previously inexplicable phenomena like haunted houses and the abilities of spirit mediums with the methodology of science; Felkin and Tuckey were part of an arcane ceremonial magic group, the Hermetic Society of the Golden Dawn. Another connection which links Bramwell and Felkin was attendance at medical school in Edinburgh, where animal magnetism remained on the syllabus long after Elliotson's humiliation had suppressed its consideration in England.

The New Hypnotists were also united by the separate visits they had made between 1888 and 1889, to Ambrose Liébeault and Hippolyte Bernheim in Nancy and the Amsterdam hypnotic clinic of Frederik van Eeden and Albert van Renterghem. The work of the Nancy school was

G. D. L. Bates, *The Uncanny Rise of Medical Hypnotism, 1888–1914*, Mental Health in Historical Perspective,
https://doi.org/10.1007/978-3-031-42725-1_2

based on the self-taught hypnotic induction skills of Liébeault, a generalist country doctor with decades of practical experience, and the theoretical input of Bernheim who formulated the doctrine of suggestion to account for the effects of hypnotism. Van Eeden and van Renterghen had studied at Nancy but adapted hypnotic practice for the more sophisticated city dwellers of Amsterdam. On their return from their visits to Europe, the New Hypnotists were so enthused by what they had experienced that all four wrote books on medical hypnotism. Tuckey and Bramwell continued to practice with hypnotism and suggestive therapy and published about it over the next thirty years. Kingsbury and Felkin's lives took strange turns which I will outline but remained interested in the psychosomatic aspects of medicine throughout their professional careers.

Tuckey's 'Faith-Healing'

The first incident which marked the arrival of medical hypnotism in Britain was the publication of Tuckey's account of his holiday to Nancy in late 1888, 'Faith-Healing as a Medical Treatment'. Tuckey described his 'chance' visit to Ambrose Liébeault and the form of medical practice that he witnessed in the lay journal, the *Nineteenth Century*.[1] His choice of journal for submission is noteworthy. The *Nineteenth Century* was not a specialist medical nor even a scientific journal but a monthly, literary periodical aimed at the general public.[2] Set up in 1877 by Sir James Knowles, the founder of the Metaphysical Society, the publication's editorial policy seemed to be an attempt to integrate science and religion or perhaps find some form of accommodation between the two. Alongside short stories, pieces on politics and contemporary issues, it had published articles on a wide selection of scientific and spiritual subjects. To give a flavour of the variety, other contributors in 1888 ranged from the former prime minister, W. E. Gladstone and Beatrix Potter (writing on social issues) to fictions from Arthur Conan Doyle and poetry and criticism from Francis Palgrave and Algernon Swinburne.

[1] Charles Lloyd Tuckey, 'Faith Healing as a Medical Treatment', *Nineteenth Century*, 21 (1888) (pp. 839–50).

[2] 'The Nineteenth Century', in *Dictionary of Nineteenth Century Journalism in Great Britain and Ireland*, ed. by Laurel Brake and Marysa Denmore (Ghent: Academia Press, 2009).

In this context, the journal can be seen not only as a prestigious one but also one offering a sympathetic home for Tuckey's essay. He would have likely expected rejection from one of the medical journals. The SPR's hypnotism experts Edmund Gurney and Frederic Myers had also published on the related topic of mesmerism in the same journal six years earlier.[3] Having identified the right journal, it does make it hard to account for Tuckey's choice of title for the paper. An essay that focuses throughout on the medical potential of hypnotism but does not mention hypnosis in the title does seem odd. As part of my research, I uncovered the solution to the riddle: it was a printing mistake. Searching the contemporary newspaper archives provided the answer. Within a few days of publication in the *Nineteenth Century* and in response to its initial reviews, Tuckey wrote to the *Standard* newspaper and clarified that this was an editorial error. He had originally entitled it 'Psycho-Therapeutics: A New Departure in Medical Treatment' and was surprised that it had been 'rechristened without my knowledge or consent.'[4]

Within months, he followed this with his medical textbook that he titled *Psycho-Therapeutics,* which would run to seven editions over the next thirty years.[5] Both Felkin and Kingsbury acknowledged not only the importance of Tuckey's pioneering visit to Nancy but also his bravery in publishing at all, given the reactionary nature of medicine in the UK and the reception that John Elliotson had experienced. Kingsbury confirmed his intellectual debt to Tuckey and described him as a friend in his textbook of 1891.[6] Felkin, whose visits to Nancy and Amsterdam and subsequent book were seemingly triggered by his review of *Psycho-Therapeutics* for the *Edinburgh Medical Journal*, also notes the importance of Tuckey to the field.[7]

Bramwell rarely cited Tuckey's later work and appears to be reluctant to concede that Tuckey was 'apparently' responsible for the 'recent revival' of

[3] Edward Gurney and Frederic Myers, 'Mesmerism', *Nineteenth Century*, 9 (October 1883) (pp. 695–719).

[4] Charles Lloyd Tuckey, 'Correspondence—Faith-Healing', *Standard* (London, England) (3 December 1888) (p. 3).

[5] Charles Lloyd Tuckey, *Psycho-Therapeutics: Or Treatment by Sleep and Suggestion* (London: Baillière, Tindall and Cox, 1889).

[6] George Kingsbury, *The Practice of Hypnotic Suggestion, Being and Elementary Handbook for the Use of the Medical Profession* (Bristol: John Wright, 1891).

[7] Robert Felkin, *Hypnotism or Psycho-Therapeutics* (Edinburgh: Y. J. Pentland, 1890).

interest in hypnotism in Britain.[8] Conversely, Tuckey routinely cites much of Bramwell's scholarship and research in his own books. In Tuckey's private correspondence, he suggested to his friend the Dutch physician and novelist Frederik van Eeden that Bramwell would become the 'big man' of British medical hypnotism and playing on a national stereotype suggested that the Scot would be financially successful.[9]

Bramwell's Hypnotic Anaesthesia

The second incident which transformed the reputation of and the wider medical interest in hypnotism was Bramwell's exhibition of hypnotism as an agent of anaesthesia to a large medical audience in March 1890. The ability to make surgery pain-free was extremely useful as ether, chloroform and nitrous oxide, the drugs used at the time, all had potential drawbacks. It was also a clear demonstration of the practical power of hypnotism which Bramwell had started to harness in his clinical practice. He had first impressed Arthur Turner, a local dentist who was able to painlessly remove 40 teeth from a range of subjects that Bramwell had anaesthetised hypnotically.

This initial event was reported positively in the *British Dental Journal* which led to Turner arranging a further public demonstration in Leeds. Sixty medical and dental professionals attended, among them nationally known doctors like Thomas Pridgin Teale and Arthur Mayo Robson, the local professor of surgery. They performed a range of surgical operations from dental extractions to toenail and bony spur removal on children, healthy adult labourers and nervous women. The surgeons were surprisingly enthusiastic about the new development, particularly in comparison to the speciality's response to Elliotson fifty years earlier. The whole demonstration was written up in an unusually supportive manner in both the *Lancet* and *BMJ*. The previous hypnotic developments in France had warranted little interest in the medical journals and this article signals

[8] John Milne Bramwell, *Hypnotism: Its History, Practice and Theory*, 3rd ed. (London: Rider, 1921) (p. 35).

[9] Charles Lloyd Tuckey to van Eeden correspondence (24 October 1893). *Van Eeden Collection* (Amsterdam: Allard Pierson, University of Amsterdam), Hs. XXIV C 81.

hypnotism's move to a more mainstream medical discourse.[10] Bramwell's success led to referrals from all over the country and prompted him to go to Nancy himself and to learn more about the technique and methods of tackling hypnotic resistance from Bernheim and Liébeault.

Before moving on to further details of the group's fight for legitimacy and credibility, I will provide some biographical details about the New Hypnotists and consider their motivations for advocating for hypnotism.

Charles Lloyd Tuckey (1854–1925)

Tuckey was a society doctor working in London's West End, whose patients included members of the wealthy Guinness family and Alice James, the American sister of the novelist Henry James and early academic psychologist William James. He was well-connected with wide social networks. His membership of the SPR and leadership of its hypnotism committee meant that he was right at the heart of British scholarship about the mind at the turn of the century. His contemporaries credited him with bringing hypnotism to Britain (Figs. 2.1 and 2.2).

Born in Canterbury in the South of England to an Irish medical family, his father Charles Caulfield Tuckey was a general practitioner and homeopath. Charles Lloyd Tuckey was delicate, youthful-looking and charming. He was widely read and erudite, collecting Genevan bibles as a hobby. Throughout his working life, he took regular trips abroad to Spain, the United States and the West Indies, a pattern of behaviour which in this era suggested that he had chronic problems with illness. His friend Percy Allan also mentioned this fact in his obituary, saying that Tuckey sometimes complained of the impact on his health of his regular contact with 'neurotic' patients.[11] A confirmed bachelor, Tuckey married late in life to Beatrice Marsland, a friend of his sister, probably because he thought he would need nursing assistance in retirement. Tuckey's death certificate states that he had valvular heart disease and this would likely explain his long-term poor health.

[10] Anon, 'Demonstration of Hypnotism as an Anæsthetic During the Performance of Dental and Surgical Operations', *Lancet*, 135 (5 April 1890) (pp. 771–2); Anon, 'Hypnotism as an Anæsthetic in Surgery', *British Medical Journal*, 1528 (12 April 1890) (pp. 849–50).

[11] Anon, 'Obituary: Charles Lloyd Tuckey', *Journal of the Society for Psychical Research*, 22 (October 1925) (pp. 115–7).

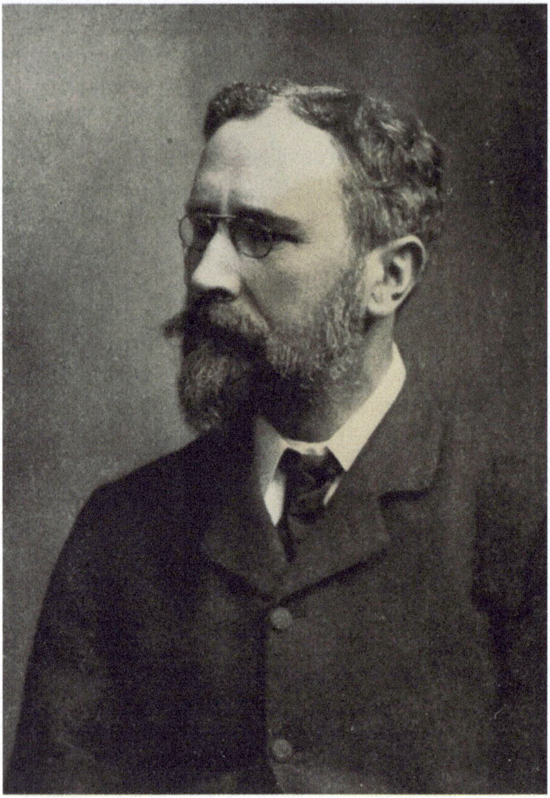

Fig. 2.1 'Charles Lloyd Tuckey, M.D.' from Psychotherapy magazine (New York: Centre Publishing, 1909)

Tuckey had been moderately successful at his local school, King's School Canterbury, becoming a probationer scholar, which had part-funded his time there. He went into medicine, attending King's College Hospital between October 1870 and July 1873.[12] As was conventional at the time, he left London after three years for Aberdeen University, to start his clinical training. Though generally accepted that the Scottish

[12] CLT entry in *Medical Graduate Schedules, 1862*, University of Aberdeen Medical Schedule (MSU 62) [with kind permission of Aberdeen University, Special Collections Centre].

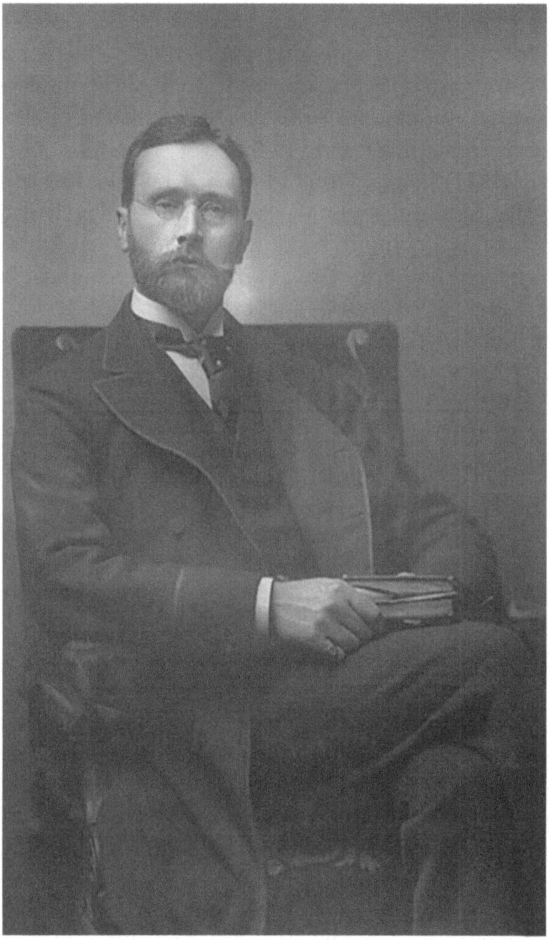

Fig. 2.2 'Dr. Lloyd Tuckey, M.D.' Photograph by Stanislaus Walery (1892) in Our Celebrities (London: Sampson, Low, Marston) [Courtesy of National Library of Scotland]

medical schools provided better clinical training and were more prestigious, this was a strange choice for the son of a medical homeopath. Less than twenty years before, the university had attracted the ire of the homeopathic community for refusing to allow medical students to graduate if they believed in homeopathy or practised it.[13] In his final year, Lloyd Tuckey returned to Kent and undertook six months medical and six months surgical training at Canterbury General Hospital.

Tuckey went on to find work at the Royal London Homoeopathic [sic] Hospital (RLHH). His father, who had held various offices within the homeopathy fraternity, was a governor there. He had also been a part of the charitable committee that had helped to fundraise for the hospital, which was built on Great Ormond Street and completed in 1858. This cannot have harmed Tuckey's chances of finding a place of work. He remained at RLHH from 1878 to 1884 as an assistant physician. Following completion of his MD in 1884, he was promoted to physician in 1885. Sadly, Aberdeen University does not have a copy or even a record of the title of his doctoral thesis. It would be interesting given that the majority of Tuckey's professional work to this point had been in the field of homeopathy.

In the late 1870s, there were only 280 medically qualified homeopaths in the UK.[14] To give some context, there were approximately five thousand medically qualified doctors in the entire country. Then, as now, homeopathy had a contested status despite its strong links with the aristocracy. The majority of homeopaths were practicing from outside the medical profession and the medical community saw them as direct competition as well as unscientific and unregulated. Social historians looking back at the nineteenth century often group together the heterodox medical disciplines of the time: phrenology, homeopathy, electrotherapy, balneotherapy or hydrotherapy and mesmerism and hypnotism.[15] This conflation is unhelpful and these fringe medicines should be considered separately as their development, contexts and outcomes were all very different. If they had nothing else in common, the orthodox medical response to them was universally negative. Though problematic, in this book the term 'fringe' is used interchangeably with 'unorthodox', 'alternative' or 'heterodox' to describe those therapeutic approaches that do not fall within allopathic medicine. 'Heterodox' or 'unorthodox' are

[13] George Atkin, *The British and Foreign Medical Homoeopathic Directory 1853* (London: Aylott, 1853) (p. 51).

[14] Phillip Nicholls, *Homeopathy and the Medical Profession* (London: Crook Helm, 1988) (p. 134).

[15] Brian Inglis, *Fringe Medicine* (London: Faber, 1964).

terms most popularly used by medical practitioners, while the terms 'natural', 'alternative' or 'fringe' medicine tend to be used by the lay population.[16]

Tuckey's strong background in homeopathy may well have contributed to his later interest in hypnosis. The medical profession's hostility had the effect of bringing together all of the non-conformists and promoted interest in each other's alternative medical practices. The fringe or heterodox practices shared metaphors of bodily and mental harmony and balancing energy. That is not to say that all phrenologists were interested, for example, in hydrotherapy but mixed treatments like phreno-mesmerism existed and influential physician homeopaths like George Wyld, elected the president of the British Homeopathic Society (BHS) in 1876, was also a phrenologist, medical mesmerist and early member of the SPR.

Certainly, homeopathy's founder Samuel Hahnemann was familiar with the therapeutic possibilities of mesmerism and mentioned it in his magnum opus *The Organon of the Healing Art*, first published in 1810 and then translated into English in 1833.[17] In the fifth edition, which would have been available to Tuckey, Hahnemann states that a medicine given in the right 'quality' but in the wrong quantity can be adjusted 'mesmerically.'[18] Tuckey would therefore be more likely to have a positive perspective towards earlier mesmeric practice than many of his contemporaries.

There is a final episode in Tuckey's early professional career, which demonstrates both his relationship to the heterodox medical therapies and gives a measure of the disputed status of homeopathy and the medical fringes at this time. This relates to the controversy around the medical staff appointments at the Margaret Street Infirmary between 1887 and

[16] Walter Wardwell, 'Orthodoxy and Heterodoxy in Medical Practice', *Social Science and Medicine*, 6 (1972) (p. 63).

[17] Samuel *Hahnemann, The Homœopathic Medical Doctrine, or "Organon of the Healing Art"*, trans. by Charles Devrient (Dublin: W.F. Wakeman, 1833).

[18] Samuel Hahnemann, *Organon of Medicine*, 5th ed., trans. by Robert Dudgeon (London: Headland, 1849).

1888. This incident was documented almost contemporaneously in John Henry Clarke's *Odium Medicum and Homoeopathy* (1888).[19]

The Margaret Street Infirmary for Consumption and Diseases of the Chest in West London, originally a parish workhouse, opened its doors in 1847 as a tuberculosis hospital. The infirmary functioned unremarkably, albeit more like a dispensary from which physicians undertook home visits.[20] However, in 1887 the hospital became the centre of a medical and newspaper storm when six members of the medical staff, backed by the executive committee, wrote to two of their colleagues, Apollinaris Victor Jagielski and Thomas Charles Marsh, and accused them of 'practising homoeopathically'. They were asked to stop using homeopathic treatments and 'to resign any appointments held in homoeopathic institutions' or face dismissal.[21]

It seems likely that Jagielski and Marsh earned the disapproval of their colleagues for reasons other than just their homeopathic interests, though both were clearly affiliated with the alternative therapy. Jagielski was made a fellow of the BHS in 1882.[22] Marsh had worked at the RLHH since 1884 and would have been a contemporary of Tuckey.[23] Little is known about Marsh but Jagielski continued to come into conflict with the medical authorities and appeared in trials before the Censors of the Royal College of Physicians no less than six times, as a result of his promotion of therapeutic use of water baths and electrotherapy, but not his homeopathic practice.[24]

Whatever the nature of the medical work of Jagielski and Marsh, the dispute been medical colleagues at a small London hospital quickly came

[19] John Henry Clarke, *Odium Medicum and Homoeopathy: "The Times" Correspondence, Reprinted by Permission of the Proprietors of "The Times"* (London: Homoeopathic Publishing, 1888).

[20] Anon, 'Margaret Street Infirmary', *Medical Review*, 31 (1887) (p. 309).

[21] Anon, 'Liberty of Opinion in the Art of Therapeutics', *Monthly Homoeopathic Review*, 31 (March 1887) 168–9 (p. 168).

[22] Giles Goldsbrough, 'Members of the British Homoeopathic Society', *Journal of the British Homoeopathic Society, New Series*, 13 (1904–5) (pp. vi–xxiv).

[23] Felix Reiswitz, *'Globulizing' the Hospital Ward: Legitimizing Homoeopathic Medicine Through the Establishment of Hospitals in 19th-Century London and Madrid*, Appendix E. (PhD thesis, University College London, 2012).

[24] Alexander Cooke, *A History of The Royal College of Physicians of London*, vol. 3 (Oxford: Clarendon Press, 1972) (pp. 904–8).

to represent something more. In the words of the *Medical Press and Circular*, it had become 'a pitched battle between the orthodox practitioners and the homoeopaths!'[25] There was considerable support for the pair from their homeopathy colleagues and well-connected lay advocates.

Through the simple expediency of making a large financial donation, the physician and homeopath Robert Ellis Dudgeon and the long-time supporter of homeopathy, Edmund Beckett, 1st Baron Grimthorpe bought their way on to the governing body of the infirmary.[26] The change of membership of the governing body of the hospital meant that the proposal to dismiss Jagielski and Marsh was never passed by the board. In fact, the board took a further turn towards homeopathy so that in February 1887, seven of the remaining medical staff took the decision to resign rather than accept a new resolution from the board that would 'make it lawful for a professed homeopath to take and hold office on the staff.' One of the physicians who had resigned, Thomas Hawksley, wrote to the *BMJ* attempting to explain the motives of the seven, claiming that to:

> accept the brazen blare of the trumpeter of one sect would open the door for others, so that any institution proposing to work in the quiet and laborious field of true scientific knowledge and experience would find itself invaded and broken up by all sorts of wild theorists and hunters after notoriety.[27]

The hospital appointed three new doctors to replace the ones who had resigned. Provocatively, at Lord Grimthorpe's suggestion, they chose two physician homeopaths to fill three vacancies. These members of the BHS were John Roberson Day and the 33-year-old, Charles Lloyd Tuckey. The *BMJ* account of the minutes of the appointments committee stress that 'it was stated in reply to a question that a candidate was not [my emphasis] ineligible on account of being a homoeopath.'[28] Strangely, it was the least

[25] Anon, 'The Margaret Street Infirmary for Consumption', *London Medical Press and Circular* (9 March 1887) (p. 3).

[26] Anon, 'Robert Ellis Dudgeon, M.D.', *Monthly Homoeopathic Review*, 48 (October 1904) (p. 577).

[27] Anon, 'Resignation of the Medical Staff from the Margaret Street Infirmary for Consumption', *British Medical Journal* (5 March 1887) (p. 541).

[28] Anon, 'Resignation'.

controversial appointment, that of Kenneth Millican, who had no obvious links to homeopathy, which exacerbated the situation further. His other employer, the Jubilee Hospital chose to dismiss him in May 1888, purely because of his position at Margaret Street which now had homeopathic associations. Millican decided to fight for unfair dismissal in the courts. He argued that the hospital had no right to sack a medical officer on account of his medical beliefs. The court found in favour of Millican but the hospital took the matter to the Appeals court where the verdict was reversed.[29]

The whole sorry affair made its way from the medical press to the national press. There then followed a month-long heated debate about quackery and the scientific authenticity of homeopathy in the correspondence section of the *Times*. This is an example of 'boundary work', a concept pioneered by the American sociologist, Thomas Gieryn. In 1983, Gieryn introduced this helpful geographical metaphor as a way of illuminating the ways that the 'domain' of a professional or disciplinary group is first discovered, established, demarcated from others and then policed.

Gieryn suggested that considerable advantages accrue from belonging to established professional groups like medicine and that the difference between members and non-members is socially created not intrinsic. Members select attributes that are characteristic of their institution, 'its practitioners, methods, stock of knowledge, values and work organization for purposes of constructing a social boundary.'[30] He identified a specific ideological style that he found in scientists' attempts to create a public image for science by contrasting it favourably to non-scientific intellectual or technical activities. One of the historical episodes that Gieryn used in his original paper, was the Edinburgh anatomists' battle for the scientific credibility of phrenology, the study of skull shape and mental attributes: 'The debate over phrenology illustrates how one group of scientists draws a boundary to exclude another also claiming to be scientific.'

The sense of orthodox medicine angrily and unreasoningly closing ranks against the heterodoxy of homeopathy was not lost on the leader writer of the *Times*. George Buckle suggested that the conventional practitioners were doing themselves a disservice by the bitterness of the

[29] Anon, 'Millican v. Sulivan and Others', *Times* (16 December 1887) (p. 3).

[30] Thomas Gieryn, 'Boundary-Work and the Demarcation of Science from Non-Science: Strains and Interests in Professional Ideologies of Scientists', *American Sociological Review*, 48, 6 (December 1983) 781–795 (p. 782).

dispute with their colleagues.[31] He went on to point out that if the lay public could not understand the complexities of the argument, and the homeopathic doctors were equivalently qualified and appeared indistinguishable from their orthodox colleagues, then the quarrel could only serve to damage public trust in all doctors. The importance of the place of popular opinion was made clear by the Margaret Street Infirmary incident and the subsequent *odium medicum*.[32] The views of advocates and cultural commentators appearing in the popular press were becoming more effective in influencing medical opinion.

Tuckey never mentions or comments on these events in his later writings. Nonetheless, a further significant link between his homeopathy and his medical hypnotism was his relationship with the Hungarian physician homeopath and exercise therapist Mathias Roth. Roth was a governor at RLHH who claimed to have worked under John Elliotson at the London Mesmeric hospital. In 1887, he wrote a short pamphlet on mesmerism apparently 'with the sole purpose of rousing the interests of my younger colleagues in a branch of the healing art.'[33] Later, Roth was to claim that it was he who was responsible for encouraging Tuckey's early interest in hypnotism while at RLHH. Roth's significance to Tuckey was apparently acknowledged by Liébeault at the testimonial dinner celebrating his retirement though it was Roth himself who documented it.[34] Again, Tuckey does not mention this, but I think that the case has been made for the importance of homeopathy in his free interest in fringe medicine, his willingness to take on the medical establishment and the methods that he used to do so.

[31] An Odium theologicum was the name given to a rancorous theological debate, characterised by intense anger and hatred. George Earle Buckle, 'Editorial: Odium Medicum', *Times* (20 January 1888) (p. 9).

[32] Buckle, 'Odium Medicum'.

[33] Mathias Roth, *The Physiological Effects of Artificial Sleep with Some Notes on Treatment by Suggestion* (London: Baillee, Tindall and Cox, 1887) (p. 2).

[34] 'My thanks are particularly due to Mathias Roth who was one of the first to appreciate the principles I have taught and who it was who induced his countryman Dr. Charles Lloyd Tuckey to investigate them.' Ambrose Liébeault qtd. by Mathias Roth, 'Correspondence: Presentation of a Testimonial to Dr. Liébeault of Nancy', *Monthly Homoeopathic Review*, 9 (1891) 488–91 (p. 490).

John Milne Bramwell (1852–1925)

Of all the New Hypnotists, Bramwell probably left the greatest mark. He wrote more articles and books on hypnotism for a medical audience than the others and was included in a contemporary *Who's Who* (1899).[35] He is known to have treated Frederick Kelly, the Australian-born pianist and Olympic rower for a nervous condition of his hands.[36] Where Tuckey was slight, gentle and charismatic, Bramwell was robust and straight-talking. A proud Scot, he was to become James Braid's greatest champion, collecting an extensive personal library of all his books pamphlets and papers and even his personal correspondence (Fig. 2.3).

Bramwell was born into a medical family in Perth, the youngest of four siblings. He had attended Perth Grammar School before following his father's career path to Edinburgh Medical School. After graduation, his father had worked in hospital practice at Perth Royal Infirmary, where James Esdaile had practiced after his return from India. Esdaile's reputation was founded on his use of mesmerism to induce the trance state to anaesthetise hundreds of the poorest local Calcuttans before surgery.[37] Esdaile passed on his techniques to Fraser Thomson, another surgeon at the hospital. Although Fraser Thomson successfully performed several mesmeric operations, he was banned from continuing by his colleagues and the hospital board.[38] But not before teaching James Paton Bramwell, John's father.

As a boy, John Bramwell had witnessed his father experiment with Esdaile's methods and became fascinated. He wrote that the experiments 'deeply impressed me; and reproduced, I eagerly devoured such books on the subject as my father possessed, notably Dr. Gregory's *Animal Magnetism* and a translation of Reichenbach's work.'[39]

[35] 'Bramwell, John Milne, M.B.', p. 125 in Victor Plarr, *Men and Women of the Time: A Dictionary of Contemporaries* (London: Routledge, 1899).

[36] Frederick Kelly, *Race Against Time: The Diaries of F.S. Kelly*, ed. by Thérèse Radic (Canberra: National Library of Australia, 2004).

[37] James Esdaile, *Mesmerism in India and Its Practical Application in Surgery and Medicine* (London: Longman, Brown, Green, and Longmans, 1846).

[38] John Milne Bramwell, 'Hypnotism: An Outline Sketch', *The Clinical Journal*, 20 (May 1902) 41–5 (p. 43).

[39] Carl von Reichenbach was a brilliant German chemist who late in life (and influenced by Franz Mesmer) described a field of energy possessed by all living things which linked

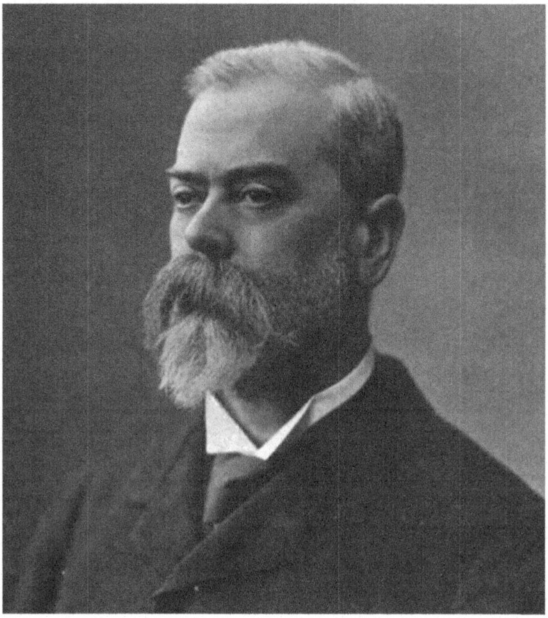

Fig. 2.3 Studio Portrait of John Milne Bramwell (1852–1925). From Begbie, Harold, "Dr. Milne Bramwell and Hypnotism", pp. 275–288 in Begbie, H., Master Workers, Methuen & Co. (London), 1905, facing page 275

Medicine was often a family business and soon after Bramwell's arrival at Edinburgh University in 1868, he befriended Charles Braid who was already a medical student there. Charles was the grandson of his hero and Britain's greatest medical hypnotist, James Braid. His friendship with Charles allowed him ongoing access to all of James Braid's papers still held by the family. Since much of his writing was in rare, hard to find pamphlets, this was a considerable advantage to him and made him one of the few Braid scholars familiar with his work after *Neurhypnology* (1843).[40]

electricity, magnetism and heat, that he called the Odic force. John Milne Bramwell, *Hypnotism: It's History, Practice and Theory* (London: Grant Richards, 1903) (p. 37).

[40] James Braid, *Neurypnology or the Rationale of Nervous Sleep* (London: Churchill, 1843).

Students at Edinburgh at this time would have found that the ideas of the Scottish common-sense realism school of philosophy were still pervasive. The school stressed the importance of sensory and mental processes in common-sense beliefs. As a result, Edinburgh was renowned for its interest in subjects relating to the mind and for investigations into practices such as mesmerism, as well as dreams and somnambulism. Influentially, the lay homeopath Spenser Timothy Hall had given an exhibition of mesmerism in Edinburgh one September night in 1844. The audience included George Combe, a local lawyer and phrenology lecturer who had set up the Phrenology Society of Edinburgh and William Gregory, a chemistry professor from the medical school. Both were so struck by what they had witnessed that they set up a scientific society and commenced their own mesmeric experiments and laid on demonstrations. Within seven years, this localised interest had become a fashionable social craze in Edinburgh.

John Hughes Bennet, another local professor of medicine, felt compelled to respond and attempted to provide a rational scientific explanation for the mesmeric phenomena. He wrote of the *Mesmeric Mania of 1851 in Edinburgh*: 'Fashionable parties have been converted into scenes of experiments on the mental functions. Noblemen, members of the learned professions, and respectable citizens, have been amusing themselves in private, whilst discourses and exhibitions to an unusual extent have been got up for the entertainment of the public.'[41]

The influence of Combe and Gregory and the medical mesmerists was long-lasting. In the first half of the nineteenth century, Edinburgh medical school had produced the majority of Britain's most prominent medical mesmerists and hypnotists. These included James Braid, John Elliotson and James Esdaile. Another Edinburgh graduate, William Engledue, was the co-editor with John Elliotson of the *Zoist*, the journal of mesmerism and phrenology which printed quarterly between 1843 and 1855. All these physicians were part of a late flowering of medical mesmerism in Britain and they published into the 1850s and some into the 1860s, long after the serious scientific consideration of animal magnetism had been terminated in London by the public disgrace of John Elliotson and rejection of his work.

[41] John Hughes Bennett, *Mesmeric Mania of 1851* (Edinburgh: Sutherland and Knox, 1851) (p. 5).

As a result of these factors, mesmerism remained in currency in Edinburgh for much longer than elsewhere in Britain.[42] Bramwell records that even around 1870 his physiology professor, the same Hughes Bennett, included a review of Braid's research as a 'regular part of his course of physiology, and he confidently asserted that one day hypnotism would revolutionise the theory and practice of medicine.'[43] Edinburgh University's strong and enduring links to animal magnetism and hypnotism were not lost on the wider public and the writer physicians Arthur Conan Doyle and Riccardo Stevens both set their tales of mesmerism, *The Parasite* (1894) and *The Cruciform Mark* (1896), respectively, among the medical students of Edinburgh.[44]

On graduation, Bramwell worked as ship's surgeon for the Liverpool, Brazil and River Plate Steam Ship Company for a year.[45] Over the year 1873, he travelled three times to Brazil before returning to Perth and taking up a post as an Assistant Surgeon at Perth City and County Infirmary. In 1875, he married Mary Reynolds, daughter of Captain Charles Reynolds, a retired Assistant-Commissioner of Assam. The couple moved to Goole in Yorkshire where Bramwell joined a general practice with Malcolm Morris. Bramwell claims to have started using Braid's hypnotic techniques in isolation in his general practice before interest in the procedure developed elsewhere: 'My success [with my first patient] encouraged me to persevere—at first cautiously amongst personal friends, and then more and more boldly amongst my patients in general.'[46] He later visited Charcot in Paris, Bernheim and Liébeault in Nancy and the Amsterdam clinic of van Eeden and van Renterghem around 1888, learning other techniques and the theory of suggestion. He was a skilled medical hypnotist and one of his medical peers, George Robertson described him as

[42] Gordon Bates, 'Arthur Conan Doyle in Mesmeric Edinburgh and Hypnotic London', *Victoriographies*, 11, 3 (2021) 314–330 (p. 318).

[43] John Milne Bramwell, *Hypnotism: Its History, Practice and Theory* (London: Grant Richards, 1903) (p. 38).

[44] Arthur Conan Doyle, 'The Parasite', *The Parasite and The Watter's Mou*, ed. by Catherine Wynne (Kansas City: Valancourt Books, 2009) (pp. 3–47); Riccardo Stevens, *The Cruciform Mark* (London: Chatto and Windus, 1896).

[45] 'Bramwell, John Milne, M.B.', p. 125 in Victor Plarr, *Men and Women of the Time: A Dictionary of Contemporaries* (London: Routledge, 1899).

[46] John Milne Bramwell, *Hypnotism: Its History, Practice and Theory* (London: Grant Richards, 1903) (p. 38).

acquiring a reputation in Goole 'resembling Professor Bernheim's in Nancy.'[47]

Bramwell would later claim that he had so many patients referred to him that he took the decision to move to London in 1892. He decided that he would be able to make a living working solely as a specialist in medical hypnotism. The move to London also made it easier for Bramwell to continue his archival and practical research into the subject, and he joined the SPR in 1890. His position in the society was reinforced by his sister's 1892 marriage to Frank Podmore, a high-ranking administrator in the Post Office and one of the more senior and prolific writers of the group. Podmore's home was the site of the first psychology laboratory in the UK, a place where hypnotic phenomena were investigated under more rigorous conditions than the parlour.

For Bramwell, his early positive experiences of hypnotism with his father and his later studies at Edinburgh University appear the critical influences on his practice of hypnotism.

George Chadwick Kingsbury (1860–1938)

There is less information available about George Kingsbury, though he was clearly a colourful figure. According to his 1938 obituary in the *Blackpool Gazette*, Kingsbury was 'the most picturesque of those who dominated local politics and social life 40 years ago.'[48] Describing his medical and hypnotic interests, they concluded that he was 'in advance of his time and he suffered the handicap of all genius' (Fig. 2.4).

Kingsbury was a bright man of many interests. Like Bramwell and Tuckey, he had visited Nancy and Amsterdam in the late 1890s before he started practising medical hypnotism and writing an influential textbook on the subject, *The Practice of Medical Suggestion* (1891).[49] Kingsbury was from a mercantile Anglo-Irish family. He trained in medicine in Dublin, graduating top of his year in 1881 and obtaining his MD in 1883. After junior positions in Dublin, he moved to Blackpool, an

[47] George Robertson, 'Psycho-Therapeutics: Another Fragment', *Lancet* (17 September 1892) (pp. 657–8) (p. 657).

[48] Anon, 'George Kingsbury', *Blackpool Gazette* (9 March 1938).

[49] George Kingsbury, *The Practice of Hypnotic Suggestion, Being and Elementary Handbook for the Use of the Medical Profession* (Bristol: John Wright, 1891).

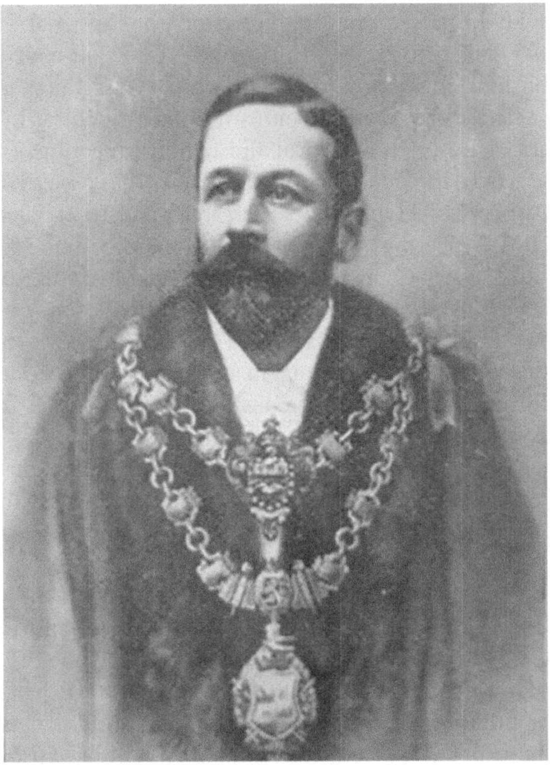

Fig. 2.4 'George C. Kingsbury, Esq., M.A., M.D. Mayor of Blackpool 1899–1900' in Blackpool Corporation. Blackpool's Progress (NP: Blackpool, 1926). Plate 25. https://www.liveblackpool.info/wp-content/uploads/2021/01/blackpools-progress-1926-from-philip-blezard.pdf

English seaside town which was a rapidly growing holiday resort with good rail links and a longstanding centre for therapeutic sea-bathing that was still fashionable among the wealthy. A good lucrative prospect for an ambitious young doctor.

In 1886, Kingsbury married a local girl Ada Edelston, daughter of a Preston cotton mill owner. He went on to secure his financial position by developing formal links with the local hotels and bathing facilities. As Blackpool grew as a holiday destination and attracted more visitors, he became the consultant physician to Blackpool's grandest new hotels: the

South Shore Hydropathic establishment and the Imperial Hydropathic Hotel. He also helped to establish Blackpool's first golf course.[50]

After publishing his book on hypnotism, Kingsbury joined both Bramwell and Tuckey in giving demonstrations of medical hypnotism to doctors at various hospitals and local and national meetings of the BMA. He wrote an article for gentleman's periodical, the *Nineteenth Century* on the legal aspects of Hypnotism.[51] He returned to Ireland to lecture at the local BMA meeting in Dublin.[52] Here he had the assistance of the unlikely ally Francis Cruise, a previous president of the Royal College of Physicians of Ireland, a urologist who had visited Nancy in 1890 and written his own book on hypnotism.

As I will describe later, Kingsbury made an important contribution to the BMA's formal evaluation of medical hypnotism. He was elected to the twelve-man committee investigating the subject by the Psychology section of the BMA after their national meeting in Birmingham in 1891. He was an active member of that committee, visiting asylums, liaising with the geographically distant members and helping to coordinate the final report.

In addition to his commitments and travel with his hypnotism campaign, Kingsbury continued to work in Blackpool and used hypnotism in his own medical practice. In December 1897, one of his patients, Mrs Harriet Howard, left him an estimated £30,000 in her will.[53] Her son would dispute this in the probate courts, suggesting that as Kingsbury had used hypnotism in his treatment of her, he might have used this nefarious power to influence her decision. The court heard that Mrs. Howard had fallen out with her family and Kingsbury was not only her medical attendant but also her friend of ten years standing. He reassured the court that he had stopped using hypnotism in her treatment several years before. Tuckey was called as an expert witness. As was William Broadbent who had sat on the original BMA Committee on hypnotism. In July 1898, the court found the will valid and he received the 'residuary estate'.

[50] Anon, 'Blackpool Golf Course Proposal', *Sheffield Daily Telegraph* (23 February 1894).

[51] George Kingsbury, 'Hypnotism, Crime and the Doctors', *The Nineteenth Century*, 29, 167 (January 1891) (pp. 145–153).

[52] George Kingsbury, 'Should We Give Hypnotism a Trial?' *Dublin Journal of Medical Science* (May 1891) 396–406 (p. 396).

[53] Anon, 'Kingsbury v. Howard', *British Medical Journal*, 2 (23 July 1898) (p. 253).

It seems likely that this huge legacy, worth around £4 million today, made a big difference to Kingsbury and his family. Within a year, he went into politics, a notoriously expensive career move. He was the mayor of Blackpool from 1899 to 1900 and remained an alderman after this. He also made an attempt at national politics, standing as the Conservative candidate for Rossendale in 1900, narrowly losing to the Liberal candidate William Mather who campaigned from St. Moritz due to illness.[54]

A notable aspect of Kingsbury's personality was his combination of litigiousness and self-assurance. He sued the editor of the *BMJ*, Ernest Hart for libel in 1896 when he believed that had been accused anonymously in the journal of self-advertisement, which was (and remains) a professional medical misconduct in the UK. He claimed that the new owners of a Blackpool hotel had used his name in their prospectus to promote themselves rather than him and without his permission. He was awarded damages of £150. After his success in court, he raised a motion against Hart at the next BMA annual meeting about this lawsuit, despite Hart's presence at the meeting. Hart was a powerful opponent to take on. He had single-handedly ensured the success of the financial stability of the BMA and the *BMJ* over his 30-year editorship. Yet Kingsbury raised the motion at the national meeting and circulated a pamphlet publicising the details of his libel case.

After standing for parliament unsuccessfully, he moved to London and started to practice law as a barrister specialising in medicolegal cases. According to his obituary, he also worked as a faith healer over this period though there are no records of this.[55] However, the rapid growth of the church of Christian Science was the source of regular work for him. He defended many Christian Scientists prosecuted for neglect or manslaughter because they had not sought orthodox medical help. One of these was Robert Chisholm, the father of a 10-year-old who had died of diphtheria despite the prayers of his Christian Science nurse.[56]

In 1906, Kingsbury defended George Adcock, a medical doctor who had converted to Christian Science, renounced his medical training and

[54] Anon, 'Rossendale By-Election', *Times* (12 February 1900) (p. 6).

[55] Anon, 'Obituary—George Kingsbury', *Blackpool Gazette and Herald* (9 March 1938).

[56] Anon, 'A Christian Science Case', *Times* (10 November 1906) (p. 8).

practiced as a healer. The doctrine of the newly popular Church of Christian Science was that physical existence was a God-given illusion. It followed that sickness was illusory and represented spiritual malaise rather than physical illness. Consequently, traditional medicine was worthless and prayer and faith-healing were the only possible approaches. Adcock was charged with the manslaughter 'by wilful neglect' of Major J. N. Whyte, who had broken his back in a riding accident three years previous.[57] He had had back surgery but remained unable to walk and developed severe bedsores. Initially, he had made some progress but before his death, Adcock attended him for several months using 'prayer rather than antiseptic'. It had been Major Whyte's decision to stick with Christian Science because it had helped his pain and he had died of his sepsis.

Kingsbury was most unusual in defending Christian Science through his knowledge of faith-healing, as most orthodox doctors were most concerned by the threat of the new church. However, Kingsbury clearly had a strong belief in himself which allowed him to challenge the medical authority and orthodoxy of the time.

Robert William Felkin (1853–1926)

Felkin's life was so extraordinary and eventful that the problem comes in remaining relevant and doing it justice. This task is not helped by the fact that the most contemporary biography we have, was written by his second wife and was at least partly fictionalised as Felkin believed his dreams and visions to be real.[58] He was a medical missionary, tropical medicine physician, explorer, ethnologist and a significant mystic and occultist who practiced and wrote about hypnotism and medical hypnotism. One of the striking things about his conventional medical biographies is the omission

[57] Anon, 'The Christian Science Case' *British Medical Journal* (2 June 1906) (p. 1321).

[58] Various, *The Lantern Volume I (A Wayfaring Man Part I)* (New Zealand: Sub Rosa Press, 2012).

or fleeting reference to these last important aspects of his life.[59] His mysticism is an important feature as there are significant connections between hypnotism and the occult which will be explored later (Figs. 2.5 and 2.6).

Felkin was born in Beeston to a wealthy Nottinghamshire family in 1853. His grandfather and father owned a famous lacemaking factory. When the business failed disastrously in 1864, the family moved to a smaller house in Wolverhampton and Robert attended the grammar school there. The explorer David Livingstone visited the school and apparently inspired Felkin with his romantic stories of Africa and it's peoples. The family did not have enough money to send both their sons to University and Felkin knew that he would have to support himself if he wished to achieve his dream of going to medical school and becoming a medical missionary.[60]

He was a prolific reader as a teenager and remembered reading medical texts including one that covered Braid and Mesmer. In *A Wayfaring Man* he recalls that he experimented with hypnotism with the teenage children of local family friends, the Bartons. On one occasion, Mr Barton came home to discover that Felkin had hypnotised his daughter Madge. He angrily demanded that Felkin brought her back out of the trance state and after this episode, he was barred from seeing the teenage girls of the family for many years.[61] There were longstanding suspicions about the misuse of mesmerism and hypnotism for sexual purposes. He describes another later incident while working as a German teacher to fund his medical studies. He hypnotised a schoolgirl who was disrupting his lesson with the sunlight from a paperweight.[62]

After Wolverhampton Grammar, the young Robert worked for several years in Chemnitz in Germany staying with an uncle and learning German. One of his German friends was a medical student and passed on all his lecture notes. In 1875, he started at Edinburgh medical school, a few years after the medical hypnotist John Bramwell. However, a couple of years into his course, he met A. M. Mackay, a Christian missionary

[59] Anon, 'Obituary: Robert William Felkin, M.D., F.R.S.Ed.', *BMJ*, 1 (12 February 1927) (p. 309); Peter Dunn, 'Robert Felkin MD (1853–1926) and Caesarean delivery in Central Africa (1879)', *Archives of Disease in Childhood—Fetal and Neonatal Edition* (1999) 80, F250–F251.

[60] Various, *A Wayfaring Man Part I* (p. 54).

[61] Various, *A Wayfaring Man Part I* (pp. 57–8).

[62] Various, *A Wayfaring Man Part I* (p. 75).

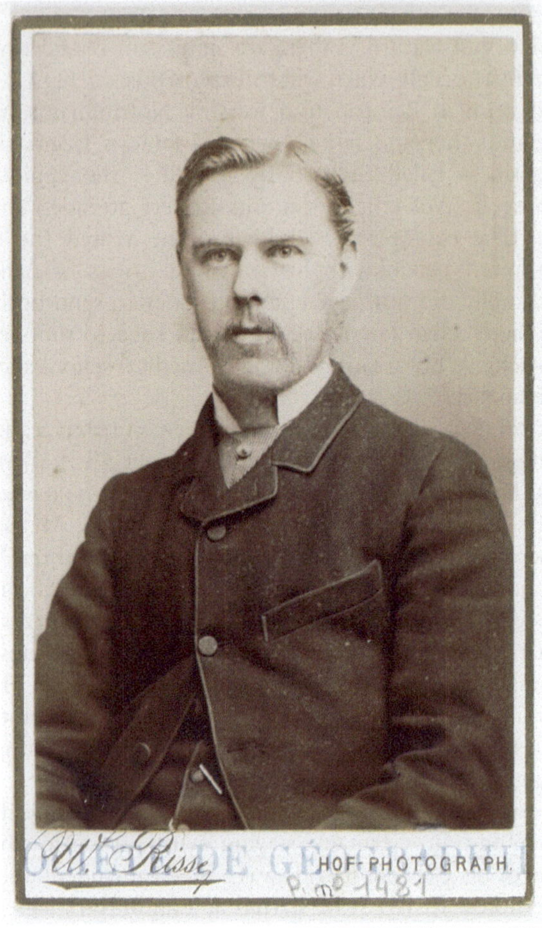

Fig. 2.5 Felkin at 22, Risse, Wilhelm Photographer. Robert Felkin 1885. Courtesy of Bibliotheque Nationale de France https://gallica.bnf.fr/ark:/12148/btv1b8452942h

to Africa. He was reinspired, and the following year accepted a posting to Uganda from the Church Missionary Society, before completing his medical studies.

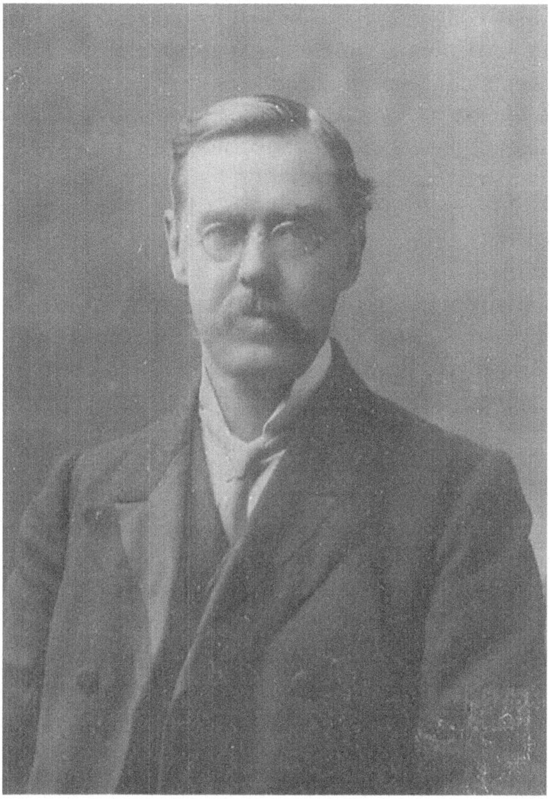

Fig. 2.6 Older Felkin picture https://commons.wikimedia.org/wiki/File:2989_Dr_Felkin.jpg

He travelled by boat up the Nile to Khartoum, where he met General Gordon, and from there travelled to unexplored and unmapped Central Africa. In the Great Lakes region, near today's countries of Uganda and South Sudan, he met and befriended Emin Pasha, the Governor of the Anglo-Egyptian Equatorial Province, and was presented to King Muteesa of Buganda, now Uganda. He became his personal physician in 1879. In Uganda, he pursued his interests in tropical medicine, obstetric practice and ethnography collecting the data that would underpin his later publications.[63] His BMJ obituary highlights the perils of his missionary work and medical research, 'He left Uganda with the envoys of King M'tesa [Muteesa] to Queen Victoria, and returned with them safely to the Nile, thus destroying an old superstition that no white man could journey to the Great Lakes and back without losing his life.'[64] However, his African travels did put a strain on his health, and in 1881, after a few further years in Zanzibar, he returned to Edinburgh to recuperate and complete his medical studies.

Felkin married Mary Manders, the daughter of his father's boss in 1882. He wrote prolifically and was a precocious medical student becoming a Fellow of the Royal Society of Edinburgh, a Fellow of the Royal Geographical Society, a member of the Anthropological Institute of Great Britain and a corresponding Fellow of the Berlin Anthropological Society. In his final year, he gave a lecture to Edinburgh's Obstetrical Society entitled 'Notes on Labour in Central Africa.'[65] On graduation, he continued his medical studies in Heidelberg and then Marburg, receiving an MD from there in 1885.

Felkin returned to Edinburgh in 1886 and was appointed a lecturer in tropical medicine, a post he retained for the next ten years. He and his wife had always been devout Anglican Christians but after exposure to Hinduism through a Bible study group, they joined the local Theosophy Society.[66] Theosophy had been founded in New York in 1875. Its synthesis of Eastern and Western religion and spiritualism had been increasing in popularity in Britain in the 1880s and 1890s. It promoted equality between sex and races and encouraged research into the occult and the powers latent in mankind. These aspects became increasingly important to the Felkins.

[63] Robert Felkin, *On the Geographical Distribution of Tropical Diseases in Africa* (Edinburgh: Clay, 1895); Charles Wilson and Robert Felkin, *Uganda and the Egyptian Soudan*, vols. 1 and 2 (London: Sampson Low, Marston, Searle, Rivington, 1882).

[64] Anon, 'Obituary: Robert William Felkin, M.D., F.R.S.Ed.', *British Medical Journal*, 1 (1927) (p. 309).

[65] Robert Felkin, 'Notes on Labour in Central Africa', *Edinburgh Medical Journal* (1884) 29 (pp. 922–930).

[66] Robert Ellwood, *Islands of the Dawn: The Story of Alternative Spirituality in New Zealand* (Honolulu: University of Hawaii Press, 1993) (p. 162).

In his biography, Felkin suggests that it was his Edinburgh medical school colleague, Dr. Joseph Bell, Conan Doyle's inspiration for Sherlock Holmes, who suggested that he investigate hypnotism further. In 1889, Felkin had been invited to review two books for the *Edinburgh Medical Journal*. These were Tuckey's *Psycho-Therapeutics* and an English translation of Rudolf Heinehan's *Hypnotism or Animal Magnetism*.[67] Instead of providing the two brief notices commissioned by the editor, Felkin thought the subject was too important. Overstepping his brief, he went to observe the work of van Eeden and van Renterghem at the Amsterdam hypnotic clinic and wrote an extensive but thoughtful summary of the international literature, particularly the French and German papers. He concluded that the Europeans had proven that there was something useful in hypnotism and that it warranted serious scientific study by the British. The journal contributions were collected and published by Young Pentland in a short book which ran to 84 pages. He kept the new coinage of the word 'psycho-therapeutics' from Tuckey's book giving it the title: *Hypnotism or Psycho-Therapeutics*.

Felkin did not write further on hypnotism but according to his biography remained interested in psychosomatic medicine throughout his career. There is evidence that he continued to use hypnotism. He was an early member of the MSSST, which formed in 1908 to support medical practitioners interested in the therapeutic use of suggestion. He also translated the Wilhelm Hilger's *Hypnosis and Suggestion* from German which was published in 1912.[68] This does suggest an ongoing scholarship in suggestion for over 20 years. The book includes an excellent foreword from van Renterghem which provides an excellent summary of the progress and debates in hypnotism and clearly follows the Nancy school.

There is insufficient evidence to know whether Felkin did use hypnotism in his medical practice, though he does make clear his fascination for the interplay between mind and body. He moved to London in 1896, where he undertook specialist work in nervous diseases and gynaecology which may well have responded to hypnotic interventions. He also made use of his experiences with infectious diseases in Africa becoming the

[67] Rudolf Heinehan, *Hypnotism or Animal Magnetism: Physiological Observations*, 2nd ed., trans. L. Wooldridge (London: Paul, Trench, 1888).

[68] Wilhelm Hilger, *Hypnosis and Suggestion: Their Nature, Action and Importance Among the Therapeutic Agents*, trans. Robert Felkin (London: Rebman, 1912).

consulting physician to various London companies with tropical colonial interests. His biography suggests that he moved due to ill health and overwork in Edinburgh but others have proposed that the relocation to England was the result of Felkin's involvement in the arcane ceremonial magic group, the Hermetic Order of the Golden Dawn (hereafter the Golden Dawn).

One of the most interesting developments in cultural life at the end of the nineteenth century was the resurgence of occultism and the resulting expansion of mystical and esoteric societies among the middle class. This had significant implications for hypnotism and its uncanny rise. Hypnotism was subject to as much attention from the occultists as the physicians. The most important of the occult orders was the Golden Dawn which was founded in 1888 by Dr. William Robert Woodman, Dr. William Wynn Westcott and Samuel Liddell MacGregor Mathers. They were all originally Freemasons and members of Societas Rosicruciana in Anglia (S.R.I.A), a Masonic esoteric Christian order formed by Robert Wentworth Little in 1865.

The Golden Dawn was a ceremonial magical group, with the aim of personal spiritual development. Membership was open to both men and women and the system of progression was modelled on the hierarchy, training and initiation of the Masonic Lodges. The organisation was divided into three orders; the First taught esoteric philosophy grounded in the Hermetic Qabalah and personal development through study and awareness of the four Classical Elements as well as the basics of astrology, tarot divination and geomancy. The Second or 'Inner' Order taught more uncanny magic, including scrying (distant vision), astral travel (projection of the spirit) and alchemy. The Third Order was that of the 'Secret Chiefs' who were said to be highly spiritually developed beings; they supposedly directed the activities of the lower two orders by spirit communication with the Chiefs of the Second Order.

Even materialist physicians have spiritual needs and medical doctors were well-represented in the Golden Dawn. Two of the founders, Woodman and Westcott were both medical. Tuckey too, was nominated and initiated at the Isis-Urania temple in 1894. Felkin's membership of the Golden Dawn was to have a profound and far-reaching influence on his life. He and his wife had initially joined the Amen-Ra temple in Edinburgh in 1894. It seems likely that he came to London from Edinburgh in 1896 to join its Isis-Urania temple, the order's centre of power, as he had achieved a place in the Second Order. Shortly after arriving in London,

Felkin started to become convinced that he was in direct communication with the Secret Chiefs of the Golden Dawn whom he referred to as 'Sun Masters'.

When the order splintered in 1900, there was a schism. A. E. Waite led those more interested in Christian mysticism while Felkin and those more curious about occultism like the writer William Butler Yeats and the lawyer John Brodie-Innes formed the Stella Matutina (Morning Star). Given Felkin's wanderlust it is no surprise that his preferred mystical practice was astral projection. In 1906, the new order established their mother temple, Amoun Temple, at Felkin's house in North London. As the new leader of the group, Felkin established several more temples: one in New Zealand and three in England. He also visited Germany searching for evidence or relatives of the original Anna Sprengel (the German Secret Chief whose letters apparently authorised the founding of the original Golden Dawn).

Felkin was in Germany in 1914 at the outbreak of the Great War. According to his biography, they had been charged with an urgent mission and ignored the warnings of war though this may represent one of the more fictional sections.[69] They managed to avoid arrest and escaped to the Netherlands, with the help of German Masons.[70] After a short time in the British National Guard, Felkin's health broke down and in 1916 he and his family decided to emigrate to New Zealand. He spent the remainder of his life there, practising as a physician and ceremonial magician between bouts of ill health.

Felkin's interest in medical hypnotism, suggestion and what came to be known as psychosomatic medicine may only have represented a small aspect of his overall multi-faceted career. Nevertheless, his timely book served to reinforce both the use of the term psycho-therapeutics as a catch-all term for psychological therapies and for treatment by suggestion.[71] Additionally, his subsequent immersion in ceremonial magic demonstrates another important aspect of the technique. Hypnotism was closely allied to the occult and medical doctors would have to tackle this

69 Various, *The Lantern Volume 2 (A Wayfaring Man Part II)* (New Zealand: Sub Rosa Press, 2012).

70 Robert Ellwood, *Islands of the Dawn: The Story of Alternative Spirituality in New Zealand* (Honolulu: University of Hawaii Press, 1993).

71 Sonu Shamdasani, '"Psychotherapy": The Invention of a Word', *History of the Human Sciences*, 18 (2005) 1–22 (p. 4).

to ensure its acceptability to the general public and more particularly, to the medical institutions.

The four New Hypnotists displayed a variety of reasons and motivations for investigating and promoting hypnotism. Although it had fringe status and sanctions for working outside, the medical orthodoxy could be severe, these doctors were convinced of its healing properties. Bramwell had encountered Braid's hypnotism at a young age from his father. He and Felkin had trained in Edinburgh where mesmerism and then hypnotism had remained more credible and acceptable over the Victorian era. Tuckey came from a family of physician homeopaths and had trained at the LHH. He was accustomed to using contested medical belief systems and through homeopathy encountered others more familiar with hypnotism like Martin Roth. The rise of scientific materialism had led to a resurgence in spirituality to which doctors were not immune. Tuckey and Felkin's membership of the Golden Dawn demonstrates that they were willing to explore both scientific and mystical approaches to understand hypnotism. Kingsbury's motivations appear to stem from his ambition, scientific curiosity and unusual self-assurance.

All were characterised by a peculiarly Victorian medical attitude of service and self-righteousness. This ethos is perhaps best encapsulated by the book dedication for the autobiography of a late convert to hypnotism, the psychiatrist and M.C.C. cricketer L. Forbes Winslow:

> This book is dedicated to every true Englishman who, having the courage of his opinions and convictions, is not ashamed to express the same, and who in every way acts up to what he thinks is right, with a view to benefiting humanity doing good in the world by preventing harm, heedless of public opinion and the consequences of jealousy, and who hits "straight out from the shoulder," as every true-born Englishman should do without fear of consequences.[72]

Bibliography

Anon. 1887a. 'Margaret Street Infirmary', *Medical Review*, 31: 309.

Anon. 1887b. 'Liberty of Opinion in the Art of Therapeutics', *Monthly Homoeopathic Review*, 31: 168–9.

[72] L. Forbes Winslow, *Recollections of Forty Years* (London: John Ouseley, 1910).

Anon. 1887c. 'The Margaret Street Infirmary for Consumption', *London Medical Press and Circular* (9 March): 3.
Anon. 1887d. 'Resignation of the Medical Staff from the Margaret Street Infirmary for Consumption', *British Medical Journal* (5 March): 541.
Anon. 1887e. 'Millican v. Sulivan and Others', *Times* (16 December): 3.
Anon. 1890a. 'Demonstration of Hypnotism as an Anæsthetic During the Performance of Dental and Surgical Operations', *Lancet*, 135 (5 April): 771–2.
Anon. 1890b. 'Hypnotism as an Anæsthetic in Surgery', *British Medical Journal*, 1528 (12 April): 849–50.
Anon. 1898. 'Kingsbury v. Howard', *British Medical Journal*, 2 (23 July): 253.
Anon. 1900. 'Rossendale By-Election', *Times* (12 February): 6.
Anon. 1904a. 'Blackpool Golf Course Proposal', *Sheffield Daily Telegraph* (23 February).
Anon. 1904b. 'Robert Ellis Dudgeon, M.D.', *Monthly Homoeopathic Review*, 48 (October): 577.
Anon. 1906a. 'A Christian Science Case', *Times* (10 November): 8.
Anon. 1906b. 'The Christian Science Case', *British Medical Journal* (2 June): 1321.
Anon. 1925. 'Obituary: Charles Lloyd Tuckey', *Journal of the Society for Psychical Research*, 22 (October): 115–7.
Anon. 1927. 'Obituary: Robert William Felkin, M.D., F.R.S.Ed.', *British Medical Journal*, 1 (12 February): 309.
Anon. 1938. 'George Kingsbury', *Blackpool Gazette and Herald* (9 March).
Atkin, George. 1853. *The British and Foreign Medical Homoeopathic Directory 1853.* London: Aylott. 51.
Bates, Gordon. 2021. 'Arthur Conan Doyle in Mesmeric Edinburgh and Hypnotic London', *Victoriographies*, 11, 3: 314–30.
Bennett, John Hughes. 1851. *Mesmeric Mania of 1851.* Edinburgh: Sutherland and Knox. 5.
Braid, James. 1843. *Neurypnology or the Rationale of Nervous Sleep.* London: Churchill.
'Bramwell, John Milne, M.B.' 1899. *Men and Women of the Time: A Dictionary of Contemporaries*, ed. by Victor Plarr. London: Routledge. 121.
Bramwell, John Milne. 1902. 'Hypnotism: An Outline Sketch', *Clinical Journal* 20: 43.
Bramwell, John Milne. 1903. *Hypnotism: It's History, Practice and Theory*, 1st ed. London: Grant Richards. 37.
Bramwell, John Milne. 1921. *Hypnotism: It's History, Practice and Theory*, 3rd ed. London: Rider. 35.
Buckle, George Earle. 1888. 'Editorial: Odium Medicum', *Times* (20 January): 9.

Clarke, John Henry. 1888. *Odium Medicum and Homoeopathy: "The Times" correspondence, reprinted by permission of the proprietors of "The Times."* London: Homoeopathic Publishing.

Cooke, Alexander. 1972. *A History of the Royal College of Physicians of London*, vol. 3. Oxford: Clarendon Press. 904–8.

Doyle, Arthur Conan. 2009. 'The Parasite', in *The Parasite and The Watter's Mou*, ed. by Catherine Wynne. Kansas City: Valancourt Books. 3–47.

Dunn, Peter. 1999. 'Robert Felkin MD (1853–1926) and Caesarean Delivery in Central Africa (1879)', *Archives of Disease in Childhood—Fetal and Neonatal Edition* 80: F250–F251.

Ellwood, Robert. 1993. *Islands of the Dawn: The Story of Alternative Spirituality in New Zealand*. Honolulu: University of Hawaii Press. 162.

Esdaile, James. 1846. *Mesmerism in India and Its Practical Application in Surgery and Medicine*. London: Longman, Brown, Green and Longmans.

Felkin, Robert. 1884. 'Notes on Labour in Central Africa', *Edinburgh Medical Journal*, 29: 922–30.

Felkin, Robert. 1890. *Hypnotism or Psycho-Therapeutics*. Edinburgh: Y. J. Pentland.

Felkin, Robert. 1895. *On the Geographical Distribution of Tropical Diseases in Africa*. Edinburgh: Clay.

Gieryn, Thomas. 1983. 'Boundary-Work and the Demarcation of Science from Non-Science: Strains and Interests in Professional Ideologies of Scientists', *American Sociological Review*, 48, 6: 781–95.

Goldsbrough, Giles. 1905. 'Members of the British Homoeopathic Society', *Journal of the British Homoeopathic Society, New Series*, 13: vi–xxiv.

Gurney, Edwards, and Myers Frederic. 1883. 'Mesmerism', *Nineteenth Century*, 9 (October): 695–719.

Hahnemann, Samuel. 1833. *The Homœopathic Medical Doctrine, or "Organon of the Healing Art"*, trans. by Charles Devrient. Dublin: W.F. Wakeman.

Hahnemann, Samuel. 1849. *Organon of Medicine*, 5th ed., trans. by Robert Dudgeon. London: Headland.

Heinehan, Rudolf. 1888. *Hypnotism or Animal Magnetism: Physiological Observations* 2nd ed., trans. L. Wooldridge. London: Paul, Trench.

Hilger, Wilhelm. 1912. *Hypnosis and Suggestion: Their Nature, Action and Importance Among the Therapeutic Agents*, trans. Robert Felkin. London: Rebman.

Inglis, Brian. 1964. *Fringe Medicine*. London: Faber.

Kelly, Frederick. 2004. *Race Against Time: The Diaries of F.S. Kelly*, ed. by Thérèse Radic. Canberra: National Library of Australia.

Kingsbury, George. 1891a. *The Practice of Hypnotic Suggestion, Being and Elementary Handbook for the Use of the Medical Profession*. Bristol: John Wright.

Kingsbury, George. 1891b. 'Hypnotism, Crime and the Doctors', *Nineteenth Century* 29, 167 (January): 145–53.

Kingsbury, George. 1891c. 'Should We Give Hypnotism a Trial?', *Dublin Journal of Medical Science* (May): 396–406.

Nicholls, Phillip. 1988. *Homeopathy and the Medical Profession.* London: Crook Helm. 134.

Reiswitz, Felix. 2012. *'Globulizing' the Hospital Ward: Legitimizing Homoeopathic Medicine Through the Establishment of Hospitals in 19th-Century London and Madrid,* Appendix E. Unpublished PhD thesis, University College London.

Robertson, George. 1892. 'Psycho-Therapeutics: Another Fragment'. *Lancet* (17 September): 657–8.

Roth, Mathias. 1887. *The Physiological Effects of Artificial Sleep with Some Notes on Treatment by Suggestion.* London: Baillee, Tindall and Cox. 2.

Roth, Mathias. 1891. 'Correspondence: Presentation of a Testimonial to Dr. Liébeault of Nancy', *Monthly Homoeopathic Review*, 9: 488–91.

Shamdasani, Sonu. 2005. '"Psychotherapy": The Invention of a Word', *History of the Human Sciences*, 18: 1–22.

Stevens, Riccardo. 1896. *The Cruciform Mark.* London: Chatto and Windus.

'The Nineteenth Century', in *Dictionary of Nineteenth Century Journalism in Great Britain and Ireland.* 2009, ed. by Laurel Brake and Marysa Denmore. Ghent: Academia Press.

Tuckey, Charles Lloyd. 1888a. 'Faith Healing as a Medical Treatment', *Nineteenth Century*, 21: 839–50.

Tuckey, Charles Lloyd. 1888b. 'Correspondence—Faith-Healing', *Standard*, London, England (3 December): 3.

Tuckey, Charles Lloyd. 1889. *Psycho-Therapeutics: Or Treatment by Sleep and Suggestion.* London: Baillière, Tindall and Cox.

Tuckey, Charles Lloyd. 1893. Letter to van Eeden, October 24th, 1893. In *Van Eeden Collection.* Hs. XXIV C 81. Amsterdam: Allard Pierson, University of Amsterdam.

Tuckey, Charles Lloyd. Entry in *Medical Graduate Schedules, 1862.* University of Aberdeen Medical Schedule (MSU 62).

Various. 2012a. *The Lantern Volume I (A Wayfaring Man Part I).* New Zealand: Sub Rosa Press.

Various. 2012b. *The Lantern Volume 2 (A Wayfaring Man Part II).* New Zealand: Sub Rosa Press.

Wardwell, Walter. 1972. 'Orthodoxy and Heterodoxy in Medical Practice', *Social Science and Medicine* 6: 63.

Wilson, Charles, and Felkin, Robert. 1882. *Uganda and the Egyptian Soudan*, vols. 1 and 2. London: Sampson Low, Marston, Searle, Rivington.

Winslow, L. Forbes. 1910. *Recollections of Forty Years.* London: John Ouseley.

CHAPTER 3

The Limits of the Imagination

To understand the full scale of the task faced by the New Hypnotists and the methods they used to achieve success I will need to provide considerable context: historical, contemporary and cultural. In this next section, I will outline some historical figures linked to trance, several contextual medical and cultural factors as well as unpacking some technical language and concepts. The first of these will be the conceptual model or 'doctrine' of the imagination. The description of this is quite convoluted and complex, in part because that which the imagination represented changed over time.

The idea of the imagination was ancient but also mystical and spiritual and therefore quite at odds with the physical and materialist turn of European nineteenth-century medicine. The French and German schools of medicine emphasised the practical sciences of anatomy and physiology as the way to understand illness. This approach had revolutionised medical practice across Europe. It provided great insights into diseases of the heart, lungs and abdomen. It was the parts of medicine that did not give up their mysteries easily to dissection and experimentation, like psychiatry, obstetrics and psychosomatic illness that still required the doctrine of imagination.

G. D. L. Bates, *The Uncanny Rise of Medical Hypnotism, 1888–1914*, Mental Health in Historical Perspective,
https://doi.org/10.1007/978-3-031-42725-1_3

It is hard to adequately describe the concept which was holistic and non-Cartesian, viewing mind and body equivalently in disease and treatment. It was still used by alienists like Daniel Hack Tuke in his classic *Illustrations of the influence of the Mind upon the Body in Health and Disease* (1870) and initially by the New Hypnotists. Tuckey observed in his first edition of *Psycho-Therapeutics* that diseases ascribed to the imagination 'may be as real as typhus and entail a thousand times more suffering on the patient.'[1] In other words, psychosomatic symptoms are experienced as real by the patient and require some form of treatment just as much as those that have an objective physical basis.

Today's narrow conception of the imagination as the creative and mostly visual aspect of the human mind does not do justice to the complex range of beliefs conveyed by the doctrine of the imagination by the end of the nineteenth century. The Swiss historian of science, Esther Fischer-Homberger has helpfully summarised that the imagination was not always seen as 'imaginary' but rather as a real physical force, which could operate at a distance. It was regarded as a respectable scientific and philosophical principle, related to certain older concepts of phantasy, creativity and memory.[2]

Within the field of medicine, the concept of the imagination was used in three separate areas. Primarily, it was a general mechanism for understanding the effects of the mind upon the body from faith-healing and the effects of curses to outbreaks of hysterical illness. As the *maternal* imagination, it accounted for the well-known observation that events occurring to a mother in pregnancy could influence the physical appearance of the delivered child. Finally, it was understood as an important part of the mind which when overstimulated could lead to madness (Fig. 3.1).

[1] Charles Lloyd Tuckey, *Psycho-Therapeutics or Treatment by Sleep and Suggestion* (London: Balliere, Tindall and Cox, 1889).

[2] Esther Fischer-Homberger, 'On the Medical History of the Doctrine of Imagination', *Psychological Medicine,* 9 (1979) (pp. 619–628) (p. 620).

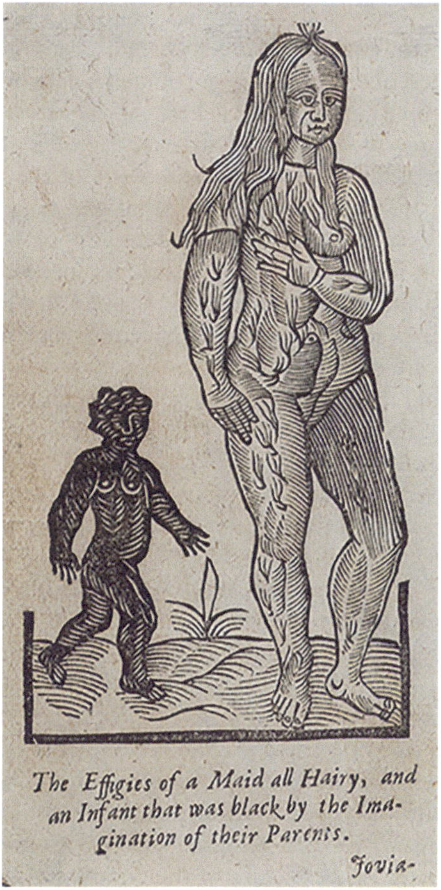

Fig. 3.1 Aristoteles Master-piece, or, The secrets of generation displayed in all the parts thereof. 1684. Cushing Collection, Yale University Medical School Library. EEBO. https://medicalhealthhumanities.com/2018/02/04/monstrous-and-mindful-births-policing-the-pregnant-imagination/

The Imagination: A Prehistory

'The Power of Imagination is exceeding great.'[3] Pierre Charron, *De la Sagesse* (1601)

[3] Pierre Charron, *Of Wisdom Three Books,* Vol 1, trans by George Stanhope (London: Printed for R. Bonwick, 1707) (p. 158).

Sleep and the trance state had enjoyed a close association with many healing practices which predate modern medicine. Classical sources describe a wide range of therapeutic customs in which sleep plays an important element. There were healing temples to divinities like Isis in Ancient Egypt and to Aesculapius in Greece and Rome. The healing procedures at the most famous of the temples to Isis at Memphis had many similarities to those of the temple to Aesculapius at Epidaurus. Both traditions employed healer-priests who interceded with the gods on behalf of the sick. Using incantation, ritual and animal sacrifice, the healer-priests would prepare them for healing. They would then ask the gods for guidance with diagnosis and treatment. At both sites, patients were encouraged to take a healing sleep or *incubatio* both for divinatory and therapeutic purposes. Sometimes the god would appear in the dreams of the patient with instructions for a cure or sometimes the healing would be the result of the sleep itself. The environments of these healing temples were dramatic and theatrical: crepuscular and thick with incense and in the case of the temple at Epidaurus, home to hundreds of snakes, symbols of regeneration and rebirth.[4]

However, from the Renaissance onwards, the mode of action for the transformative healing power of sleep and trance was no longer universally believed to be miraculous in origin nor to be directly mediated by the gods. Instead, it was theorised by some scholars to be the result of the imagination (the creative aspect of the mind) acting upon the body. The imagination was a credible construct of philosophy and natural science that had applications wider than medicine and which lasted from classical antiquity, well beyond the Enlightenment period. It has been described by the cultural historian George Rousseau as 'the greatest advance ever made in the history of the "body-mind" problem'.[5]

The Renaissance model of the imagination was a rediscovery of the classical beliefs of the Greeks. Humans were believed to have three faculties or souls which were simultaneously unitary and tripartite: the vegetative faculty, the sensitive faculty and the rational faculty.[6] Mankind

[4] Károly Kerényi, *Asklepios: Archetypal Image of the Physician's Existence,* Ch 2 *Epidauros* trans by Ralph Manheim (Princeton: Princeton University Press, 1959) (pp. 18–46).

[5] George Rousseau, 'Science and the Discovery of the Imagination in Enlightened England', *Eighteenth Century Studies,* 3 (1969) (pp. 108–35) (p.112).

[6] Stanley Jackson, 'The Imagination and Psychological Healing', *Journal of the History of Medicine and Allied Science,* 26 (1990) (pp. 345–58).

alone had a rational soul which was constituted of three further faculties: imagination, reason and memory. The souls each communicated their effects through the *pneuma*, the spirit or more literally, the breath. Each soul was seen as situated in its own organ (the liver, heart and brain respectively) which could then act through the pneuma. These were not simply metaphors but seen as physically based attributes. For example, the imagination was thought to be located in the lateral ventricles of the brain. The idea of the three-part, rational soul came from Aristotle but was promoted by the influential Galen (129–210 A.D.), the Greek physician and philosopher who described the rational as the most important of the different souls. This same structural physical schema can be found in the work of the English physician Robert Burton and his *The Anatomy of Melancholy* published in 1621.

Another Classical idea to be found in Burton's work but emerging from the Greek Stoic philosophers was the idea of the *passions*. The stoics developed a system of ethics based upon personal development through self-restraint, cooperating with others and understanding the world. Extremes of emotions or *passions* were dangerous as they resulted in errors of judgement. Stoics viewed distress as the result of an incorrect judgement concerning a present evil and the resulting passions to be a potent cause of mental illness. Consequently, the imagination, as an important component of the rational soul, also had a major role in the development or prevention of disturbed behaviour and mental illness.

In the Renaissance period, the boundaries between scientific and mystical thought were not well-demarcated and many of the writers who shaped subsequent scientific thinking were also alchemists. It was quite possible to hold both scientific and magical beliefs simultaneously. It is only the passage of time which has revealed which side of the divide any given idea will fall. The alchemists wrote about the imagination in ways that were useful and later resurfaced, repeated by subsequent natural philosophers and physicians. Probably the most famous of these alchemists was the Swiss physician and mystic Paracelsus (1493–1541) who identified and named zinc, promoted clinical observation in medicine as well as used astrological methods to make prophecies.

While his writings are often opaque and frequently mix allegory and observation, Paracelsus made several important contributions to the medical doctrine of imagination. He credited the imagination as the cause of many invisible diseases and as a mediator between the body and soul. He suggested that curses, which cause illness, and blessings and talisman for cures operate not through some inherent power of the words but through the power of the imagination. This could operate internally on oneself but also externally on another. The imagination was powerful enough to kill as well as cure.[7] Another important aspect of Paracelsian thought was his belief in a connection or 'magnetism' between the stars, minerals, beasts and humans. This appears to be more of a mystical, astrological idea of spiritual connection than the modern concept of physical ferromagnetism. However, he believed that this magnetism could be manipulated by the healthy to enhance the feeble magnetism of the sick.[8] These theories were re-worked and appeared more than 250 years later in the ideas of another physician Franz Mesmer.

Of all the medical aspects of the imagination that Paracelsus described, one of the most powerful and intellectually persistent examples was the doctrine of maternal imagination. This referred to the possible influence of the pregnant mother's emotional experiences on the physical appearance of her unborn baby:

> The imagination of a pregnant woman is so strong that it can influence the seed and change the fruit in her womb in many directions. [...] For the child in the mother's womb is exposed to the mothers influence, and is as though entrusted to the hand and will of its mother, as the clay is entrusted to the hand of the potter, who creates and forms out of it what he wants and what he pleases.[9]

Perhaps strangely for modern readers, this belief endured for centuries and remained the received wisdom for physicians and philosophers well into the eighteenth and nineteenth centuries. Perhaps, its persistence lay in the way it answered questions about birth defects and deformities, and any similarities or dissimilarities between the child and its parents. It came to symbolise a widespread belief in the importance of the mind's influence on the body as well as increasing the culpability of women who could not bear healthy and physically attractive children. Traces of this concept can

[7] Frantz Hartmann, *Life of Paracelsus (1493–1541)* (New York: Theosophical Publishing, 1918) (p. 179).

[8] Arthur Waite, *The Occult Sciences: A Compendium of Transcendental Doctrine and Experiment* (London: Paul Keagan, Trench, Trübner & Co., 1891) (p. 230).

[9] Jolande Jacobi, *Paracelsus Selected Writings* (Trans. Norbert Guterman) (London: Routledge and Kegan Paul, 1951) (p. 106).

still be found in contemporary English. The likely etymology of the term harelip, for the malformation above the upper lip, is derived from the idea that an expectant mother's encounter with a hare was the cause of this facial midline closure defect.[10]

The holistic and mystical doctrine of the imagination was further developed and refined by the Belgian alchemist and chemist, John Baptista van Helmont (1577–1644), perhaps the most innovative of Paracelsus' successors. While he rejected Paracelsus' more astrological theories, van Helmont incorporated many Paracelsian and alchemical ideas in the formation of human physiology based on various *archei* or spiritual energy centres. These were psychological and spiritual at the same time and anatomically based in the major organs. Van Helmont viewed disease as the result of a morbid thought causing the archei to fail to regulate the body properly. The morbid image or thought was first imagined into being by the archeus but could assume a physical form and manifest as illness in certain parts of the body. He gives examples of plagues being caused by 'stupid imagination and fright'. Convulsions, jaundice and paralysis after an animal bite or poison were the result of a transmission of an image of frenzy.[11] For Van Helmont, illness was simultaneously and equally physically real and 'imagined.'

The second important idea developed by van Helmont, was the importance of the site of the archeus. The supreme archeus was seen as the stomach and spleen. All of the other organs from blood to oesophagus were minor archei and could also hold the imagination. However, he saw the uterus as an equivalent to the stomach/spleen which resulted in an increased rate of illness in women. Van Helmont had envisioned two separate models for disease: 'as if Eve had sinned doubly.'[12] This is the origin of the link of 'imaginary' diseases to the terms, hypochondria and hysteria. In hypochondria (literally below the cartilage of the sternum, the upper part of the abdomen), the imagination is operating from the stomach/spleen archeus to cause real somatic disease. In the

[10] Fischer-Homberger, *Imagination* (p. 625).

[11] J. B. van Helmont, *Aufgang der Artzney-Kunst,* trans. by F. M. van Helmont (Sulzbach: Endters Söhne: 1683) qtd. in Fischer-Homberger, *Imagination* (p. 622).

[12] J. B. van Helmont, *Artzney-Kunst* (qtd in Fischer-Homberger, *Imagination*) (p. 621).

case of hysterical diseases, the womb is the location of the disturbed imagination which upsets the proper functioning of the body again producing genuine illness.

These ideas spread rapidly and were taken up more generally than solely by those who would consider themselves followers of Paracelsus. In the sixteenth and seventeenth centuries, the use of enchanted and blessed items (like amulets) or magical incantations (like spells and charms) in physical healthcare was widespread. They were readily available from quacks, folk medicine practitioners and more orthodox physics. Over this period, the mode of action of these talismans and charms came to be understood by scholars as the result of the patient's imagination. In Keith Thomas' social history, *Religion and the Decline of Magic,* he examines contemporary pamphlets and the work of minor writers to explore why people between 1500 and 1700 gradually stopped using the supernatural to understand their lives. He describes the changes in healing practices over this time away from invoking magic and highlights the healer's ingenious methods to find the best ways of influencing the patient's imagination as a way of encouraging mental and physical cures.[13]

Before the Enlightenment, religious belief and the Church also had a major role in healing which continued but diminished into the nineteenth century. Most healers made it clear that they were not directly responsible for the physical cures they could accomplish but were merely the instruments of God. Probably the most famous of these British examples was the 'great stroker' Valentine Greatrakes (1628–1682). In 1666, the Irish war veteran came to London and created 'Greatrakes-mania' by performing public healing on a grand scale. Initially, he was able to cure scrofula, a common tuberculous neck-swelling, but over time was able to widen his repertoire. His healing powers were witnessed and authenticated by the nation's elite including the physicist Robert Boyle and the poet Andrew Marvell. He was even asked to show his work to King Charles II.

A contemporary witness described the response to Grearakes: 'So great was the confidence in him, that the blind fancied they saw the light which they did not see – the deaf imagined they heard – the lame that they

[13] Keith Thomas, 'Magical Healing' Ch 7 in *Religion and the Decline of Magic: Studies in Popular Belief in Sixteenth and Seventeenth Century England* (London: Penguin, 2003).

walked straight, and the paralytic that they had recovered the use of their limbs. An idea of health made the sick forget for a while their maladies.'[14]

With King Charles permission (since healing by stroking was the King's prerogative), Greatrakes remained in England and continued to lay hands on prodigious numbers of the sick. While his only intervention was the stroking of the affected part, many collapsed or had fits before they actually saw him (a further example of the importance of trance or altered consciousness in this form of healing). Greatrakes was a deeply religious man and contemporary accounts describe him as having 'a grave but simple countenance that shewed no signs of his being a cheat.'[15] He interpreted the fits as evidence of demonic possession and saw his treatment as a kind of exorcism. Indeed, he thought all illness to be caused by evil spirits.

The other name for scrofula was the 'King's evil'. This was because this unsightly lymphatic inflammation was believed to be cured by the touch of the British sovereign. This ability was seen as a demonstration of their God-given right to rule. In fact, the condition is self-limiting and will often remit spontaneously. Henry I was believed to be the first to use his talent in England, but the procedure was formalised by Henry VII (reign 1485–1509). He introduced a four-part ceremony which found its way into the Anglican *Book of Common Prayer* (1634). English monarchs varied in their enthusiasm for the ceremony and generally the Catholic ones participated more than the protestant ones. Popular fervour and regal inclination coincided in the reign of Charles II who personally touched 92,000 people over his lifetime. In religious mass ceremonies, he sometimes touched several hundred in a day.[16] It was not until the early eighteenth century that George I discontinued the practice and it was finally removed from the *Book of Common Prayer* in 1732.

By the start of the nineteenth century, scholars could see the similarities been religious faith-healing, charismatic quacks and even the cures of physicians with neutral agents. They were able to explain the phenomenon in all cases with the doctrine of imagination. For example, in

[14] Charles Saint-Evremond, *The Works of Saint-Evremond,* 2 Vols. (London: Jacob Tonson, 1705) (p. 81).

[15] Charles Saint-Evremond, *The Works of Saint-Evremond,* 2 Vols. (London: Jacob Tonson, 1705) (p. 79).

[16] Stephen Brogan, 'Introduction' in *The Royal Touch in Early Modern England: Politics, Medicine and Sin* (Woodbridge, Suffolk: Boydell, 2015) (pp. 1–22).

1841, the journalist and writer Charles McKay observed in *Extraordinary Popular Delusions and the Madness of Crowds*:

> The influence of the imagination in the cure of diseases is well known. A motion of the hand, or a glance of the eye, will throw a weak and credulous patient into a fit: and a pill made of bread taken with sufficient faith, will operate a cure better than all the drugs in the pharmacopeia.[17]

Testing the Imagination

The next incidents, which further shaped and helped define the doctrine of the medical imagination, arose from two popular and highly fashionable but controversial medical therapies which appeared inexplicable to contemporary science. They urgently required an explanation different to that proffered by their inventors and the imagination was the conceptual model that was called upon by scientists and physicians. The first was the meteoric rise of Franz Mesmer's animal magnetism and its sensational reception in pre-revolutionary Paris. The second therapy was Elisha Perkins' patent tractors and their impact in Britain at the end of the eighteenth century. Both were well-known to late Victorian physicians and featured in contemporary texts.

The story of the Austrian physician, Franz Mesmer (1734–1815) and mesmerism is an integral part of the story of therapeutic trance as well as the development of imagination.[18] He theorised a form of energy transfer between both animate and inanimate objects mediated by magnetism. He believed that this process could be utilised in healing through the

[17] Charles McKay, 'The Magnetisers' in *Extraordinary Popular Delusions and the Madness of Crowds* (Ware: Wordsworth Editions, 1995) (pp. 304–345) (p. 304).

[18] Mesmer's story remains contested and has been appropriated by many academics for their own ends. Robert Darnton, 'Mesmerism and Popular Science', in *Mesmerism and the End of the Enlightenment in France* (New York: Schocken Books, 1970) (pp. 2–45); Marie Tatar, 'Preface' in *Spellbound: Studies on Mesmerism and Literature* (Princeton: Princeton University Press, 1978) (pp. ix–xvi); Adam Crabtree, *From Mesmer to Freud: Magnetic Sleep and the Roots of Psychological Healing* (New Haven: Yale University Press, 1993); Henri Ellenberger, *The Discovery of the Unconscious, the History and Evolution of Dynamic Psychiatry* (London: Allen Lane, 1970); Alan Gauld, *A History of Hypnotism* (Cambridge: Cambridge University Press, 1992); Robin Waterfield, *Hidden Depths: The Story of Hypnosis* (London: Pan, 2004); Leon Chertok and Mikkel Borch-Jacobsen, *Hypnose et Psychanalyse: Reponses a Mikkel Borch-Jacobsen* (Paris: Dunod, 1987).

magnetic physician creating an 'artificial tide' to correct the imbalance of the patient. Mesmer's theory of animal magnetism owes an obvious debt to both Classical and alchemical ideas: the invisible fluid that he hypothesised was similar to ether and his idea of rebalancing the body linked it to the humoral theory of disease. His technique of 'passes', exaggerated gestures above the body part would have been familiar to many as it was so close to the touch-healing of Greatrakes and thaumaturgy (magical or religious healing) more generally. However, Mesmer viewed himself as a physician scientist and in his writings linked his healing to a kind of magnetism that he viewed in physical terms similar to Newton's theory of gravitation which he had studied to a doctoral level in Vienna.

Graduating in 1766, Mesmer stayed in Vienna and married a local wealthy widow. He started to attract a widening interest in his healing techniques and developed a healthy practice. However, he was hounded out of the city, ostracised by the Viennese medical establishment, ostensibly the result of a scandal involving a young woman named Maria Paradis. She was a young concert pianist with hysterical blindness whom he had advised to stay at his house for treatment. After staying for several months, Maria refused to leave with her parents who had become worried that her successful treatment might lead to the loss of her musical pension from Empress Maria Theresa. Both her long stay with Mesmer, an impressionable unmarried young woman with a powerful influential older man, and the suggestive and intimate appearance of his mesmeric passes led to medical and societal disapproval. The associations between mesmerism, hypnotism and sexual impropriety started very early and will repeat in the historical narrative.

In 1778, Mesmer headed for Paris, the cultural centre of Europe in the late eighteenth century. He rapidly achieved fame and notoriety, as a result of his sensational new medical treatment. For his cures, Mesmer used *baquets*, wooden tubs filled with metal and glass tubes that were supposed to focus and conduct the invisible forces of animal magnetism which promoted the healing process. Mesmer craved respectability and the acceptance of the medical and scientific fraternity but failed to have his theories approved by the French Royal Academy of Sciences. The Austrian *émigré* would probably have been ignored altogether, by the establishment, were it not for phenomenal uptake of his treatment by not only the wealthy and fashionable but also several eminent Parisian physicians. As a result of the contemporary zeal for popular science in Paris at that time, he rapidly became very wealthy which did not endear him to his medical colleagues either. He was accused of being a charlatan and a fraud.

In 1784, Louis XVI, established a public investigation into animal magnetism and Franz Mesmer's work.[19] Mesmer refused to take part but his follower Charles d'Eslon agreed to demonstrate his own practice, learned directly from Mesmer. The royal commission included several scientific notables such as the American polymath, Benjamin Franklin, the chemist Antoine Lavoisier and the physician Joseph-Ignace Guillotin who became infamous for the instrument of execution that bears his name.

During the investigation, members of the commission bathed in the *baquets* separately from the patients themselves but also witnessed the mass treatments. The male commissioners remained quiet and unruffled while the subjects, usually women, screamed and shook in their tubs. Mesmer called these convulsions, or episodes of altered consciousness, 'crises' and viewed them as an important part of the healing process. The investigators were bemused by the difference between the negligible effect on themselves and the convulsions of the other patrons which they saw as evidence of the participants' diseased imaginations.[20]

In another part of their investigation, they blindfolded the subjects so they could not see the directions of the mesmerist or whether or not the water was 'magnetised'. These subterfuges produced a random response demonstrating that animal magnetism was not the causal factor. They wrote in their report to the King that animal magnetism did produce genuine effects but these were through the combined effects of 'contact, imitation and imagination but mostly ***imagination*** [my emphasis].' The report went on to break down which aspects of the process might enhance the action of the imagination suggesting the anticipation of cure, the financial investment, the ceremonial aspect and the involvement of a prestigious doctor.

It is easy to misinterpret the findings of the commission and many physicians and commentators have done this subsequently. It must be emphasised that describing the cause of the cures to be the result of the imagination was not the same as saying that they were 'imaginary', that

[19] *Anonymous Report of Dr. Benjamin Franklin, and Other Commissioners: Charged by the King of France, with the Examination of the Animal Magnetism, As Now Practised at Paris* (London: J. Johnson, 1785).

[20] Lorraine Daston, 'Fear and Loathing of the Imagination in Science', *Daedalus*, 27 (1998) (pp. 73–95) (p. 80).

is non-existent, feigned by the subjects or invented by the physician. The members of the Commission were drawing on the long tradition of the imagination that I have been presenting in this chapter.

Mesmer and his work rapidly fell out of fashion after the commission's findings were published and he left Paris. However, his legacy was the formation of several Societies of Universal Harmony, groups that continued to practice and investigate animal magnetism across continental Europe. The most important branch was the Strasburg branch founded by the Armand de Chastenet, the Marquis de Puységur (1751–1825). Puységur's contributions to the scientific study of mesmerism were highly significant. If Mesmer did much to bring popular and cultural attention to the phenomenon of animal magnetism, the formal features of what became called mesmerism were actually described and delineated by Puységur. They include the ideas of an intimate rapport between operator and somnambule, post-hypnotic suggestion and changes of personality and the uncovering of extraordinary mental powers in the subject.

Puységur's books closely documented his practical experiences with mesmerism but did include some theoretical points. He freely acknowledged his intellectual debt to Mesmer but moved away from Mesmer's idea of an invisible magnetic fluid or the importance of a hypnotic, convulsive crisis. He felt that Mesmer had been unfairly treated by the first royal commission and disputed its findings. He accepted that the imagination might be involved in the phenomena but:

> If...the effects of the imagination are of value, the academie will be forced to agree that the imagination is the most important doctor on earth.[21]

Enhancing the association of hypnotism with the imagination, Puységur had described his belief that the curative effects of animal magnetism occurred through a form of induced somnambulism. This discovery had inextricably tied 'magnetic sleep', Puységur's own term, to the phenomenon of somnambulism, which was understood in both

[21] Marie Jacques de Chastenet, Marquis de Puységur, *An Essay of Instruction on Animal Magnetism* trans. by John King (New York: J C Kelley, 1838).

the public and medical spheres to be a manifestation of the imagination.[22] For Puységur, the idea of induced sleep called on renaissance ideas which saw the act of sleeping as an intrinsic part of life which was essential in balancing the humours and therefore vital for the maintenance of health.[23] However, the ideal of sleep was a passive restorative process thus problematising sleepwalking. Robert Burton, for example, saw night-walking as the result of a diseased imagination but saw the imagination, the soul, the mind and the body as interlinked and capable of affecting each other in illness:

> For as the Body works upon the minde, by his bad humours, troubling the spirits, sending grosse spirits into the Braine; and so per consequens disturbing the Soule and all the faculties of it.[24]

These ideas were also played out culturally in Shakespearean plays like *MacBeth* and in Italian operas by Verdi and Bellini, somnambulism signified that the sleeper's passions had been roused by powerful events in waking life and it was believed that it was the imagination that mediated the disturbance of natural sleep process.

Somnambulism may have been conceived by Puységur as a natural health-promoting state but it was simultaneously viewed in the medical literature as profoundly abnormal and a disruption of the natural order. Also known as *oneirodynia activa*,[25] somnambulism was a new Latin word coined in French but first used in English in 1786 and used to mean 'walking in one's sleep or *under hypnosis*.' The Collins English dictionary has kept this two-part definition to the present day.[26] Animal magnetism,

[22] Sharda Umanath, Daniel Sarezky, and Stanley Finger, 'Sleepwalking Through History: Medicine, Arts, and Courts of Law', *Journal of the History of Neuroscience*, 20 (2011) (p. 4) (pp. 253–76).

[23] William MacLehose, 'Sleepwalking, Violence and Desire in the Middle Ages', *Culture, Medicine and Psychiatry*, 37 (2013) (pp. 606–17).

[24] Robert Burton, *The Anatomy of Melancholy* (New York: New York Review of Books, 2001) (p. 247).

[25] John Watts, *Medical Dictionary, Containing an Explanation of the Terms in Surgery, Medicine, Midwifery, Anatomy*, Chemistry 2nd Ed. (London: Printed for Highley and Son, 1813).

[26] Somnambulism. Dictionary.com. *Dictionary.com Unabridged*. Random House, Inc. http://www.dictionary.com/browse/somnambulism (accessed 25 September 2017).

somnambulism (or the trance state) and the imagination were inextricably linked.

Elisha Perkins (1741–1799) was a physician from Plainfield, Connecticut who experienced international success with his patented 'tractors'.[27] These were pairs of metallic rods that, when stroked over the afflicted part of man or beast, would allegedly heal. Their name was taken from the Latin *trahere*, to draw or pull out. Perkin's advertised that the device would draw off the 'noxious electrical fluid' that was the cause of the illness in a process that he inelegantly called 'tractoration'. His invention came at a time when there was great interest in electromagnetism as a therapeutic agent. The forces were usually invisible like the magnetism of animal magnetism but the machines used to create the forces could be quite large and theatrical which could add to the drama for the travelling quack or 'nostrum-vendor'.[28]

Perkins' tractors themselves were something of an exception. The rods themselves were relatively modest measuring only three inches in length. They were flat on one aspect and round on the other, tapering to a point. Crucially, his patent describes the use of different metals for the pair of rods: one was an alloy of platinum, silver and iron, the other zinc copper and gold. It was this specific combination which he claimed was responsible for the therapeutic effects. In reality, they were usually made of brass and steel but the small size, patented status and ease of manufacture and distribution made for an excellent business model.

He registered the patent for his device in 1796 and it was such a word of mouth sensation that it had spread to Europe by 1798. Its broadening appeal was the result of an early international advertising campaign. Perkin's son, Benjamin, was a bookseller who published his *The Influence of Metallic Tractors on the Human Body* in London in 1798.[29] In the book, he made an early effort at celebrity endorsement by announcing that George Washington the US president had bought a set. He also publicised the equipment in *The Times* newspaper where they sold in England

[27] Geoff Watts, 'Histories: Elisha Perkins and his Medical Tractors', *New Scientist,* 2481 (2005) (p. 25).

[28] Jacques Quen, 'Elisha Perkins, Physician, Nostrum-Vendor, or Charlatan?', *Bulletin of the History of Medicine,* 37 (1963) (pp. 159–166).

[29] Benjamin Perkins, *The Influence of Metallic Tractors on the Human Body* (London: Printed for J. Johnson, 1798).

for five guineas a pair; restricting their affordability to the wealthy but maximising profits.[30]

Perkin's treatment was controversial from the outset and early on he was expelled from the Connecticut Medical Society as a quack and user of nostrums. The doubts and criticisms from other medics followed him to Europe. In 1799, the English physician John Haygarth and his friend and mentor William Falconer conducted a series of experiments to assess the efficacy of the tractors.[31] Haygarth was an eminent and accomplished doctor who discovered the importance of isolation in preventing the spread of fever.[32] For his work in reducing the rate of smallpox in Chester by inoculation and public health initiatives, he had been made a fellow of the Royal Society.

Like the Franklin commission into animal magnetism he used a 'double-blinding' procedure to keep the subjects and assistants unaware of the real treatment and a sham treatment: 'Let the secret be kept inviolable not only from the patient, but every other person.'[33] He had prepared painted, wooden tractors to resemble metal ones and compared the effectiveness of the Perkins tractors against the wooden ones in five subjects with chronic rheumatism on consecutive days. Four of the five patients reported symptomatic improvements with both the real and the sham treatments. Essentially, both were equally effective. He went on to persuade his colleagues in Hull and Bristol to use the same protocol with the same results. This was a multiple-site trial: another experimental innovation for Haygarth.

Haygarth was an insightful physician and critically did more than just say that the tractors were bogus. He wrote that the results 'prove to a degree which has never been suspected what powerful influence on diseases is produced by mere imagination.'[34] Haygarth was also quick to draw parallels between his results, those of animal magnetism and the findings of the Franklin commission. He linked the power of imagination

[30] Anon, *The Times*, 10 October, 1799.

[31] John Haygarth, *On the Imagination As a Cause & As a Cure of Disorders of the Body* (Bath: Crutwell, 1800).

[32] Christopher Booth, 'John Haygarth FRS (1740–1827)', *Journal of the Royal Society of Medicine*, 107 (2014) (p. 12) (pp. 490–493).

[33] Haygarth, *Imagination* (p. 2).

[34] Haygarth, *Imagination* (p. 15.).

to the strength of faith that the patient has in the doctor and went on to make more general comments about the role of imagination in other medical encounters: 'on this principle we may account for the marvellous recoveries frequently ascribed to empirical remedies, which are commonly inert drugs.'[35]

The Limits of the Imagination

By the end of the nineteenth century, the scientific revolution of clinical observation, experimental physiology and post-mortem examination had radically changed the theory and practice of medicine in Britain and Europe. Doctors were both healers and scientists. The increasingly respectable profession had closely allied itself to the objectivity and respectability of science and the scientific method and drew its authority from this association. Infectious diseases like scarlet fever and heart diseases like dropsy were observed, named and delineated. Routine pathological examination revealed the secrets of the body in disease. The alliance of medicine to science and its claims to scientific truth was successful. As a result, British physicians were able to successfully lobby parliament to draft and pass 'The Medical Act' of 1858. This helped to secure the social and financial aspects of the practise of medicine by effectively creating a professional monopoly on healthcare based on agreed standards in medical education and apprenticeship. It also excluded legitimacy from all other forms of healers.

However, the ancient and rather mystical doctrine of the medical imagination did not fit well in this new scientific paradigm. Common longstanding conditions, such as the 'vapours' and hypochondria, which had been conceptualised in the seventeenth and eighteenth centuries as diseases of the imagination, became trivialised. Over the nineteenth century, they were no longer considered serious physical diseases. The holistic and psychosomatic aspects of the concept of imagination meant that the illnesses changed their meaning from physical to primarily psychological disturbances. The vapours became linked to dramatic displays of psychological distress via hysteria and women's health problems and hypochondria came to describe a patient's over-reaction to minor or irrelevant symptoms. The medical historian Stanley Jackson has

[35] Haygarth, *Imagination* (p. 32).

observed a clear decline in the references to the imagination in textbooks of *Materia medica* and general therapeutics over the course of the nineteenth century.[36]

The two areas of medicine that were slowest to benefit from the application of the scientific method and pathological observation were psychiatry and obstetrics and gynaecology. As a result, imagination remained the explanatory model in these fields for the longest. In the field of mental health, the work of the French physicians Phillipe Pinel (1745–1826) and Georges Cabanis (1757–1808) was influential on British alienists like William Tuke and his moral therapy at 'The Retreat' in York. While Pinel is better known for advocating treatment of the mentally ill without the use of physical restraint, Jan Goldstein has convincingly demonstrated the important contributions of Cabanis to the moral hygiene movement.[37] Cabanis was a physiologist and materialist who was interested in early psychology and developed an outline of the physiology of the mind. He was convinced of the importance of the imagination, which he saw as a crucial reciprocal pathway between the mind and the body. However, in keeping with contemporary views, he also saw the imagination as the weak link in the psychic apparatus between the two that represented a danger to the individual as well as the wider society. Aware of the alchemical origins of the concept, he cited Montaigne's 'excellent' essay on the imagination and gave examples of the pathology caused by the imagination: 'How many men have been killed or cured by imagination?'.[38]

Cabanis described his approach as a 'medicine of the imagination' which entailed a concern for the emotional state of the patients that could be achieved by soothing, reassurance and sustaining hope. It can be seen how this viewpoint evolved into a more practical, 'moral treatment' espoused by Pinel. Goldstein has argued that, by connecting a commonsensical humane treatment to a sophisticated medical and philosophical framework, Cabanis gave imagination legitimacy as an approach to mental

[36] Stanley Jackson, 'The Use of the Imagination', Ch. 10 in *Care of the Psyche* (New Haven; London: Yale University Press, 1999) (pp. 221–35) (p. 232).

[37] Jan Goldstein, *Console and Classify: The French Psychiatric Profession in the Nineteenth Century* (Chicago: University of Chicago Press, 2002) (pp. 49–54).

[38] Michel de Montaigne, '*The Essays*' Ch 20, 'Of the Force of Imagination' (Trans. Charles Cotton) (1877). http://www.gutenberg.org/files/3600/3600-h/3600-h.htm.

illness and shifted it 'from the shadowy periphery to the center [sic] of medical orthodoxy'.[39]

Another aspect of the imagination that I have previously touched upon, was the idea of the maternal imagination. Some writers have suggested that this idea had either died out by the end of the eighteenth century or was at least viewed as superstition by the nineteenth century.[40] However, Lars Andersen has clearly demonstrated that the idea of maternal imagination was not obsolete in the nineteenth century, appearing no less than 37 times in the *Lancet* between 1823 and 1875.[41] While these references both support and critique the concept, it shows that the idea still held currency, recognised in medical and lay culture if no longer seen as orthodox.

Typically, physicians would share case reports from their own practice, in articles and letters published in medical journals. In one letter to the *Lancet* from 1850, Dr. MacCormack relates the story of a man whose mother was making redcurrant jam when she was two months pregnant with him. MacCormack ascribes the appearance of the child to this antenatal incident utilising the concept of the maternal imagination. He describes an

> ...extraordinary mark all down his left thigh and leg, (which strange as it may seem is nevertheless true) is much more vivid and prominent during the summer than at any other time. The appearance it then presents is that of a red currant-tree [sic] branch in all fruit...[42]

Even as late as 1892, the physician hypnotist Tuckey had contributed to an edition of *Baby* magazine which had a special edition covering 'Maternal Impressions and their influence on the Offspring' which advised that 'expectant mothers cannot be too carefully shielded from distressing sights and painful emotions and their lives should be surrounded by

[39] Jan Goldstein, *Console and Classify* (pp. 52–54).

[40] Margrit Shildrik, 'Maternal Imagination: Reconceiving First Impressions', *Rethinking History*, 4 (2000) (pp. 243–60).

[41] Lars Andersen, 'Before the Placebo Effect: Discussions on the Power of the Imagination in 19th Century Medicine—With Perspectives to Present Discussions on the Mind's Influence upon the Body', *Tidsskrift for Forskning i Sygdom og Samfund*, 12 (2016) (pp. 31–52).

[42] M. J. MacCormack, 'Influence of Maternal Impressions on the Foetus: Letters to the Editor', *The Lancet*, 2 (1850) (p. 697).

sympathy, love and kindness'. This excerpt demonstrates the tenacity of the complex body–mind interactions that were understood through the lens of the imagination.

In the Victorian era, the more holistic or psychosomatic aspects of the imagination were still widely known within and outside the field of medicine but lacked a materialist or physical mechanism. Both the philosopher poets Samuel Coleridge (1772–1834) and William Wordsworth (1770–1850) were better known for their work on the poetic imagination but were also influential in their use of the concept of the medical faculty of the imagination. In his preface to their jointly authored *Lyrical Ballads* (1798), Wordsworth writes: 'I wished to draw attention to the truth, that the power of the human imagination is sufficient to produce such changes even in our physical nature as might almost appear miraculous.'[43]

For the Romantic writers, poets and philosophers, the imagination was a precious gift that could intercede between body and soul, mediate between nature and mind, and reconcile subjective and objective experience. As the shared aspect of body and spirit, the imagination was therefore capable of profound and wonderful changes to the human form and health, as well as the mind. The critic, Jasmine Jagger has suggested that as a result of their shared belief that 'the imagination was both corporeally connected and all-powerful,' both men assumed that poetry could feasibly have a physical effect on the body.[44] As the most practical example of their shared psychosomatic beliefs, Wordsworth attempted to treat his friend Coleridge, when he was sick with a variety of bodily and nervous afflictions, by readings of his verse.

The Victorian peak in the use of the doctrine of the medical imagination was probably Daniel Hack Tuke's *Illustrations of the influence of the Mind upon the Body in Health and Disease* ([1872] hereafter *Illustrations*).[45] Hack Tuke was an alienist and prolific writer on psychological medicine. He came from a family of medical doctors. His father, brother

[43] William Wordsworth, *William Wordsworth*, ed. Stephen Gill, 21st-Century Oxford Authors Series (Oxford: Oxford University Press, 2012) (p. 74).

[44] Jasmine Jagger, 'Wordsworth, Coleridge, and the Healing Powers of the Imagination', *Romanticism*, 22 (2016) (pp. 33–47).

[45] Daniel Hack Tuke, *Illustrations of the influence of the Mind upon the Body in Health and Disease, Designed to Elucidate the Action of the Imagination* (London: J. & A. Churchill, 1872).

and grandfather and great-grandfather had all worked with the mentally ill. His grandfather, Henry, and great-grandfather, William, had been responsible for the establishment of the hospital, *The Retreat* in York which had fundamentally changed the approach to treating those with mental health needs. For 17 years, he was the editor of the *Journal of Mental Science* (*JMS*), the major English-language mental health journal, and he was also president of the Medico-Psychological Association (MPA), the precursor to the British Royal College of Psychiatrists (Fig. 3.2).

Illustrations is probably the most sophisticated development and articulation of the ideas of medical imagination in the English language. Tuke initially wrote it for the *JMS* in the form of eight separate interlinked articles, published in 1870.[46] He expanded and refashioned it for publication as a book which was printed two years later.[47] Though the initial reception was mixed it remained one of his favourite books and he revised it for a second edition in 1884.[48] However, its worth was recognised in Europe and it was translated into both French and German in the 1880s where such luminaries of psychiatry as Hippolyte Bernheim, Paul Dubois, Pierre Janet and Jean-Martin Charcot all cited this work. Such was its continuing popularity that it had two further English reprints in the 1890s.

Illustrations is a well-written work that demonstrates considerable scholarship for a man whose school days were hampered by his delicate constitution. Tuke uses a multitude of diverse though admittedly repetitious case histories from his own experience, contemporary and older sources to illustrate the impact of the mind on the body. Over nearly 500 pages he constructs a history of the imagination covering many of the major writers and incidents that I have already mentioned in this chapter. The book is divided into four sections. The first three examine the effect of the intellect, the emotions and the will (or volition) on the body and the last part looks at the therapeutic uses to which the mind can be put. Although he worked as a psychiatrist, it is clear that his intention in this

[46] Daniel Hack Tuke, 'Illustrations of the influence of the Mind Upon the Body in Health and Disease, Part 1', *Journal of Mental Science,* 16 (1870) (pp.166–95).

[47] Daniel Hack Tuke, *Illustrations of the influence of the Mind upon the Body in Health and Disease, Designed to Elucidate the Action of the Imagination* (London: J. & A. Churchill, 1872).

[48] Henry Rollin, 'Obituary: Daniel Hack Tuke', *British Journal of Psychiatry,* 166 (1995) (pp. 403–5).

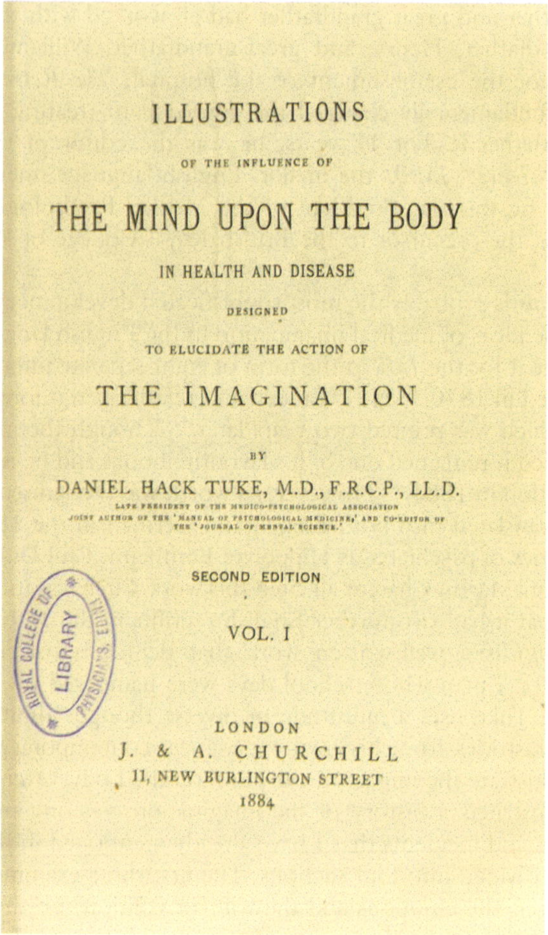

ILLUSTRATIONS

OF THE INFLUENCE OF

THE MIND UPON THE BODY

IN HEALTH AND DISEASE

DESIGNED

TO ELUCIDATE THE ACTION OF

THE IMAGINATION

BY

DANIEL HACK TUKE, M.D., F.R.C.P., LL.D.

LATE PRESIDENT OF THE MEDICO-PSYCHOLOGICAL ASSOCIATION
JOINT AUTHOR OF THE 'MANUAL OF PSYCHOLOGICAL MEDICINE,' AND CO-EDITOR OF THE 'JOURNAL OF MENTAL SCIENCE.'

SECOND EDITION

VOL. I

LONDON
J. & A. CHURCHILL
11, NEW BURLINGTON STREET
1884

Fig. 3.2 Tuke, Daniel Hack. Illustrations of the Influence of the Mind upon the Body in Health and Disease (London: Churchill, 1884) Front page

book was to highlight the importance of the mind to the bodily health and to bring the study of mental health closer to general medicine.

The idea of harnessing the person's mind in the treatment of both their physical and mental illness also represented a shift away from prevailing beliefs in the physiology and psychology of reflex inhibition. The evolving discoveries of the electrical operation of the nervous system had helped to maintain a highly materialistic view of mental functioning in Britain and resulted in a rather static, deterministic view of mental illness.[49] Tuke's eminent peer Henry Maudsley, for example, saw mental illness as essentially hereditary and fixed. With his book, Tuke was deliberately exploiting an earlier but more optimistic model of a dynamic psychology. This corresponded with his personal experience of the importance of benign treatment of the mentally ill and of encouraging them to exercise self-control. Indeed, one of the critics of the book, writing in the *Lancet*, focussed on the arguments about treating mental illness and mindful of Tuke's family history and experiences at 'The Retreat' announced that his 'psycho-therapeutics' was merely 'moral therapy' by another name.[50]

Tuke, like the Romantics saw the imagination as a powerful and special creative force: 'those ideas which arise without any direct external stimulus.'[51] Specifically, he understood it as the route for the mind's undeniable influence on the body. He viewed the imagination as a life force and the mechanism by which a patient's mind could lead to 'certain (bodily) phenomena' when there was no other cause to explain the changes.[52]

By the time of his second edition of *Illustrations*, published in 1884, Tuke was aware of the growing profile of hypnotism in Europe and reviewed the relationship between hypnotism and the imagination in some detail. He preferred the French term 'Braidism' to hypnotism and both to mesmerism in the text but in a footnote reveals himself to be a pragmatist arguing that it is better to 'Cure disease under a name which is associated with an unproved theory, than refuse on that account to employ it.'[53] Tuke repeated the clinical histories of eight patients who had consulted James Braid (the originator of the term Braidism) and were cured of conditions ranging from deafness to cataracts and stroke by hypnosis. He accepted Braid's contention that the hypnotic state is one

[49] Roger Smith, *Inhibition: History and Meaning in the Sciences of Mind and Brain* (Oakland: University of California Press, 1992).

[50] Anon, 'Reviews and Notices of Books', *Lancet,* 101 (1873) (p. 2576) (pp. 52–3).

[51] Tuke, *Illustrations* (p. 180).

[52] Tuke, *Illustrations* (p. 180).

[53] Tuke, *Illustrations* (p. 441).

in which the patient is able to intensify the power of the mind's influence on the body and quoted Braid's agnosticism as to the mechanism:

> Whether these extraordinary physical effects are produced through the imagination chiefly, or by other means, it appears to me quite certain that the imagination has never been so much under our control, or capable of being made to act in the same beneficial and uniform manner, by any other mode of management hitherto known.[54]

In the closing summary of *Illustrations*, Tuke seemed wary of committing himself to one causal mechanism for hypnotism. He also remained careful to ascribe limits to the therapeutic possibilities of the imagination and did not attribute all of the therapeutic effects of hypnotism to the imagination or to the hypnotic sleep. Like the Franklin commission, he commented on the importance of faith and expectation in the healing process. He also thought that attention might be an important component. Drawing on the work of English physiologist William Carpenter on expectant attention and reflexes in *Principles of Mental Physiology* (1876), he proposed it might act by directing the patient's focus towards the affected part which may work physiologically by increasing the blood supply or more directly though he does not specify the process involved.[55] It could also be that distracting the attention from the affliction might be therapeutic.

In summary, the imagination has a long history as an explanatory model for a variety of physical, medical and psychological phenomena. However, as I have demonstrated it had several meanings both in general and medical usage. In fact, its amorphous nature and lack of clear definition served to sustain its versatility and usefulness within philosophical and scientific discourses. At the start of the nineteenth century, the imagination was still referred to in the medical literature as both the cause and potential cure of mental and physical illness. Associated features such as maternal imprinting as a cause of foetal abnormality continued to appear in reputable medical journals despite their alchemical origins. However, by the middle of the century, the popularity of this construct was on the wane. Medicine was a science and physiology and anatomy were the

[54] Braid, James, *Neurypnology or the Rationale of Nervous Sleep* (London: J. Churchill: 1843). qtd in Tuke, *Illustrations* (1884) (p. 445).

[55] William Carpenter, *Principles of Mental Physiology* (London: King, 1876).

central pillars of that science. It is indicative of the absence of other coherent models for hypnosis that the imagination continued to be used in this context so late into the century.

References

Andersen, Lars. 2016. 'Before the Placebo Effect: Discussions on the Power of the Imagination in 19th Century Medicine - with Perspectives to Present Discussions on the Mind's Influence upon the Body' *Tidsskrift for Forskning i Sygdom og Samfund*, 12: 31-52.

Anon. 1785. *Anonymous Report of Dr. Benjamin Franklin, and other commissioners: charged by the King of France, with the examination of the animal magnetism, as now practised at Paris*. London: J. Johnson.

Anon. 1799. Advertisement, *The Times*, 10 October.

Anon. 1873. 'Reviews and Notices of Books', *The Lancet* 101 2576: 52-3.

Booth, Christopher. 2014. 'John Haygarth FRS (1740-1827)' *Journal of the Royal Society of Medicine* 107 12: 490-493.

Brogan, Stephen. 2015. 'Introduction' in *The Royal Touch in Early Modern England: Politics, Medicine and Sin*. Woodbridge, Suffolk: Boydell. 1–22.

Burton, Robert. 2001. *The Anatomy of Melancholy*. New York: New York Review of Books. 247.

Carpenter, William. 1876. *Principles of Mental Physiology*. London: King.

Charron, Pierre. 1707. *Of Wisdom Three Books,* Vol 1, trans by George Stanhope. London: Bonwick. 158.

Chertok, Leon and Borch-Jacobsen, Mikkel. 1987. *Hypnose et Psychanalyse: Reponses a Mikkel Borch-Jacobsen*. Paris: Dunod.

Crabtree, Adam. 1993. *From Mesmer to Freud: Magnetic Sleep and the Roots of Psychological Healing*. New Haven: Yale University Press.

Darnton, Robert. 1970. 'Mesmerism and Popular Science', in *Mesmerism and the End of the Enlightenment in France*. New York: Schocken Books. 2-45.

Daston, Lorraine. 1998. 'Fear and Loathing of the Imagination in Science', *Daedalus,* 27: 73-95.

de Chastenet, Marie Jacques. Marquis de Puységur. 1838. *An Essay of Instruction on Animal Magnetism,* trans. by John King. New York: J C Kelley.

de Montaigne, Michel. 1877. '*The Essays*' Ch 20, 'Of the Force of Imagination' trans. Charles Cotton. http://www.gutenberg.org/files/3600/3600-h/3600-h.htm

Ellenberger, Henri. 1970. *The Discovery of the Unconscious, the History and Evolution of Dynamic Psychiatry*. London: Allen Lane.

Fischer-Homberger, Esther. 1979. 'On the Medical History of the Doctrine of Imagination', *Psychological Medicine* 9: 619-628.

Gauld, Alan. 1992. *A History of Hypnotism*. Cambridge: Cambridge University Press.

Goldstein, Jan. 2002. *Console and Classify: The French Psychiatric Profession in the Nineteenth Century*. Chicago: University of Chicago Press.

Hartmann, Frantz. 1918. *Life of Paracelsus (1493-1541)*. New York: Theosophical Publishing. 179.

Haygarth, John. 1800. *On the Imagination as a Cause & as a Cure of Disorders of the Body*. Bath: Crutwell.

Jacobi, Jolande. 1951. *Paracelsus Selected Writings* trans. Norbert Guterman. London: Routledge and Kegan Paul. 106.

Jackson, Stanley. 1990. 'The Imagination and Psychological Healing', *Journal of the History of Medicine and Allied Science* 26: 345-58.

Jackson, Stanley. 1999. 'The Use of the Imagination', Ch 10 in *Care of the Psyche*. New Haven; London: Yale University Press. 221-35.

Jagger, Jasmine. 2016. 'Wordsworth, Coleridge, and the Healing Powers of the Imagination' *Romanticism* 22: 33–47.

Kerényi, Károly. 1959. *Asklepios: Archetypal Image of the Physician's Existence*, Ch 2 *Epidauros*, trans by Ralph Manheim. Princeton: Princeton University Press. 18-46.

MacCormack, M J. 1850. 'Influence of Maternal Impressions on the Foetus: Letters to the Editor' *The Lancet* 2: 697.

MacLehose, William. 2013. 'Sleepwalking, Violence and Desire in the Middle Ages', *Culture, Medicine and Psychiatry* 37: 606-17.

McKay, Charles. 1995. 'The Magnetisers' in *Extraordinary Popular Delusions and the Madness of Crowds*. Ware: Wordsworth Editions.304–345.

Perkins, Benjamin. 1798. *The Influence of Metallic Tractors on the Human Body*. London: J. Johnson.

Quen, Jacques. 1963. 'Elisha Perkins, Physician, Nostrum-Vendor, or Charlatan?' *Bulletin of the History of Medicine* 37: 159-166.

Rollin, Henry. 1995. 'Obituary: Daniel Hack Tuke', *British Journal of Psychiatry* 166: 403-5.

Rousseau, George. 1969. 'Science and the Discovery of the Imagination in Enlightened England', *Eighteenth Century Studies* 3: 108-35.

Saint-Evremond, Charles. 1705. *The Works of Saint-Evremond*, 2 Vols. Jacob Tonson: London.

Shildrik, Margrit. 2000. 'Maternal Imagination: Reconceiving First Impressions' *Rethinking History* 4: 243-60.

Smith, Roger. 1992. *Inhibition: History and Meaning in the Sciences of Mind and Brain*. Oakland: University of California Press.

Tatar, Marie. 1978. 'Preface' in *Spellbound: Studies on Mesmerism and Literature*. Princeton: Princeton University Press. ix-xvi.

Thomas, Keith. 2003. 'Magical Healing' Ch 7 in *Religion and the Decline of Magic: Studies in Popular Belief in Sixteenth and Seventeenth Century England*. London: Penguin.

Tuckey, Charles Lloyd. 1889. *Psycho-Therapeutics: Or Treatment by Sleep and Suggestion*. London: Baillière, Tindall and Cox.

Tuke, Daniel Hack. 1870. 'Illustrations of the influence of the Mind upon the Body in Health and Disease, Part 1', *Journal of Mental Science* 16 74:166-95.

Tuke, Daniel Hack. 1872. *Illustrations of the influence of the Mind upon the Body in Health and Disease, Designed to Elucidate the Action of the Imagination*. London: Churchill.

Umanath, Sharda, Sarezky, Daniel and Finger, Stanley. 2011. 'Sleepwalking through history: medicine, arts, and courts of law'. *Journal of the History of Neuroscience* 20 4: 253-76.

van Helmont, J.B. 1683. *Aufgang der Artzney-Kunst*, trans. by F. M. van Helmont. Sulzbach: Endters Söhne.

Waite, Arthur. 1891. *The Occult Sciences: A Compendium of Transcendental Doctrine and Experiment*. London: Paul Keagan, Trench, Trübner & Co. 230.

Waterfield, Robin. 2004. *Hidden Depths: The Story of Hypnosis*. London: Pan.

Watts, John. 1813. Medical Dictionary, Containing an Explanation of the Terms in Surgery, Medicine, Midwifery, Anatomy, Chemistry 2nd Ed. London: Printed Highley and Son.

Wordsworth, William. 2012. *William Wordsworth*, ed. Stephen Gill, 21st-Century Oxford Authors Series. Oxford: Oxford University Press. 74.

CHAPTER 4

The Power of Suggestion

In the previous chapter, I described the complexity and protean nature of the idea of the medical imagination. I have argued that this conceptual framework for the mind's influence on the body was losing traction in the late nineteenth century. The rapid progress in clinical sciences had led to an increasingly materialistic and reductionist turn in medicine and its teaching. The archaic Romantic and alchemical notions of the imagination required an urgent overhaul. Recent ideas about the workings of the nervous system, based on the physiological observation of and experimentation on reflexes and inhibition, were of limited use in explaining more complex behaviours or interpersonal effects.[1] This had led to rather static ideas about mental illness which was by now understood to be brain-based.

Later, I will propose that by the 1890s a tipping point was reached and that both medical and lay culture were ready for an alternative model to understand non-material doctor-patient effects, psychosomatic medicine and the effectiveness of hypnotism. At the time of the transition between imagination and suggestion, there was a fertile interplay and exchange of ideas between the medical community and lay culture. The general

[1] William Carpenter, *Principles of Mental Physiology*, 3rd ed (London: Henry S. King, 1875).

G. D. L. Bates, *The Uncanny Rise of Medical Hypnotism, 1888–1914*, Mental Health in Historical Perspective,
https://doi.org/10.1007/978-3-031-42725-1_4

public could readily understand the novel concept of suggestion and its simplicity and intuitive nature helped to secure its rapid dissemination and acceptance. It also provided a powerful way of understanding other phenomena such as faith-healing and would be used to account for the behaviour of groups of people and crowds.

The Oxford English Dictionary describes suggestion as 'the action of prompting one to a particular course of action; the putting into the mind of an idea, an object of thought, a plan or the like; an instance of this, an idea a thought suggested, a proposal.' It dates this usage between 1382 and 1885, illustrating with examples from Milton and the King James Bible. The more technical usage, meaning 'the action of influencing a person to accept an idea or belief uncritically, especially as a technique in hypnosis', arose quickly between 1887 and 1903.[2] However, the etymology is interesting as outside of a clinical context, suggestion has had a slightly negative moral quality which it has retained to this day particularly in the adjectival form as *suggestive*. In middle English suggestion was 'a prompting to evil' and can be found in Chaucer and Milton's work.[3]

Suggestion in Nancy

The psychological concept of suggestion as an explanatory model for hypnotism is closely associated with the Nancy school and the names of the country doctor, Ambroise-Auguste Liébeault (1823–1904) and the hospital physician Hippolyte Bernheim (1840–1919). Liébeault was a rural general practitioner who had taught himself medical hypnosis in isolation. After hearing a French translation of the Scottish surgeon James Braid's work read at the French Academy of Sciences in 1860, he

[2] 'Suggestion'. Oxford English Dictionary. https://en.oxforddictionaries.com/definition/suggestion [accessed 8 October 2018].

[3] 'Suggestion'. https://www.etymonline.com/word/suggestion [accessed 26 March 2018]. Geoffrey Chaucer helped to establish Middle English vernacular with *The Canterbury Tales* written in the fourteenth Century. In stanza 331 of *The Parson's Tale* he writes 'Deedly synne hath first suggestion of the feend.' John Milton was a seventeenth century poet whose *Paradise Lost* influenced centuries of British writers: 'The first sort by thir own suggestion fell, Self-tempted, self-deprav'd', Book 3, line 129.

obtained and studied Braid's textbook *Neurypnology*.[4] Braid's work had been published at the end of the rather limited period of medical interest in mesmerism in the UK and had been rapidly forgotten there. In France, the procedure was so linked to the work of James Braid that the term 'Braidism' was used in medicine rather than Braid's preferred coinage, hypnotism (Figs. 4.1 and 4.2).

Liébeault had worked independently in rural practice developing his hypnotic technique for nearly twenty years before he became something of a medical celebrity and father figure to the entire medical hypnotic movement. When Professor Bernheim, from the local medical school in Nancy, discovered that Liébeault had cured one of the patients with severe sciatica that he had failed to help, Bernheim wanted to know more and arranged a meeting and demonstration. Liébeault had published his own book on hypnotism in 1866, but it was long, running to 534 pages and densely written, containing in addition Liébeault's views on psychology and philosophy.[5] The book was not widely read selling only five copies in five years.[6] So, in 1882 when approached by Hippolyte Bernheim, he readily agreed to collaborate. Bernheim enthusiastically took up the new mode of treatment by suggestion and together they established the Nancy school of hypnotism.

Bernheim himself published on the rediscovered therapy in 1884 and his book was far better received than Liébeault's.[7] He expanded it and renamed it, *De la Suggestion et de ses Applications a la Therapeutique*.[8] Within a year, by 1888, the book had been so successful it had gone into a second edition. The following year was also translated into English with the more memorable title, *Suggestive Therapeutics*. In this book, Bernheim made clear his debt to Liébeault, describing his methods in detail

[4] James Braid, *Neurypnology* or the Rationale of Nervous Sleep (London: J. Churchill, 1843); Robin Waterfield, *Hidden Depths* (London: Pan, 2002) (p. 214); George Kingsbury, *The Practice of Hypnotic Suggestion, Being and Elementary Handbook for the Use of the Medical Profession* (Bristol: John Wright, 1891) (p. 12).

[5] Ambroise-Auguste Liébeault, *Du Sommeil et des Etats Analogues, Considérés surtout du Point de Vue de l'Action du Moral sur le Physique* (Paris: Victor Maisson, 1866).

[6] Waterfield, *Hidden Depths* (p. 214).

[7] Hippolyte Bernheim, *De la suggestion dans l'état hypnotique et dans l'état* de veille, 1st ed (Paris: Doin, 1884).

[8] Hippolyte Bernheim, *De la Suggestion et de ses applications a la therapeutique*, (Paris: Doin, 1886).

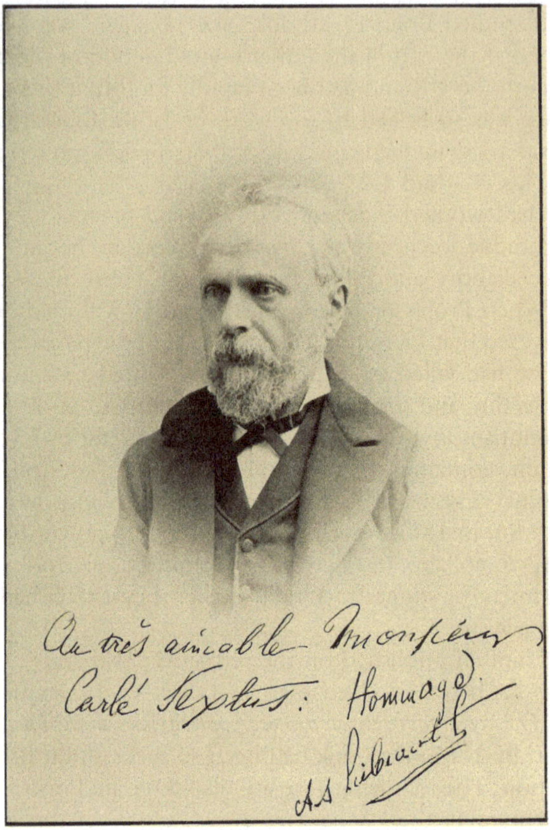

Fig. 4.1 Portrait of A.A. Liébeault (Courtesy of Wellcome Collection)

and describing Liébeault's original text as 'the most important work that has ever been published on Braidism.'[9]

The early editions and translations of *Suggestive Therapeutics* were highly influential across most of Europe where the seeds fell into fertile soil. German, Dutch, Swedish and Russian physicians visited Nancy to learn about the practice of hypnotism and the theory of suggestion. There was a rapid uptake of the Nancy school ideas across Europe with two

[9] Hippolyte Bernheim, *Suggestive Therapeutics* (London: G.P. Putnam, 1888) (p. 117).

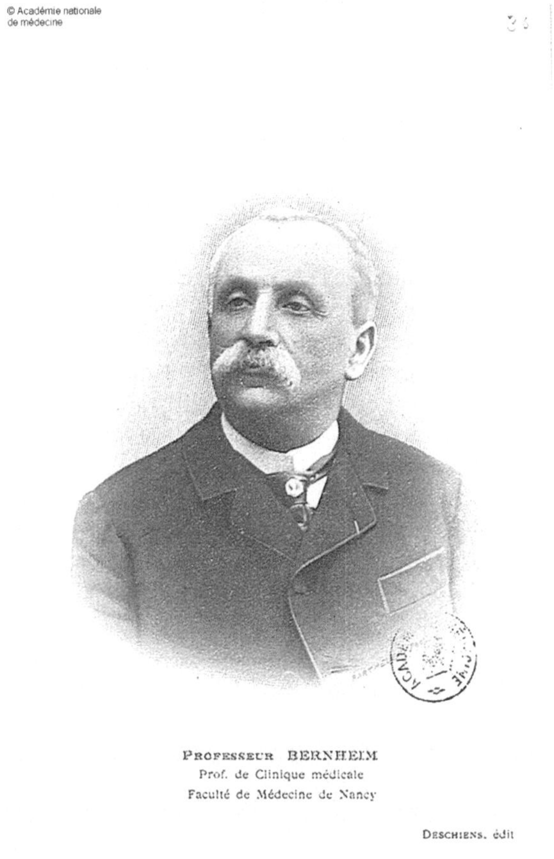

Fig. 4.2 Hippolyte Bernheim https://en.wikipedia.org/wiki/Hippolyte_Bernheim#/media/File:Bernheim.jpg

principal exceptions: Britain and France.[10] In France, this was because Bernheim and Liébeault's views came into conflict with those of the great Jean-Martin Charcot, the most eminent neurologist of his day. While in Britain, few physicians were brave enough to go against the medical establishment after the very public fall from the grace of John Elliotson, nearly

[10] Alan Gauld, *A History of Hypnotism* (Cambridge: Cambridge University Press, 1992) (p. 327).

fifty years before. Despite his previous achievements and recognition in the UK, the ideas of Charcot on hypnotism and hysteria were already viewed with great suspicion in the medical and lay press and so the Nancy school had nothing to build upon.

This may have been partly due to a longstanding conservatism among the medical profession and a deep-rooted general mistrust of foreign ideas. In the words of John Stuart Mill, the prominent Victorian philosopher: 'England [...was] usually the last to enter into the general movement of the European mind.'[11] This had been equally true at the start of the century when Mesmer's ideas had never been accepted by the main body of the medical community in the UK.

Suggestion was not just a new way of explaining hypnotism, it was also understood as being in opposition to the theories of Charcot and his colleagues, sometimes known as the Salpêtrière School. Charcot was the chief physician at the hospital which was home to over 5000 disturbed or destitute patients with a range of conditions from senility to severe and enduring mental illness and progressive neurological complaints. He used this huge group of subjects to describe and separate different clusters of illnesses and then housed them in different wards. He and his staff would routinely examine the brains and central nervous systems of these patients after death and described the clinical features, prognosis and pathology of many new neurological conditions such as multiple sclerosis and motor neurone disease.

Both a skilled clinician and a pathologist, Charcot was also an effective administrator. As his fame grew in France and then Europe, he helped to finance the running of the enormous hospital with clinical demonstrations for the public and visiting physicians. He had a reputation as an excellent teacher and demonstrator of pathology. Positions at the hospital were sought after and his colleagues included some of the most celebrated neurologists of their day: Paul Richer, Georges Gilles de la Tourette and Joseph Babinski. Charcot himself was made a new chair of neurological diseases and elected to the Academy of Sciences. In later life, he became an Officer and then Commander in the French Legion of Honour.

The Salpêtrière was the home of 'Le Grand Hypnotisme', as well as the academic centre for neurology in Europe. According to Charcot, only those with severe hysteria or neurosis could be hypnotised and this

[11] John Stuart Mill, *A System of Logic, Raciocinative and Inductive,* 8th ed., *Book 6: The Logic of the Moral Sciences* (London: Longman and Green, 1925) (p. 643).

propensity could be demonstrated objectively, without fear of simulation or deception, by the presence of distinct physical signs. These signs of hysteria were regularly displayed alongside other neurological disorders at the public demonstrations for which Charcot and the Salpêtrière were renowned. Charcot and his assistants typically used a small number of 'star patients', female subjects who showed the three discreet stages of Charcot's hypnotic progression: lethargy, catalepsy and somnambulism.[12]

The doctors or demonstrators would usually use light eyeball compression to induce the initial lethargic state in which the patient, who usually had a diagnosis of hystero-epilepsy, became passive, motionless and unaware. Opening the patient's eyes at this point would result in the development of catalepsy, the prolonged maintenance of whichever posture the patient was placed in by the demonstrator. The final stage of somnambulism could be reached by rubbing the top of the head. In this phase, awareness seemed to return and the patient could walk and talk freely. However, they were in a state of heightened suggestibility and would freely act out the instructions of the hypnotiser or operator. They could convincingly show specific emotions or act out bizarre scenarios. By the finale, Charcot's scientific presentations and the shows of Europe's premier travelling stage hypnotists like the Dane Carl Hansen and the Belgian-born, Donato (Alfred Edouard D'Hont) were virtually indistinguishable.

Charcot's concept and use of hypnotism was in no way therapeutic. He saw hypnotism as a technique to reveal objective clinical proof of hysteria, a condition that he tried to understand as a brain disorder rather than a mental one. His colleague Charles Féré described Charcot's use of hypnotism to George Robertson, a British medical visitor in disturbing and graphic terms: 'the hypnotised hysterical woman is to be regarded as "the psychological frog" and what the frog has done for physiology, the hysterical woman is to do for psychology.'[13]

If the Salpêtrière was famed for its displays of 'Le Grand Hypnotisme', Nancy was the home of 'Le Petit Hypnotisme'. Physician visitors to both centres of hypnotism, and there were many in the 1880s, were immediately struck by the difference. In Nancy, hypnotism was used

[12] Gauld, Hypnotism (p. 311).

[13] George Robertson, 'Hypnotism at Paris and Nancy: Notes of a Visit', *Journal of Mental Sciences*, 38 (1892) (pp. 494–531).

universally, therapeutically and with spectacular results. However, the drama surrounding the trance state was almost entirely absent. There was no sign of the three-stage procedure and often, the onlooker could not even discern that the patient was hypnotised. One of the first British doctors to visit was Tuckey, in 1888. He recorded the unpretentious one-storied building in which Liébeault saw his patients and prosaically hypnotised them.[14] He noted the wide variety of working-class men who attended his surgery and responded to hypnotism. The difference between the two centres was stark (Fig. 4.3).

To the visiting physicians, there were several aspects of the Nancy approach that seemed readily applicable and transferable to conventional medical practice. Firstly, their direct witnessing of near-miraculous cures of pain and sleep disturbance and for other conditions without clear treatments like drug and alcohol abuse. Second, the Nancy school view was

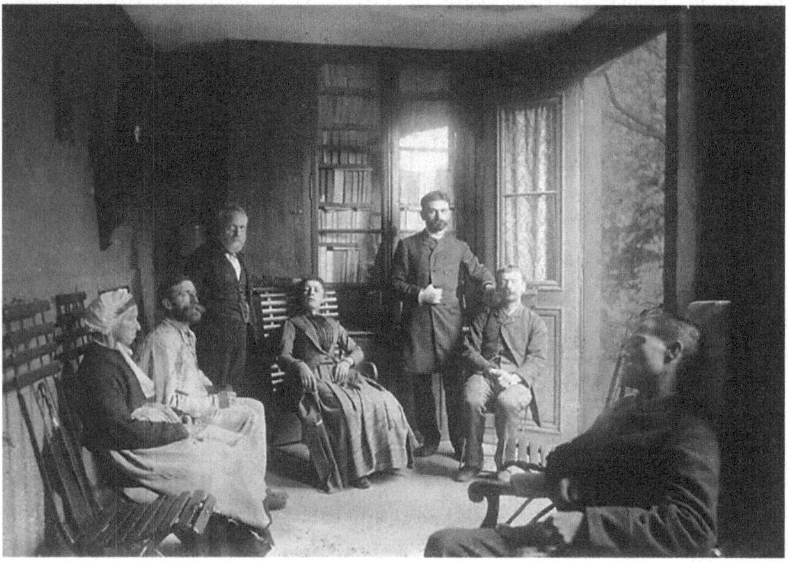

Fig. 4.3 Liébeault in his clinic, 1873. (Collection D. Morque Conservatoire Régional de l'Image)

[14] Charles Lloyd Tuckey, 'Faith-Healing', *Nineteenth Century*, 21 (1888) (pp. 839–50) p. 842.

that everyone would respond to suggestion and the trance state, not just those with severe hysteria and neurosis. Suggestibility to hypnotism and suggestive therapy was normal though it varied in the population. Third, hypnotic sleep was not essential to the therapeutic effects because the state merely enhanced the active ingredient of the procedure which was suggestion. Hypnosis acted as a way of enabling the patient to enter a mental state of exaggerated suggestibility to the health-promoting suggestions of their physician. Bernheim also rejected all the mystical aspects of Mesmer's animal magnetism, demonstrating that since magnetised rods were unnecessary for the effects, so was the idea of an intangible magnetic fluid between healer and patient focussed by the rod. Overall, the Nancy school shifted the understanding of the mode of action of hypnotism from something mystical or even intrinsic to the physiology of the trance state to a process dependent upon the relationship between patient and healer.

The debate between the schools lasted for nearly a decade, until Charcot's death in 1893. Court cases like the 1890 Eyraud-Bompard murder trial meant this rarefied academic dispute had real-world implications and reached a wider lay audience. The case had seized the public imagination both in France and Britain. It was reported in the *Times* that over 5000 people applied for the 80 available tickets to witness the hearing in Paris.[15] The previous year, Gabrielle Bompard had lured a wealthy Parisian bailiff named Alexandre-Toussaint Gouffé to her bedroom with promises of sex. While Gouffé was preoccupied, the waiting petty criminal Eyraud had strangled him with Bompard's silk belt. The amateur scheme quickly unravelled when the couple found little cash on Gouffé's person and realised they had to dispose of the body. When it was eventually found, the police successfully identified the corpse and the pair fled the country. The case stayed in the newspapers for many months because, in an early triumph for the police and forensic procedure, the victim was successfully identified and a trunk that had contained the bag and a boot linking the couple to the body were found near the crime scene. The couple fled to the United States and Cuba and, in another exciting scoop for the newspapers, were made subject to the first Interpol (international police) order and were tracked down and extradited for trial.

[15] Anon, 'The Gouffé Murder', *Times* (17 December 1890) (p. 5).

The infamous court case was closely covered by both the English and French press between December 1890 and February 1891.[16] Gabrielle Bompard was only 22 years old and faced the death penalty for murder. Her defence claimed that she could not be held responsible because 'she had acted under a post-hypnotic suggestion implanted by her former lover.'[17] Several psychiatrists examined her and decided that while she was mildly hysterical, she was perfectly capable of knowing what she was doing. A law professor Jules Liégeois, who identified with the Nancy school, gave lengthy testimony to the effect that Bompard had been hypnotised and was no more than an automaton. Eyraud went to the guillotine while Bompard was imprisoned for 20 years. Her lesser sentence reflected the fact she had separated from Eyraud and had given herself up in the United States, rather than the success of the arguments of Liégeois. The issues of criminal responsibility and the competing theories of the rival schools of hypnotism were discussed at length in the daily press and periodicals on both sides of the channel.[18]

It is hard to get a measure of the level of scientific literacy in the general reading population at this time but it appears much greater than today. The Victorian gentleman's journals were full of articles concerning the scientific and medical developments of the day. Another indicator is the extent to which significant scientists and theories are mentioned in the contemporary fiction. At least three different English language stories from this era involve hypnotism in their plotting and mention Charcot's name directly suggesting an expectation by the author of a wider knowledge in the readership. These include Bram Stoker's *Dracula* (1897),

[16] Robert van Plas, 'Hysteria, Hypnosis, and Moral Sense in French 19th-century Forensic Psychiatry. The Eyraud-Bompard Case', *International Journal of Law and Psychiatry*, 21 (1998) (pp. 397–407); Steven Levingston, *Little Demon in the City of Light* (New York: Doubleday, 2014); Dorothy Hoobler and Thomas Hoobler, *The Crimes of Paris: A True Story of Murder, Theft, and Detection* (Lincoln, NE: Bison, 2010).

[17] Ruth Harris, 'Murder Under Hypnosis in the Case of Gabrielle Bompard: Psychiatry in the Courtroom in Belle Époque Paris', Ch.10 in *The Anatomy of Madness: Essays in the History of Psychiatry* II, ed. by William Bynum, Roy Porter and Michael Shephard (London: Tavistock, 1987) (pp. 197–241).

[18] These are a fraction of the publications: Jean-Martin Charcot, 'Hypnotism and Crime', *Forum of New York*, 9 (1890) (pp. 159–68); A. Taylor Innes, 'Hypnotism in Relation to Crime and the Medical Faculty', *Contemporary Review*, 58 (1890) (pp. 555–66); George Kingsbury, 'Hypnotism, Crime and Doctors', *Nineteenth Century*, 29 (1891) (pp. 145–53).

Arthur Conan Doyle's *The Parasite* (1894) and J. Maclaren Cobban's *Master of his Fate* (1890).[19] All writers implied in their texts that Charcot's work had allowed hypnotism to become mainstream and accepted into the medical orthodoxy. The role of fiction in representing hypnotism, explaining and expanding it will be examined later.

Hypnotism offered the possibility of the experimental examination of hidden mental processes. This development helped to shift psychology from a branch of philosophy to a scientific discipline and coincided with the building of the first psychology laboratories at French, German and American universities. The first international congress on physiological (or experimental) psychology was held in Paris in 1889 and papers on hypnotism represented almost half of the programme. After Bernheim's paper, there was a challenge that suggestion could account for all aspects of hypnotic phenomena from Joseph Babinski of the Salpêtrière. He disagreed that the three phases of grand hypnotism seen at their hospital and witnessed by many could be purely the result of suggestion and suggested that there must be a physical basis.[20] Bernheim argued that there was nothing special about the stages or postures and he could teach or suggest to his patients to adopt them.

Although Charcot remained a figurehead, much of the scholarly work on hypnotism at the Salpêtrière was conducted and theorised by two of his colleagues there, Alfred Binet and Charles Féré. The historical depiction of two competing schools with binary opposing ideas is just a convenient simplification. Binet and Féré did not completely reject the role of suggestion in hypnotism, instead, they saw it as one of several contributing factors. In *Animal Magnetism* (1888) they conducted an extensive historical review of hypnotism and mesmerism. Ironically, one of their conclusions was the proposition that the therapeutic effects observed in many notable and notorious cases which had previously been ascribed to the imagination should more properly be seen as the result

[19] James Maclaren Cobban, *Master of his Fate* (Edinburgh: William Blackwood and Sons, 1890). In this topical novel, Cobban introduces a charming and urbane vampire of spiritual energy whose plans are thwarted by a British physician who trained under 'Charbon' [sic].

[20] Carlos Alvarado, 'Nineteenth-Century Suggestion and Magnetism: Hypnosis at the International Congress of Physiological Psychology (1889)', *Contemporary Hypnosis*, 27 (2010) (pp. 48–60).

of 'suggestive therapeutics'.[21] Their historical review included instances of miraculous healing attributed to either magic or religion, known as thaumaturgy. This retrospective projection of suggestion to bolster the credibility and legitimacy of the new approach was repeated in Britain by the New Hypnotists and will be covered in greater depth.

While I am arguing that there was a transition or tipping point when the explanation for medical hypnotism moved from the imagination to suggestion, this was a step further than Bernheim himself, would go. In all editions of *Suggestive Therapeutics*, he still attributed the somatic effects of suggestion to the doctrine of the imagination. The European hypnotists and British New Hypnotists' views did shift over time. Kingsbury deliberately omitted any discussion of hypnotic theory from his manual and Felkin mentions the physiological theories of brain inhibition as well as referring to Hack Tuke's work on the imagination.[22] Employing the idea of the imagination in his first edition, Tuckey's successive editions of *Psycho-Therapeutics* mention the word less and less, until the idea disappears altogether.

However, the problem still remained: what was the mechanism that caused the objective physical changes in the body initiated by the immaterial aspects of hypnotism and suggestion, belief and relationship. Bramwell was aware of the inadequacies of the suggestion theory: 'Suggestion no more explains the phenomena of hypnotism than the crack of a pistol explains a boat race. Both are simply signals—mere points of departure, and nothing more. In Bernheim's hands the word suggestion has acquired an entirely new signification [...] It has become mysterious and all-powerful, and is supposed to be capable, not only of evoking and explaining all the phenomena of hypnotism, but also of originating—nay, even of being—the condition itself.'[23]

Other members of the SPR like Frank Podmore and the chemist William Crookes continued to write about medical hypnotism, invoking the older classical concept of the *vis medicatrix naturae*. Literally, this meant the healing power of nature, an idea which referred to the human

[21] Alfred Binet and Charles *Féré*, *Animal Magnetism* (New York: Appleton, 1888) (pp. 352–5).

[22] George Kingsbury, *Hypnotic Practice*; Robert Felkin, *Hypnotism or Psycho-Therapeutics* (Edinburgh: Y. J. Pentland, 1890).

[23] John Milne Bramwell, *Suggestion, Its Place in Medicine and Scientific Research* (London: Grant Richards, 1903) (p. 27).

body's inherent ability to heal itself.[24] This was a Hippocratic theory but resurfaced in Paracelsus writings and was widely used in heterodox medicine. Consequently, this was little better than the imagination itself for the New Hypnotists. As a result, the New Hypnotists did not have an answer for the conundrum of the mechanism and remained between imagination and suggestion. We are a little further forward today in explaining the way that immaterial aspects influence physical illness.

Bibliography

Alvarado, Carlos. 2010. 'Nineteenth-Century Suggestion and Magnetism: Hypnosis at the International Congress of Physiological Psychology (1889)', *Contemporary Hypnosis*, 27: 48–60.

Anon. 1890. 'The Gouffé Murder', *Times* (17 December): 5.

Bernheim, Hippolyte. 1884. *De la suggestion dans l'état hypnotique et dans l'état* de veille. Paris: Doin.

Bernheim, Hippolyte. 1886. *De la suggestion et de ses applications a la therapeutique*. Paris: Doin.

Bernheim, Hippolyte. 1889. *Suggestive Therapeutics: A Treatise on the Nature and Uses of Hypnotism*. London: G.P. Putnam.

Binet, Alfred and *Féré*, Charles. 1888. *Animal Magnetism*. New York: Appleton. 352–5.

Braid, James. 1843. *Neurypnology or the Rationale of Nervous Sleep*. London: J. Churchill.

Bramwell, John Milne. 1903. *Suggestion, Its Place in Medicine and Scientific Research*. London: Grant Richards.

Carpenter, William. 1876. *Principles of Mental Physiology*, 3rd ed. London: King.

Charcot, Jean-Martin. 1890. 'Hypnotism and Crime', *Forum of New York*, 9: 159–68.

Chaucer, Geoffrey. 2003. *The Canterbury Tales*. London: Penguin Classics.

Cobban, James Maclaren. 1890. *Master of his Fate*. Edinburgh: William Blackwood.

Crookes, William. 1898. 'Address of the President Before the British Association for the Advancement of Science, Bristol, 1898', *Science*, 8, 200: 561–75.

Felkin, Robert. 1890. *Hypnotism or Psycho-Therapeutics*. Edinburgh: Y. J. Pentland.

Gauld, Alan. 1992. *A History of Hypnotism*. Cambridge: Cambridge University Press.

[24] William Crookes, 'Address of the President Before the British Association for the Advancement of Science, Bristol, 1898.' *Science*, 8, 200 (1898) (pp. 561–75).

Harris, Ruth. 1987. 'Murder under Hypnosis in the Case of Gabrielle Bompard: Psychiatry in the Courtroom in Belle Époque Paris', Ch 10 in *The Anatomy of Madness: Essays in the History of Psychiatry* II, ed. by William Bynum, Roy Porter, and Michael Shephard. London: Tavistock. 197–241.

Hoobler, Dorothy and Hoobler, Thomas. 2010. *The Crimes of Paris: A True Story of Murder, Theft, and Detection*. Lincoln, NE: Bison.

Innes, Alexander Taylor. 1890. 'Hypnotism in Relation to Crime and the Medical Faculty', *Contemporary Review*, 58: 555–66.

Kingsbury, George. 1891. 'Hypnotism, Crime and the Doctors', *Nineteenth Century*, 29, 167 (January): 145–53.

Kingsbury, George. 1891. *The Practice of Hypnotic Suggestion, Being and Elementary Handbook for the Use of the Medical Profession*. Bristol: John Wright.

Levingston, Steven. 2013. *Little Demon in the City of Light*. New York: Doubleday.

Liébeault, Ambroise-Auguste. 1866. *Du Sommeil et des Etats Analogues, Considérés surtout du Point de Vue de l'Action du Moral sur le Physique*. Paris: Victor Maisson.

Mill, John Stuart. 1925. *A System of Logic, Raciocinative and Inductive*, 8th ed., *Book 6: The Logic of the Moral Sciences*. London: Longman and Green. 643.

Milton, John. 2003. *Paradise Lost*. London: Penguin Classics. 61.

Robertson, George. 1892. 'Hypnotism at Paris and Nancy: Notes of a Visit', *Journal of Mental Sciences*, 38: 494–531.

'Suggestion'. Oxford English Dictionary. https://en.oxforddictionaries.com/definition/suggestion [accessed 8 October 2018].

'Suggestion'. https://www.etymonline.com/word/suggestion [accessed 26 March 2018].

Tuckey, Charles Lloyd. 1888. 'Faith Healing as a Medical Treatment', *Nineteenth Century*, 21: 839–50.

van Plas, Robert. 1998. 'Hysteria, Hypnosis, and Moral Sense in French 19th-Century Forensic Psychiatry. The Eyraud-Bompard Case', *International Journal of Law and Psychiatry*, 21: 397–407.

Waterfield, Robin. 2004. *Hidden Depths: The Story of Hypnosis*. London: Pan.

CHAPTER 5

A Very British History of Hypnotism

If we understand history as the story we tell about the past for present purposes, then rereading medical histories can tell us something useful about the views and motivations of the writers in the time that they were written. This form of study is called historiography. The medical historians Roy Porter and Mark Micale have outlined the important role that histories can serve in securing the knowledge base for disciplines like psychiatry, helping to delineate boundaries for the new speciality: 'science histories, by memorialising the proper lineage of figures, texts and ideas serve to legitimate particular theories and methodologies and to delegitimate others.'[1] The artifice of a carefully constructed history for a specialty or profession is also known as a founding myth or *mythe d'origine*.

As we read the Victorian histories of hypnotism, we can ask why the New Hypnotists presented John Elliotson and James Braid as critical figures in their new lineage of hypnotism. Bramwell, for example, credited James Braid with the independent development of hypnotism from mesmerism and the invention of the theory of suggestion as its principal mode of action, anticipating the Nancy school by over thirty years. There

[1] Roy Porter and Mark Micale, 'Introduction: Reflections on Psychiatry and Its Histories', in *History of Psychiatry*, ed. by Micale and Porter (Oxford, Oxford University Press, 1994) 3–26 (p. 5).

G. D. L. Bates, *The Uncanny Rise of Medical Hypnotism, 1888–1914*, Mental Health in Historical Perspective,
https://doi.org/10.1007/978-3-031-42725-1_5

are likely to be several reasons for this very British version of hypnotic history.

James Braid can be seen as a pivotal figure in this narrative. Before Braid, it was recognised that therapeutic trance processes had occurred, but they were not properly understood. Indeed, they were linked to occult or spiritual concepts that predated the Age of Reason. The New Hypnotists argued that there was an aspect of mesmerism that was beneficial but until Braid, the trance state was being used implicitly or unknowingly. Placing Braid as the founding father of scientific trance, then allowed a retrospective projection of the discipline back to the Enlightenment and even earlier. Braid's version of hypnotism was mechanistic and rather prosaic: a long way from the mystical theatre of the mesmerists. In his obituary, he was described as professionally skilled and of 'high personal character'.[2] These were both important characteristics for a mythical figure to 'legitimise' the contested features of trance and hypnotism that were in the public domain.

John Elliotson was also proposed as an earlier transitionary figure and we must consider what he might offer to the New Hypnotists. Elliotson was a British medical Olympian before he dabbled in mesmerism. Despite the notoriety that followed, there was no doubting his eminence and scientific credentials as a professor of medicine. In my reading, the New Hypnotists could portray Elliotson as a great doctor who was unaware of the 'reality' of hypnotism but still acted honourably and beneficently towards his patients using prototype hypnotism. As such, the New Hypnotists would need to rehabilitate his reputation, reassess his medical contributions and remember his true achievements. As an 'expert' in human physiology and a philanthropist (he never charged for mesmeric treatments), Elliotson had offered proficiency, authority and humanity.

Finally, both Braid and Elliotson were British establishment figures. Surprisingly perhaps, mesmerism was viewed as dangerously revolutionary in its potential to transform society. As the cultural historian Robert Darnton has shown mesmeric ideas were commonly used in the language and metaphors of pre-revolutionary France: ideas that the country was sick and its energies unbalanced.[3] The revolutionaries proposed that that

[2] John Milne Bramwell, *Hypnotism: It's History, Practice and Theory* (London: Grant Richards, 1903) (p. 29).

[3] Robert Darnton, 'A Radical Political Theory', Ch 4 in *Mesmerism and the End of the Enlightenment in France* (New York: Schocken Books, 1970) (pp. 106–25).

the 'head' (that is the monarchy) needed treatment (removal) in order for the country to rebalance the magnetic flow. When mesmerism eventually came to the UK in the mid-nineteenth century, these rebellious associations came with it. Some of its staunchest advocates were among the working-class radicals and reformists. Mesmerism was seen by the Chartist, Thomas Cooper, as not only the intellectual property of the common people but a means by which the will of the workers could be reinforced which would be necessary in any class struggle.[4] Placing middle-class professionals Braid and Elliotson, who had both advocated for a specialist monopoly of the technology, at the heart of this timeline had the effect of deflecting the hostility and suspicion against the foreign and national radical thinking. It was also a time of great British scientific advance, and hypnotism could be employed in a wider narrative of national scientific superiority.

In spite of the important European developments in mesmerism in the early part of the nineteenth century, particularly the mesmeric ground rules established by Puységur, there was little discussion or mention of medical mesmerism in Britain. This situation started to change in 1830s London with the legacy of Percy Shelley's writings and his coterie of intellectuals and the approving report of the second committee set up to re-evaluate animal magnetism by the French *Académie* de *Médecine*, whose report was translated by Colquhoun in 1833.[5] However, probably the most important driver for the massive cultural shift that followed in Britain was the collaboration of the ambitious London physician, John Elliotson, with the French magnetist, Charles Dupotet de Sennevoy in 1837 and the subsequent publicity given to the pair's experiments by the new medical journal, the *Lancet* under the editorship of Thomas Wakley. It was these events that led to the central role that mesmerism played in British mid-Victorian life, documented by Alison Winter, the cultural historian.

This chapter will focus on the salient aspects of the stories of both men to highlight the medical and cultural impact of mesmerism in Britain and

[4] Alison Winter, *Mesmerized: Powers of Mind in Victorian Britain* (Chicago and London: University of Chicago Press) (p. 131).

[5] John Campbell, *Colquhoun, Report of the Experiments on Animal Magnetism Made By a Committee of the Medical Section of the French Royal Academy of Sciences* (Edinburgh: Robert Cadell, 1833).

to demonstrate the new historical framing of the New Hypnotists.[6] It is important to show John Elliotson's eminence and ability as a conventional physician, in order to show the full scale of his fall from grace. The medical establishment emphatically rejected mesmerism and it was the humiliating public and medical opprobrium that followed which effectively suppressed the consideration of mesmerism from British medicine for fifty years. It also explains why his colleagues repeatedly refer to Tuckey's bravery in endorsing hypnotism so publicly fifty years later. The *Lancet* played an important role in advancing Elliotson but it and other new medical journals also played an important role in policing the borders of established medical practice from new heterodox innovations. These events closely mirror the New Hypnotist's battle with Ernest Hart, the editor of the *BMJ* in the 1890s.

Unlike Elliotson, who was well-known but for the wrong reasons, James Braid was much more of a peripheral and forgotten figure. He had worked as a surgeon outside of London and struggled to gain attention for his ground-breaking research. Braid had found that he could not get his work on hypnotism published in the orthodox London-based medical journals. He also struggled to find approval with Elliotson, becoming unable to disseminate his discoveries in Elliotson's journal the *Zoist*. He self-published some of his work but his later pamphlets and books had very small print runs. After his death, he was better known in France than in Britain. The New Hypnotists would need to both rehabilitate Elliotson's reputation and credibility and to rediscover and publicise Braid and his work. In this way, they advanced a new *mythe d'origine* of pure British hypnotism, for their new discipline.

[6] These events have been well told by biographers like Wendy Moore, historians of hypnosis such as Robin Gauld, Robin Waterfield and William Hughes as well as cultural critics like Winter. Wendy Moore, *The Mesmerist, the Society Doctor who held Victorian London Spellbound* (London: Weidenfield and Nicholson, 2017); Robin Gauld, *A History of Hypnotism* (Cambridge: Cambridge University Press, 1992); Robin Waterfield, *Hidden Depths* (London: Pan, 2004); William Hughes, *That Devil's Trick: Hypnotism and the Victorian Popular Imagination* (Manchester: Manchester University Press, 2015); Winter, *Mesmerized*.

The Rise and Fall and Rise of John Elliotson (1791–1868) (Fig. 5.1)

The extraordinary career of John Elliotson and the response of the medical establishment to his promotion of mesmerism shows the conservative and reactionary nature of British medicine at the time. Even its brightest lights could be sacrificed to secure the link of the profession to materialist science. Elliotson was born in 1791 into a family of chemists and apothecaries in Southwark, South London. His father's successful business allowed him to embark on undergraduate medical training in Edinburgh, Guy's Hospital in London and later Cambridge. He had an ambition to become a physician from an early age despite the significant handicap of his mercantile background and the absence of a medical

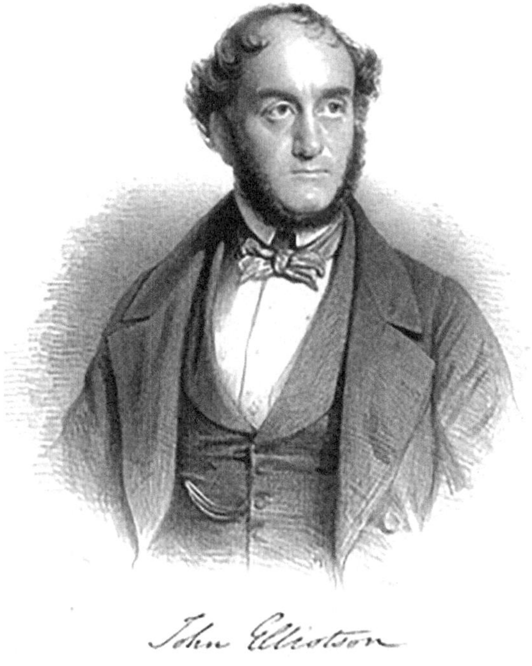

Fig. 5.1 An engraving, taken from the life, of John Elliotson (1791–1868). Unknown Artist. http://www.ucl.ac.uk/library/exhibitions/innovators-educators

family or mentors. After three years at Cambridge, he travelled to the medical schools of Europe, learning French and German and developing a professional network in the international medical community. He was most impressed by what he found and viewed Continental medicine as considerably more advanced than British medicine.

By the age of 24, Elliotson was so ambitious that he decided not only to translate but also make corrections to *Institutiones Physiologicae*, the standard physiology text of the day. Johann Blumenbach was a professor of physiology at Göttingen University in Germany. He had published *Institutiones* in Latin in 1787 and it soon became recognised in Germany and later Europe as the primary reading for the subject.[7] The merit of Blumenbach's work was even recognised in parochial Britain and he had been elected a Fellow of the Royal Society in 1793. Elliotson's English first edition was published anonymously in 1815. It was well-reviewed, even by Blumenbach himself, and Elliotson went on to write and take the credit for four further editions, increasingly supplementing the original text with his own and more contemporary scholarship.[8] There was no sixth edition from Elliotson: by 1840 he had retitled his book *Human Physiology* and replaced Blumenbach's name with his own.[9] The new work quickly replaced *Institutiones* as the standard UK textbook of physiology.

At this early stage of his career, Elliotson demonstrated many of the features that come to characterise him and his later work: an enthusiasm for novel European medical approaches; an impatience with reactionary British medicine; a prodigious talent, combined with scholarship, industry and vaulting ambition. With an old Edinburgh friend, the physician and eminent chemist, William Prout, he started a new medical journal, *The Annals of Medicine and Surgery*. They used this as a vehicle to promote novel therapies. Most notably this included the prescription of potassium iodate which Prout had formulated as a treatment for goitre, a cause of neck-swelling resulting from thyroid gland overgrowth.[10] This

[7] Johann Blumenbach, *Institutiones Physiologicae* (Gottingae: Jo. Christ. Dieterich, 1787).

[8] There are no copies of the first edition extant Johann Blumenbach, *The Institutes of Physiology*, 2nd ed., trans. by John Elliotson (London: Bensley, 1817).

[9] John Elliotson, *Human Physiology*, 5th ed. (London: Longman, Orme, Brown, Green and Longmans, 1840).

[10] William Brock, 'The Life and Work of William Prout', *Medical History,* 9 (1965) (pp. 101–26).

proved very effective and a modified preparation of iodine remains current treatment for hypothyoidism: an early ground-breaking advance for the precocious doctor.

In 1822, Elliotson's immediate superior at St. Thomas's George Currey died unexpectedly on his honeymoon. Elliotson replaced him, appointed a hospital consultant in January 1823 at the relatively young age of 31. Having secured his goal, Elliotson did not rest on his laurels like most others. He worked long days, using his position to treat and learn from his patients as well as to promote some of his unconventional views. He was among the first and probably the most influential of British physicians to adopt the newly invented, stethoscope as a clinical aid. The first prototypes were on sale in Britain in 1819. They looked like old-fashioned ear trumpets and consisted of a wooden tube attached to a single microphone at one end and earpiece at the other. It would be twenty years before they were more universally adopted in the UK.[11] He became interested in the new treatment system of acupuncture and the diagnostic approach of phrenology. Soon after his appointment, he founded the Phrenological Society of London.

Elliotson was clearly attracted by novelty and at the vanguard of innovation. An 1845 biography in the *Medical Times* observed, 'Elliotson's motto was everlastingly "Onward!" If he did not look with hate, he did with distrust, on all that was old – the past seemed nothing to him, the future boundless.'[12] He was one of the first doctors to wear trousers rather than breeches and stockings and to grow an 'under the chin' beard. Recording this, the *Dictionary of National Biography* noted, 'His desire to be original led Elliotson into many eccentricities.'[13] The implication was that in conservative medical circles, this was not a good thing. He was also self-assured and impatient of other's differing opinions. However, his enthusiasms were influential in both the medical and non-medical worlds. As a result, he was able to popularise the use of quinine for malaria and worked out the likely cause of hay-fever. The extent of his authority

[11] Melissa Dickson, 'Hats, Cloaks, and Stethoscopes: The Symbolic Fashions of the Nineteenth-Century Medical Practitioner', in *Fashion and Material Culture in Victorian Fiction and Periodicals*, ed. by Nickianne Moody and Janine Hatter (Brighton: Edward Everett Root, 2019) (pp. 105–20).

[12] Anon, 'Pencillings of Eminent Men', *The Medical Times* (1 February 1845) (p. 392).

[13] 'John Elliotson' in *Dictionary of National Biography*, Vol 17, ed. by Robert Hunt (London: Smith and Elder, 1885–1900).

among medics was partly the result of his very public endorsement by Thomas Wakley and the *Lancet* journal. This association initially was to help Elliotson to make his name. Later, his lay reputation stemmed from his friendships with writers like Charles Dickens and William Thackeray and politicians like Benjamin Disraeli.

In 1825, St Thomas's medical school formally split from Guy's, when Guy's set up its own anatomy school. This meant that there was no reason for the governors to protect the monopoly of the Guy's doctors and the contractual constraints on Elliotson's teaching came to an end. This meant he could finally teach the way he wanted. Elliotson introduced many techniques that he had observed in Europe. These included the routine use of the thermometer and stethoscope, bedside teaching of clinical skills, the post-mortem to clarify diagnosis after death and the use of illustrations and pathology specimens in his classroom lectures. These changes in teaching style combined with a clear and systematic approach were revolutionary. One of his pupils writing over forty years later described him as 'the greatest clinical teacher of his time.'[14] The *Lancet* was highly supportive, publishing his clinical case notes from 1827 and his lectures from 1829 and comparing them very favourably to the 'miserable compilations of medical and surgical dictionaries' of other medical school lecturers.[15] With the assistance of the *Lancet*, his reputation and private practice both took off dramatically. A contemporary pupil and contributor to the *Lancet*, James Clarke described him in his memoirs as becoming 'the talk of the town' between 1827 and 1828 observing that at the same time, his private income rocketed, multiplying tenfold.[16]

In 1829, Elliotson was elected a fellow of the Royal Society and by 1831 he had left St Thomas's to become Professor of Medicine at the new secular London University. Though he was not the only complimentary voice in medical journalism, Wakley continued to sing his praises following his appointment writing that 'Elliotson is not surpassed by any physician in the metropolis.'[17] In 1833, he was elected as president of the

[14] James Fernandez Clarke, *Autobiographical Recollections of the Medical Profession* (London: J. and A. Churchill, 1874).

[15] Thomas Wakley, 'Editorial', *Lancet* (17 April 1830) (p. 86).

[16] Clarke, *Autobiographical Recollections* (p. 180).

[17] Anon, 'Lancet Gallery of Medical Portraits: John Elliotson, M.D.', *Lancet* (8 June 1833) (pp. 341–44).

Medical and Chirurgical Society, the forerunner of the Royal Society of Medicine, which temporarily met at his grand new mansion house, located just off Regent Street and previously owned by the Prime Minister George Canning. The self-styled cockney and self-made man had well and truly arrived. It was to be a long fall. But as Clarke later reflected in his reminiscences: 'It is somewhat curious that the journal [the *Lancet*] which in 1828 had laid the foundation of his fame and fortune, should just ten years afterwards do so much to effect his ruin; but it was so.'[18]

Elliotson first became interested in mesmerism after witnessing the demonstrations of the Irish chemist, Richard Chenevix at St Thomas's hospital in 1829. He was sufficiently convinced and brave enough to publicly back the mesmerist, endorsing him in an article for the *London Medical and Physical Journal:* 'From this time I was satisfied that mesmerism exists, and hope some day to inquire into it.'[19] The *Lancet*, on the other hand, was typically scathing of Chenevix. Wakley portrayed him as a quack and described mesmerism, particularly used fraudulently for material gain, as 'a wretched and disgraceful piece of deception.'[20] Chevenix returned to France and died the same year, leaving the majority of Britain unconvinced by mesmerism.

Elliotson did not take his interest any further for another eight years till the arrival of Jules Denis, the Baron Dupotet in 1837. Dupotet had practised mesmerism in France for many years and developed a reputation for successfully treating epilepsy and hysteria. Having moved to London, he failed to attract an audience for his lectures and demonstrations of animal magnetism, in part due to his conspicuous inability to speak any English. Undeterred, he offered his services to all of the London hospitals. He sought an audience with Elliotson at University College Hospital (UCH) and despite his problems communicating directly was able to 'charm to sleep' a 24-year-old groom, Thomas Orton, who had been admitted to UCH with seizures that had not responded to six months treatment with acupuncture, electricity or metallic salts. Orton was treated daily with mesmerism and his frequency and severity of seizures reduced. He was discharged as cured three months later.

[18] Clarke, *Autobiographical Recollections* (p. 180).

[19] John Elliotson, 'Addendum', *London Medical and Physical Journal*, 62 (1829) (pp. 315–24).

[20] Thomas Wakley, 'The Medical and Physical Journal', *Lancet* (13 June 1829), 341–5 (p. 344).

Elliotson was intrigued and embraced the new therapy with his characteristic enthusiasm. He closely studied the techniques or 'passes' of Dupotet and initially experimented on patients with him. Later, he trained his clinical clerk William Wood and started to offer animal magnetism or 'mesmerism' as he preferred to call it, routinely to his patients at UCH. Although mesmerism was ineffective for some patients, it worked sensationally within days or weeks for others previously unresponsive to conventional treatments.

By May 1838, such was the interest in mesmerism from the medical students that he moved from his traditional bedside teaching to the hospital's lecture theatres which had benches for 250 but still could not seat all of the crowds. He went on to draw such large audiences from the general public that he was accused of actively seeking publicity by some of his colleagues like the surgeon, Robert Liston, and the hospital governors. At this stage, he was still enjoying the support of the *Lancet* which had decided to reserve judgement about mesmerism. The journal respectfully reported one of his spring lectures on mesmerism quite positively, which was then carried to the general public by the popular lay journals. Within his own hospital, there were quite vocal critics of his new work like the Liston. Elliotson hit back in a typically radical and forthright manner: 'the hospital was not founded to fill the pockets of the professors, but to throw light on truth and nature, and to expose fallacies.'[21]

Elliotson's best experimental subjects were the Irish Okey sisters, Elizabeth and Jane. They were housemaids, originally identified and recruited by Baron Dupotet as very responsive to mesmerism and he was able to cure their seizures. The 'Celtic' heritage was supposed to indicate creativity, spirituality and heightened sensitivity to mesmerism and later hypnotism. These racial stereotypes and the link to hypnotism were still widespread in popular culture at the end of the century.

The Okeys were so susceptible that they were mesmerised on a daily basis and became Elliotson's preferred patients for his public displays, too. After a few mesmeric passes Jane became quite insensible to pain but it was her sister's behaviour that was most remarkable and drew the crowds. A quiet, shy girl normally, under the influence of mesmerism she completely changed character. While in her 'sleep-waking' state she was

[21] Thomas Wakley, 'University College Hospital: Animal Magnetism', *Lancet* (26 May 1838) 282–7 (p. 283).

highly amusing.[22] She could sing and dance, mimic her fellow patients and would mock Dr Elliotson and members of the audience regardless of their social status. With a longer historical viewpoint, some of the things she said may be seen as strangely prophetic: 'I say, Dr. Ellison [sic], 'spose I was to knock you off your perch; how funny you'd look.'[23]

The scientific demonstration of mesmerism had become a public spectacle and a most entertaining one at that. Elliotson's 'experiments' were attended by a broad spectrum of Victorian society: eminent scientists such as Michael Faraday and Charles Wheatstone; novelists like Charles Dickens and William Thackeray; members of parliament, the clergy and the aristocracy. In the London of 1838, mesmerism had become the *mode du jour*. Unwittingly, Elliotson had ushered into Britain a novel entertainment: the mesmeric lecture, which was soon to be taken up across the country by performers as well as mesmerists.

Over the summer of 1838 the mesmerism displays at UCH became increasingly strange and soon got out of hand. The Okey sisters started to embellish their performances into something quite extraordinary. Elizabeth showed that she was able to copy the movements of Elliotson and others when hidden behind a screen of brown paper. Elliotson believed that she had 'transposition of the senses' and could use her hand as an organ of vision. She also developed a form of clairvoyance: an ability to diagnose herself, guide treatment and successfully predict her own recovery. This was unsurprising to Elliotson as it had been previously described by Puységur. Indeed, it is more than likely that in trying to test for this ability he had inadvertently fostered Elizabeth's skill. Some of the other girls developed their abilities and she then denounced four of her peers as frauds, apparently to secure her own position. The medical and popular press were suspicious: if one was faking, perhaps they all were.

In August, Wakley challenged his old friend Elliotson to provide verifiable proof of his claims. He suggested that Elliotson bring the Okeys to his house in Bedford Square for further demonstrations with independent observers. Wakley had devised a test procedure that involved 'blinding', the same method used by the Franklin commission in the investigation of animal magnetism in the previous century. This meant that Elizabeth was unaware as to whether an item used to induce trance was 'magnetic'

[22] A neologism of Elliotson's; John Elliotson, '*Human Physiology*' (1840) (p. 616).

[23] Wakley, 'UCH: Animal Magnetism' (p. 287).

or not. This was achieved by placing a pasteboard in front of her face. Elliotson had established by his previous experiments that nickel could be magnetised (hold animal magnetic energy) but the lead could not. Elizabeth responded vigorously to the first contact of her palm with nickel, becoming rigid, flushed and hyperventilating for fifteen minutes with her back arched above the couch (*opisthotonos*). In the next challenge, Wakley had palmed the nickel to a colleague who then stood at the back of the room. Wakley then rubbed his fist, which now contained a piece of lead (which was magnetically inert) against Elizabeth's hand. Both Elliotson and Okey missed the subterfuge. Simultaneously, another of Wakley's impartial observers loudly whispered, 'Don't apply the nickel too strongly.' At this, she was thrown into yet another frenzy. Later that day, Elliotson continued on his Swiss vacation as planned, but while he was away, Wakley continued to experiment on the Okeys and came to the conclusion that there was no scientific basis for a physical force of animal magnetism or mesmerism.

At first, Wakley published Herbert Mayo's fairly neutral observations of the events at Bedford House over seven pages of the *Lancet* of 1 September 1838.[24] However, in subsequent weeks, he adopted a more overtly hostile tone towards mesmerism in his journal. He did not directly censure Elliotson, instead suggesting that he was a naïve dupe who had been misled by the foreigner, Baron Dupotet and deceived by the duplicitous Okeys. Wakley was unable to account for all the strange phenomena that had been witnessed from anaesthesia to trance state and 'double consciousness' but was happy to ascribe most of them to Elizabeth's genius for acting and the deviousness of the sisters. He proposed that their motives were straightforward and understandable for uneducated servant girls: initially they 'pitied the believers panting for signs and wonders which the slightest exertion of her will could produce' then they wished to please their friends and finally to 'exert their utmost power over a large audience.'[25]

Elliotson returned from his holiday on the continent to a major scandal. The Okeys had been discharged from UCH to Dover and the *Lancet's* account of the proceedings at Bedford House had been picked

[24] Herbert Mayo, '"Animal Magnetism"; or, "Mesmerism"', *Lancet* (1 September 1838) (pp. 805–14).

[25] Thomas Wakley, 'Editorial'. *Lancet* (15 September 1838) (pp. 873–7).

up, first by the *London Medical Gazette*. This highly critical version was then reprinted verbatim by the *Times* and then reported by other popular journals.[26] The tone of the newspaper reports was mocking and salacious by turns. The frenzied writhing and opisthotonos of Elizabeth Okey and the other female patients in the trance state were too close to sexual ecstasy to go unremarked. The columnists of the *Satirist* were quick to question the origins of the girls suggesting they were from Coventry Court, a notorious red-light district.[27] The journal also questioned the integrity and motives of all the men who were experimenting with the Okeys so frequently (including Wakley himself in the accusation). By this stage, the Okeys were kept in an almost permanent trance state and acted like young children or 'idiots' in the contemporary medical lexicon. The piece used the term 'gentlemen' in inverted commas to describe the investigators and commented that they hoped that the wives were present.[28] Both the magnetic operator and the somnambule were viewed as morally suspect. As time went on, even Wakley did not shy from sensationalising the possibility that mesmerism could have a role in exploitative sex in his ironically titled 'Virtues of Animal Magnetism' (Fig. 5.2):

> Long before the days of Mesmer and his deluded followers, the effects of certain manipulations, now called 'passes', on the frames of delicate or nervous females, were known to libertines... The men-about-town [of today] avoid practising in public their mesmeric tricks, lest some common-sense view of the case might construe them into what they really are *indecent assaults* [original emphasis].[29]

Back from his holiday, Elliotson returned to his work at UCH and continued to treat his patients with mesmerism as if nothing had happened. He wrote to the *Lancet* to complain about the misrepresentations and misunderstandings but Wakley would not print his letters. He readmitted Elizabeth Okey to UCH in October 1838, putting him

[26] Anon, 'Animal Magnetism', *Times* (6 September 1838) (p. 2); Anon, 'Progress of Animal Magnetism', *The Times* (15 September 1838) (p. 3).

[27] Hughes, *Devil's Trick* (p. 119).

[28] Anon. 'Chit-Chat', *The Satirist; or the Censor of the Times* (9 September 1838) (p. 285).

[29] Thomas Wakley, 'The Virtues of Animal Magnetism', *Lancet* (8 December 1838) (p. 413).

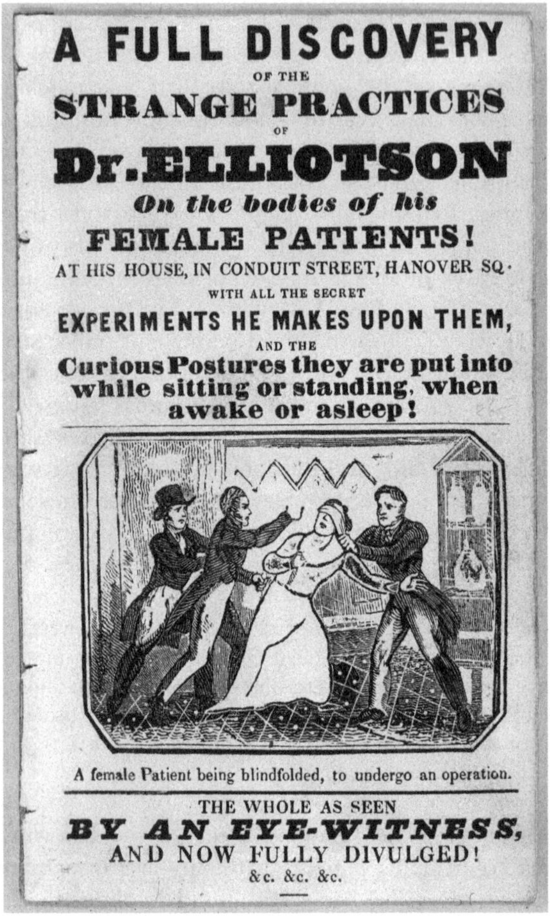

Fig. 5.2 'A full discovery of the strange practices of Dr. Elliotson' Anonymous Pamphlet (Courtesy of the Wellcome Collection)

directly at odds with his medical colleagues and the hospital management at UCH. However, the final act of the drama was imminent. In November, Okey revealed to Elliotson that, while in a trance state, she could tell when a patient was soon going to die. When standing near a chronically ill patient she felt 'a sense of great oppression, sickness, and misery' and could see a figure in a white robe standing near the patient's bed she named 'Great Jackey', who was the angel of death.[30]

Elliotson wanted to witness this new mesmeric phenomenon for himself. In December, he led Elizabeth through one of the male wards by hand, passing in front of all of the beds. He felt her give a violent shudder at two of them. She told him that she had seen the figure of Jack at the foot of both of the beds. Rumours of the escapade spread throughout the hospital. When the *Lancet* reporter learned that one of the patients identified by Elizabeth had actually died that night and that the other was expected to die very soon, there was uproar.

On Elliotson's arrival at the hospital the next day, the pandemonium continued. He immediately went to the lecture theatre and delivered an account of the science behind Elizabeth's predictions and visions to the medical students. A few days later, Elliotson was summoned by the hospital committee who wanted to know why Elizabeth was still a patient but also why she had been on the male ward. Elliotson tried to defend himself, saying that Elizabeth was not fraudulent and that there was something genuine and exceptional about what had just occurred. However, the board disagreed and decided that mesmerism should be banned at UCH and Elizabeth should be immediately discharged from its care. When the findings of the board were approved, Elliotson resigned. He demanded that his students be refunded their fees for his lectures and vowed that he would never again return to the hospital or college that he had done much to establish.

The *Lancet* congratulated UCL on its handling of the affair. Wakley suggested that their decisive action had the 'hearty approval' of medical men and supporters of the university.[31] He went on to declare that mesmerism was humbug and that 'When DR ELLIOTSON [sic] became a mesmerist, he ceased to be a "physician"'.[32] These opinions moved quickly from the medical to the popular press. They were eagerly repeated in the *Times* under the banner, 'The Humbug called "Mesmerism"'.[33] The Okeys bore the brunt of the outrage. Elizabeth was described as

[30] John Elliotson, 'John Elliotson's Letter', in *London Medical Gazette* (23 March 1839) (p. 951).

[31] Thomas Wakley, 'University College and Hospital', *Lancet* (5 January 1839) (pp. 561–2).

[32] Wakley, 'UCH' (p. 562).

[33] Anon, 'The Humbug called "Mesmerism"', *Times* (7 January 1839) (p. 6).

'a flatulent, hysterical and impudent baggage' who took strange liberties with the 'worthy doctor' and was ridiculed for predicting the action of medicines of which she was totally ignorant.[34] Elliotson's humiliation was complete. He was portrayed as either a gullible fool or as a charlatan.

However, if the medical establishment believed this to be the end of mesmerism or John Elliotson, they were mistaken. The *Lancet*, under Wakley may have successfully protected the main body of the medical profession from the taint of quackery and unconventional ideas but the publicity generated had only served to launch mesmerism and the trance state across Britain. The majority of the metropolitan elite had significant reservations about the new technology but in the provinces, it was enthusiastically adopted by the public and even some physicians. The science of the trance state was disseminated by a new wave of travelling lecturers who were already an established part of Victorian self-improvement and public science. Previously, they had been doing good business teaching the working and middle classes instructional subjects like geology and animal biology. As Alison Winter put it these new 'peripatetic lecturers created a new, nationally based experimental culture, prominently featuring mesmerism.'[35]

Over time, the mesmerism lectures developed a routine format which had clear similarities to Elliotson's public experiments at UCH. The metamorphosis from therapeutic ritual to performance piece did not require wholescale changes. Playing to lay audiences in town halls across the country, these lectures blurred the boundaries between entertainment and education, and titillation and scientific discovery even more than Elliotson. The mesmerist would usually commence with a display of anaesthesia (loss of sensation) or 'insensibility'. This was seen as the least likely aspect of trance to be feigned. The demonstration could involve a lack of response by the mesmerised to a range of noxious stimuli: smelling salts, electric shocks, fingers in candle flames or a gunshot next to the ear. All of these could be tested against ordinary members of the public for comparison. The established lecturers would often have to bring hypnotically susceptible or pain-tolerant subjects (who came to be known as 'horses' for their ability to tolerate suffering) with

[34] Anon, 'Animal Magnetism', in *Medico-Chirurgical Review* (1 October 1838) (p. 636).

[35] Winter, *Mesmerized* (p. 111).

them on tour as they could not guarantee such predictable effects from random local participants.[36] Once the *bona fide* nature of the trance had been established it was then followed by acts of clairvoyance, prophecy and 'traction', the name given to the mimicry of movement induced by the mesmerist which included writhing, opisthotonos and catatonic postures. This formula spread rapidly and reinforced specific ideas about trance across the country. The best-known lecturers such as Charles Lafontaine, William Davey and Spencer Hall were attracting audiences in their thousands. It was the entertainer, Lafontaine who was responsible for introducing the technique to James Braid, surgeon and author of *Neurypnology, or the Rationale of Nervous Sleep*.[37]

Elliotson was not one to back down or to change his views and had maintained a steady private medical practice. He persisted in employing mesmerism and continued to witness favourable results. Although he was not as busy as he had been at UCH, he had a regular stream of interested visitors and patients, partly because he did not charge if they were impoverished. He continued to mix with prominent writers and thinkers and was a close friend of Charles Dickens. Mesmerism was a cultural phenomenon and force in Victorian Britain.

Influentially, the literary critic Fred Kaplan has shown the impact of mesmerism on the literary work of Dickens among others.[38] Other authors who knew Elliotson were William Thackeray, Edward Bulwer-Lytton, and later Nathaniel Hawthorne.[39] All these authors believed in the medical power of animal magnetism and used aspects of mesmerism in their fictions. In gratitude for Elliotson's *pro bono* treatment which he believed had been life-saving, Thackeray wrote a short dedication at the

[36] Fred Nadis, *Wonder Shows: Performing Science, Magic, and Religion in America* (New Brunswick: Rutgers University Press, 2005) (p. 108).

[37] James Braid, *Neurypnology or the Rationale of Nervous Sleep* (London: J. Churchill, 1843).

[38] Fred Kaplan, *Dickens and Mesmerism: The Hidden Springs of Fiction* (Princeton: Princeton University Press, 1975).

[39] Lord Bulwer-Lytton became fascinated by mesmerism as a result of his Cambridge friendship with the leading lay mesmerist, Chauncy Hare Townshend. He corresponded with the *Zoist*, complimenting Elliotson on the elegance of his Latin and his manly appeal (*Zoist*, 8 [1850], p. 383)! He wrote several novels with mesmeric themes including *A Strange Story* (1862), *Zanoni* (1842) and *The Coming Race* (1871). The US author Nathaniel Hawthorne was also influenced. He visited Elliotson in London in 1856 and wrote the novels *The House of the Seven Gables* (1851) and *The Scarlet Letter* (1850).

start of *Pendennis* and included a thinly veiled portrait of Elliotson himself as the humane and altruistic 'Dr Goodenough' in the novel.[40]

It was Bulwer-Lytton who recommended that the influential social reformer and writer, Harriet Martineau (1802–1876) consult a medical mesmerist for her complex health problems. Her successful treatment did much to publicise and convince the general public of the efficacy of mesmerism. Martineau was unusually open about her illness, writing about her abdominal pain, constipation, frequent menstruation and discharges. She had also developed such pain on walking and standing that she became a bed-bound invalid, having previously energetically lectured and extensively travelled in the States. After her recovery in 1844, she had become a zealous convert. She wrote a series of positive letters for the *Athenaeum*, a popular Victorian gentleman's periodical which had previously criticised Elliotson and mesmerism. In her introduction to the book that followed she prophesied a not too distant time when mesmerists would cure half the illnesses in the land.[41]

Emboldened by the interest shown in mesmerism outside orthodox medical circles, in 1843, Elliotson set up his new quarterly journal, the *Zoist: A Journal of Cerebral Physiology and Mesmerism* and founded his second hospital, the London Mesmeric Infirmary in 1849. Mesmeric institutions followed in Bristol, Edinburgh and Dublin. The *Zoist* motto on the title page was taken from the writings of the German phrenologist Franz Gall and set the provocative tone, 'This is Truth, though opposed to the Philosophy of Ages'. The journal was a strange home for writing on mesmerism and phrenology as well as quite radical political views on education and the treatment of prisoners and children. In the bold prospectus of the first journal, the editors, Elliotson and the phrenologist and Edinburgh physician, William Collins Engledue, aimed to publish equally on mesmerism and phrenology. They ambitiously stated their breadth of vision and their search for 'Truth' unimpeded by outside interests. They also highlighted the significance of mesmerism in both physical treatment and the understanding of the workings of the nervous system but cannot resist the reference to the doubters and naysayers:

[40] William Thackeray, *The History of Pendennis* (London: Penguin Books, 1986).

[41] Harriet Martineau, *Life in the Sickroom: Essays by an Invalid*, 2nd ed. (London: Edward Moxon, 1845) (p. 82).

> The new science of Mesmerism is a new physiological truth of incalculable value and importance; and, though sneered at by the pseudo-philosophers of the day, there is not the less certainty that it presents the only avenue through which is discernible a ray of hope that the more intricate phenomena of the nervous system,—of Life,—will ever be revealed to man. Already has it established its claim to be considered a most potent remedy in the cure of disease.[42]

Within later editions, Elliotson was surprisingly churlish about the mesmeric craze that he had instigated. He was critical of the 'Lecture mania' that was widespread across the country and derided the lack of education of the lecturers. While he understood the democratic and progressive potential of mesmerism and was an advocate of healthcare reform, he also believed that mesmerism was best left to those with a natural science background characterised by a scientific 'inductive approach' and 'a calm, persevering nature', in other words, physicians.[43] Nonetheless, by encompassing high and low culture, the travelling lecturers and Elliotson, together ensured that by the mid-century mesmerism had become an abiding preoccupation of Victorian Britain.[44]

The Historiography of Elliotson

Frank Podmore of the SPR wrote in his 1909 history of mesmerism and hypnotism that in Britsin after Elliotson, mesmerism was increasingly interlinked with Spiritualism. He describes how the mesmeric operators transformed into spiritual healers, and their subjects became trance mediums. 'The spiritualist platforms were thronged with magnetic clairvoyants who had developed into "inspirational speakers".' The two movements were conflated in the minds of the public and shared in a 'common condemnation.' As a result, he finishes his chapter on 'Mesmerism in Britain' with his view that 'No physician who valued his professional reputation could afford to meddle with the subject.[45]

[42] John Elliotson and William Engledue, 'Prospectus', *Zoist*, 1 (1844) (p. 2).

[43] John Elliotson, 'Lecture Mania', *Zoist*, 1 (1844) (p. 99).

[44] Winter, 'Introduction: Welcome to the *Séance*' in *Mesmerized* (pp. 1–14).

[45] Frank Podmore, *Mesmerism and Christian Science* (Philadelphia: George Jacobs, 1909) (p. 150).

For the New Hypnotists, it was important that Elliotson's reputation be restored for hypnotism to have any credibility as a new therapy. In part, this was because even forty years later, his disgrace was still widely remembered, particularly among the doctors. There was sufficient interest in the story that the doctor and journalist, James Fernandez Clarke had published his account of his own involvement in the affair as recently as 1874. However, the rehabilitation of Elliotson's good name was also as part of a grander and more daring project to advance a new narrative of the British discovery and development of hypnotism.

In the fifth edition of *Psycho-Therapeutics*, Tuckey praised Elliotson as 'a physician of rare ability' and 'a man of unimpeachable probity' but criticised him for his lack of discretion and described his experimental work on mesmerism as 'superincumbent rubbish.'[46] Bramwell, on the other hand, devoted full 17 pages to Elliotson in his 37-page chapter on the entire history of hypnotism. He also allocated eight pages to the mesmeric surgeon James Esdaile and nine to James Braid.[47] In total, he devoted 34 pages or over 90% to the story of the British hypnotists.

Bramwell portrays Elliotson as a liberal and social radical, a brilliant and visionary physician who was misunderstood and unfairly maligned by his critics, peers and friends. He makes it clear that Elliotson did not consider mesmerism as 'universally applicable' to all illnesses and continued to use other conventional treatments where appropriate. He saw it as particularly useful for hysteria and other functional nervous disorders where little else made a difference. Bramwell suggests that although gullible in some ways, Elliotson was no friend of spiritualism or séances, the craze that followed mesmerism and swept the world from its humble US origins with the Fox sisters. He makes allowances for some of his views by normalising them: he did 'share the mesmeric errors of the day' believing in clairvoyancy and phrenology.[48] Bramwell suggests that over the publishing life of the *Zoist* (1834–1856), which Elliotson had edited throughout, the beliefs in clairvoyancy and phrenology were losing ground.

In his *Hypnotism, or Psycho-Therapeutics*, which was published in 1890, Robert Felkin suggested that British scientists had been slow to pick up

[46] Charles Lloyd Tuckey, *Psycho-Therapeutics: or Treatment by Hypnotism and Suggestion*, 5th ed. (London: Baillière, Tindall and Cox, 1907) (p. 128).

[47] Bramwell, 'Historical', Ch 2 in *Hypnotism* (pp. 3–39).

[48] Bramwell, *Hypnotism* (p. 10).

on hypnotism and were in danger of being left behind by their continental cousins. He attributed this to the 'unfortunate impostures which were practiced between the years of 1840 and 1850.'[49] In his overview, he separates Elliotson's name from these 'impostures' (deceptions) and places him in a clear British genealogy of hypnotic discovery. The next two physicians in this British lineage of hypnotism were James Esdaile (1808–1859), a regular contributor to the *Zoist* and superintendent of the Mesmeric Hospital in Calcutta and then London, who originally used mesmerism to undertake painless surgery as an army doctor in India and James Braid (1795–1860), the originator of the term hypnotism.

George Kingsbury started his book, *The Practice of Hypnotic Suggestion* with a chapter on the history of hypnotism.[50] Like the other New Hypnotists, he created a founding myth, suggesting an ancient lineage: 'Hypnotism is no new thing, but has in some form or other been known since the earliest times; it was practised by the Egyptians, Persians, Greeks and Indians, and employed by priests, mystics, soothsayers, fakirs, and charlatans.'[51] To do this, he conflates hypnotism, mesmerism and other ways of inducing the trance state. He covers Elliotson's achievements and the role of the *Lancet* in destroying him. Kingsbury's account separated Elliotson's other work from the Okey scandal itself. He also clarified that modern hypnotists did not use *clairvoyantes* or mesmerised assistants to diagnose.

Kingsbury observed the way that hypnotism or mesmerism was frequently denounced by the medical institution along with other fringe treatments. It was often cited in a list of other apparently fraudulent alternative therapies like balneopathy (a therapeutic regime based on copious water ingestion, bathing and steam rooms). Given Kingsbury's own positive experience of balneopathy in Blackpool, he notes how it 'has now made good its claims to be considered, and that in all modern works on therapeutics, it ranks as a legitimate and useful agent.'[52] This highly personal aside emphasises the partial and subjective facets of this history.

[49] Robert Felkin, *Hypnotism or Psycho-Therapeutics* (Edinburgh: Y. J. Pentland, 1890) (p. 3).

[50] George Kingsbury, 'Introduction', Ch 1 in *The Practice of Hypnotic Suggestion, Being and Elementary Handbook for the Use of the Medical Profession* (Bristol: John Wright, 1891) (pp. 1–16).

[51] Kingsbury, *Hypnotic Suggestion* (p. 1).

[52] Kingsbury, *Hypnotic Suggestion* (p. 7).

Kingsbury made a flattering comparison between Elliotson and the illustrious William Harvey, the English physician who first demonstrated the circulation of blood. There were several similarities: the magnitude of their discoveries, the obsession with scientific truth which drove them both, the initial rejection of their evidence by their peers and the destruction of both their reputation and their means of making a living by the medical institutions. Elliotson was not shy of making the same lofty parallel, when he received the honour of giving the Harveian oration (established by William Harvey) to the Royal College of Physicians in 1846.[53] Kingsbury clearly admired Elliotson and showed how he chose to lecture on and advocate for mesmerism, despite intense pressure to focus on his more mainstream interests and achievements. There was almost universal condemnation of his speech in the contemporary medical journals. It reignited a level of hostility that Elliotson had not experienced since the *Lancet's* exposure of the Okeys. The medical journals accused him of treating science 'like a harlot' and darkly hinted about his sexual passions 'burning strongly either in secret or notoriously'.[54] Once more mesmerism was linked to sex and impropriety.

Kingsbury admitted that Elliotson had his faults but lamented the low quality of the professional dispute: 'To us who look back to the warfare against Elliotson, it may seem that the fighting was not fair. I cannot say whether Elliotson laid his case wisely before the profession of his time, but it does appear to me that personal abuse and indecent insinuation are poor forms of argument.' Perhaps rather optimistically he added 'Let us hope that in these days scientific observation and critical examination will replace vituperation.'[55] This was to be a baseless hope as the story of the battle between the New Hypnotists and Ernest Hart reveals.

[53] At the time of his speech, Elliotson was unaware of the final poignant likeness with William Harvey: that his private practice would fall away and that he would eventually die in poverty. He expired at the home of one of his few loyal friends, Edmond Symes. John Elliotson, *The Harveian Oration* (London: H. Baillière, 1846).

[54] Kingsbury, *Hypnotic Suggestion* (p. 6).

[55] Kingsbury, *Hypnotic Suggestion* (p. 8).

The Neglect and Recovery of James Braid (1795–1860) (Fig. 5.3)

The final character in the highly partial British history of hypnotism was James Braid. For the late Victorian hypnotists, he was a critical figure for several reasons. James Braid had attempted to separate the therapeutic benefits of the trance state from the mystical frills of mesmerism. Following the Scottish 'Common Sense' school of philosophy, he had rejected Mesmer's ideas of a mysterious fluid and Puységur's vague concept of an influence passing from the operator to the subject. He had

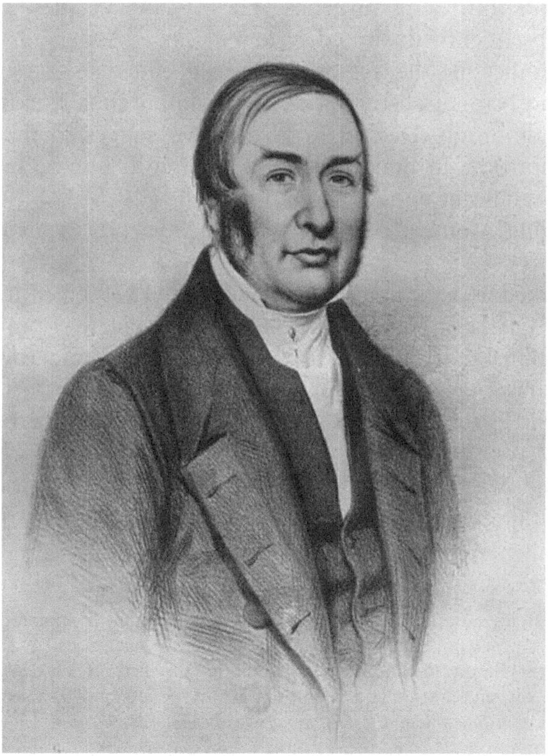

Fig. 5.3 Photograph of *Portrait of James Braid*. Before 1860, artist unknown. From an engraved portrait in the possession of the Manchester Medical School

introduced a new set of technical terms for the procedure to linguistically distance his scientific 'hypnotism' from esoteric mesmerism.[56] He also had written the book that originally introduced the French country practitioner Liébeault to the technique and could be reasonably credited with the responsibility of inspiring the therapeutic advances of the Nancy school. In fact, for many years, hypnotism was known in France as 'Braidism.' His work was known to the SPR before Tuckey's visit to Liébeault, appearing in William Preyer's German language text *History of Hypnotism* (1881).[57]

James Braid was a Scottish surgeon from Fife, who trained at Edinburgh medical school between 1812 and 1814 while apprenticed to the father and son, Leith surgeons, Thomas and Charles Anderson to whom he subsequently dedicated *Neurypnology*.[58] Anderson senior was a founding member and the vice-president of an elite scientific society called the Wernerian Natural History Society of Edinburgh, a rival to the Royal Society of Edinburgh. Donald Robertson has suggested that Anderson might have introduced Braid to the society and its library. Braid felt the connection significant enough to sign himself as 'C.M.W.S.' or 'M.W.S.' (Corresponding Member of the Wernerian Society), in his articles and books.[59]

Braid worked as a surgeon in Scotland until 1828 when he moved to Manchester. On 13th November 1841, Braid went to a public demonstration of animal magnetism and phrenology in his hometown that was to change the course of his career. The stage show was the popular form of public lecture or entertainment previously described. They were widespread across Europe at the time and known as a *séance* or *conversazione*. Braid was initially highly sceptical of the *séance* conducted through an interpreter by a Swiss demonstrator of mesmeric phenomena

[56] Although Braid was the first to use the terms hypnotism, hypnotize and hypnotist in English, the equivalent terms *hypnotique*, *hypnotisme*, *hypnotiste* had been used by the French mesmerist Baron Etienne Félix d'Henin de Cuvillers (1755–1841) at least as early as 1820. Melvin Gravitz and Manuel Gerton, 'Freud and Hypnosis: Report of Post-rejection Use', *Journal of the History of the Behavioral Sciences*, 17 (1984) 68–74 (p. 109).

[57] William Preyer, *Die Entdeckung des Hypnotismus* (Berlin: Gebruder Paetel, 1881).

[58] Braid, *Neurypnology*.

[59] James Braid, *The Discovery of Hypnosis: The Complete Writings of James Braid, the Father of Hypnotherapy*, ed. by Donald Robertson (Raleigh: Lulu.com, 2013) (pp. 19–21).

called Charles Lafontaine. However, he was intrigued enough to attend a repeat performance, six days later. He witnessed one of the mesmerised subjects insensible to pain and another unable to open their eyes and convinced himself that it was genuine if subjective phenomenon. He experimented on friends and family and his interest grew. He viewed it as his responsibility as a practising doctor to communicate his findings and started to lecture by the end of the year. He persisted throughout 1842 despite the antipathy towards mesmerism and published his first pamphlet on the subject, *Satanic Agency and Mesmerism* in response to a hostile sermon from a Liverpool preacher.[60] He was quite robust in his response to opposing views but never rude. When the Medical section of the BMA refused his offer to speak, instead he gave a *conversazione* outside the meeting to many members of the Association, in which he read his paper and showed cases (Fig. 5.4).

The following year, Braid published his influential *Neurypnology*.[61] This was a key work for late Victorian hypnotists for its new terminology, its technique and its theory. Braid proposed that the 'nervous sleep' of the title, which was induced by mesmerism or in his new nomenclature, 'hypnotism', was different from normal sleep. He described the most effective way of inducing the trance state as fixing the eyes on a small bright object held above eye level at a position which just caused strain to the eye muscles: 'the mind riveted to the one idea of the object held above the eyes.'[62] He went on to describe the movement of the operator's fore and middle fingers of the right hand from behind the bright object towards the subject's eyes: 'most probably the eyelids will close involuntarily, with a vibratory motion.'[63] Following this procedure, the subject is likely to be hypnotised, the likelihood increasing with the frequency of previous hypnotic inductions. Braid summarised the main tenets thus:

[60] James Braid, 'Satanic Agency and Mesmerism Reviewed, In A Letter To The Reverend H. Mc. Neile, A.M., of Liverpool', in *Reply to a Sermon Preached by Him in St. Jude's Church, Liverpool, on Sunday, 10 April 1842* (Manchester: Simms and Dinham; Galt and Anderson, 1842).

[61] Braid, *Neurypnology*.

[62] Braid, *Neurypnology* (p. 110).

[63] Braid, *Neurypnology* (p. 109).

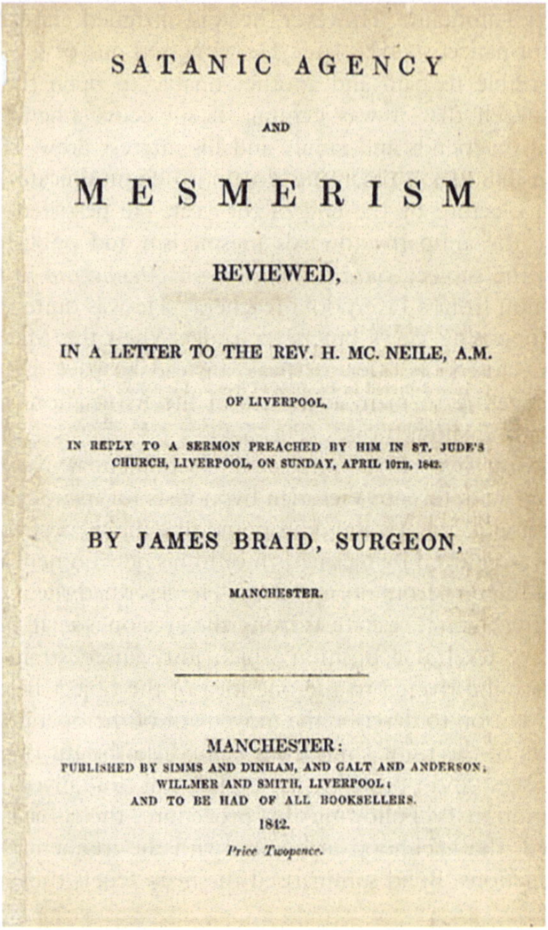

SATANIC AGENCY

AND

MESMERISM

REVIEWED,

IN A LETTER TO THE REV. H. MC. NEILE, A.M.

OF LIVERPOOL,

IN REPLY TO A SERMON PREACHED BY HIM IN ST. JUDE'S CHURCH, LIVERPOOL, ON SUNDAY, APRIL 10TH, 1842.

BY JAMES BRAID, SURGEON,

MANCHESTER.

MANCHESTER:
PUBLISHED BY SIMMS AND DINHAM, AND GALT AND ANDERSON;
WILLMER AND SMITH, LIVERPOOL;
AND TO BE HAD OF ALL BOOKSELLERS.
1842.
Price Twopence.

Fig. 5.4 James Braid. Satanic agency and mesmerism reviewed (Manchester: Simms and Dinham 1842). Title page

the phenomena of mesmerism [are] accounted for on the principle of the derangement of the state of the cerebral spinal centres, and of the circulatory, respiratory, and muscular systems, induced by a fixed stare, absolute repose of body, fixed attention and suppressed respiration, concomitant with that fixity of attention. That the whole depended on the physical and psychical condition of the patient arising from the causes referred to, and *not at all* [my emphasis] on the volition or passes of the operator, throwing out magnetic fluid, or exciting to activity some mystical, universal fluid or medium.[64]

Braid's new technique was very different from the 'passes' or stroking of the mesmerists and faith healers. While it did require some proximity between hypnotist and hypnotised, the movements were focussed on the head and were therefore less erotically charged than the gestures over the affected parts of the body, usually the abdomen and pelvis. Ever the pragmatic surgeon, Braid rejected the involvement of any mystical mesmeric fluid, on the basis that anyone could hypnotise themselves simply by following his instructions. He proposed that hypnotism was merely a physiological condition that was brought on by the strain on the attention, the overexercise of the eye muscles and the suppression of breathing. He claimed that the hypnotised voluntarily gave up their agency and autonomy creating the trance through attention and imagination. The focus of the attention was irrelevant, once the attention was fixed, the will was suspended. The physical and mental state of the subject were considered critical, the behaviour and willpower of the hypnotist irrelevant. Early in his hypnotic career, Braid made no comments to the patient. He considered that the trance itself was therapeutic.

The most far-reaching aspect of Braid's work was his introduction of a new medical lexicon. He was aware of the importance of new technical vocabulary for the technique. He explained that Greek was traditionally used for doctrinal words but accepted the need for shortening his neologism, *Neurypnology* for common parlance: 'Neurypnology is derived from the Greek words νεύρον, nerve; υπνος, sleep; λογος, a discourse; and means the rationale, or doctrine of nervous sleep, which I define to be, "a peculiar condition of the nervous system, into which it can be thrown by artificial contrivance" or thus, "a peculiar condition of the nervous system, induced by a fixed and abstracted attention of the mental and visual eye, on one object, not of an exciting nature."'.[65]

He went on to introduce the terms *hypnotise* meaning to induce nervous sleep; *hypnotism* for the state of nervous sleep; *hypnotist* for one who practises neuro-hypnotism and *hypnotised* for one who has been put into a state of nervous sleep. It should be stressed that in the 1840s

[64] John Milne Bramwell, 'James Braid', *Brain*, 19 (1896) 90–116 (p. 91).

[65] Braid, *Neurypnology* (p. 13).

hypnotism was but one of many mesmeric or trance-inducing practices. The names that Braid devised survive to this day though what they connote has changed significantly.

James Braid continued to offer surgery to his patients and use hypnosis where appropriate. Like Elliotson he was fascinated by the phenomenon and experimented with friends, servants and patients to learn its laws. As a practising doctor, he was highly critical of the 'unlearned' travelling mesmeric lecturers even when their theories were close to his own. He condemned the Mancunian lay performer Joseph Catlow, who developed a 'soporific machine' based on his similar ideas that a trance state could be induced by sensory repetition. By comparison, he was initially respectful of fellow doctors, especially John Elliotson, despite fundamentally disagreeing with his assumptions and core beliefs. Like Elliotson, he did believe in phrenology but it should be understood that this was a common belief system at the time. Like Elliotson, he struggled to get much of his work on hypnotism published in any reputable scientific journals apart from *The Medical Times,* an early rival to the *Lancet*. In his obituary, the *Lancet* emphasised Braid's surgical contributions and good results for club foot and squint rather than any mention of his considerable hypnotic work.[66]

The fact that he could not get his hypnotic experiments and clinical material published in *The Zoist* is surprising at first sight, but there appeared to develop some personal antagonism between the two of them. Elliotson described Braid's methods as 'coarse'.[67] Braid accused the 'chief of the mesmeric school' (presumably Elliotson) of hypocrisy in rejecting his work for publication and of being an 'illiberal, vindictive and persecuting mesmeric autocrat.'[68] It seems that Braid's materialist and mechanical ideas on the trance state put him somewhere between the mesmerists and the medical establishment but acceptable to neither.

Braid was never clear whether hypnotism was the same as mesmerism or a different entity. However, he was able to demonstrate that the trance state could be achieved without theatre and without previous experience of the anticipated effects through the simple method of fixing the gaze. He viewed hypnotism as a powerful therapeutic tool that should be

66 Anon. 'Obituary: James Braid', *Lancet* (31 March 1860) (p. 335).

67 Moore, *The Mesmerist* (p. 211).

68 Braid, *Discovery of Hypnosis* (p. 161).

utilised solely by the medical profession. Braid died suddenly and unexpectedly in March 1860. As a provincial surgeon with limited ability to publish in the national medical journals, his ideas had little impact in his lifetime. He left no intellectual heirs and with Elliotson's slow decline, medical interest in the trance state receded in Britain.

There is a strange postscript to Braid's story. According to Bramwell, three days before his death Braid had sent his manuscript entitled *On Hypnotism* to the French surgeon, Étienne Eugène Azam for delivery to the French Academy of Sciences.[69] Its existence was unknown in the UK at the time and there is no surviving copy. Bramwell later managed to secure a German copy from the German physician, William Preyer and publicised its importance. However, it was the French translation of this final work that was to inspire Liébeault, the Nancy school and all that followed.

The Historiography of James Braid

I have already stressed Braid's significance for the New Hypnotists. Tuckey includes a couple of references to Braid's technique but not his theory. However, his opinion of the man himself is made clear by this sentence in the 5th edition of *Psycho-Therapeutics*: 'One looks forward to a time, in a not very remote future, when Englishmen will take the leading position in the investigation and practice of hypnotism which one would expect from the compatriots of James Braid.'[70]

Kingsbury neatly summarises the position of the New Hypnotists: 'To James Braid, a Manchester Surgeon, the honour is now generally accorded of having rescued mesmerism from the region of quackery, and of endeavouring to secure it a recognised place in medicine.' He describes Braid's success in anaesthesia as well as curing various other conditions. Kingsbury comically demonstrates the hostility shown to hypnotism and mesmerism by the medical institutions of the time. He describes the rejection of Braid's paper on hypnotism for the 1842 BMA National meeting in Manchester but the inclusion of another paper on the recognition and discrimination between mature and immature spiders.[71]

[69] Bramwell, '*Hypnotism*' (1913) (p. 29).

[70] Tuckey, *Psycho-Therapeutics*, 5th ed. (1907) (p. 7).

[71] Kingsbury, *Hypnotic Suggestion* (p. 10).

Frank Podmore was not one of the New Hypnotists nor a medical doctor. However, he was a prolific writer on esoteric topics, who wrote an influential history on mesmerism and hypnotism. While he was a colleague of both Tuckey and Bramwell at the SPR, he did present a wider and more international history than the physicians. Nevertheless, in his chapter on British mesmerism, he continues with the mythologising about Braid speculating on what might have happened in Britain 'if, say, Elliotson on the one side and Wakley on the other had condescended to learn from Braid.'[72] In another passage, he describes the three kinds of medical attitude to hypnotism/mesmerism in the 1840s: 'that of contemptuous rejection, of implicit belief, and of discriminating acceptance, typified by the Lancet, by Elliotson, and by Braid respectively.'[73]

Perhaps because of his personal connection, Milne Bramwell was particularly fascinated by Braid's work and wrote prolifically about him. Partly through his friendship with Braid's son, he had collected all Braid's writings including his pamphlets and published a biography in *Brain* in 1896. In his later books, Bramwell decided that the Nancy school had merely repeated what Braid had previously discovered and credited Braid with the invention of suggestion rather than Bernheim.[74] Braid's only monograph on hypnotism was *Neurypnology; or, the Rationale of Nervous Sleep* written in 1843 but he never managed to write a second edition so his later books and pamphlets like Magic, Witchcraft, Animal Magnetism, Hypnotism and Electrobiology and The Physiology of Fascination were crucial to understanding his later thinking on hypnotism.[75] In a review of the collection of '800 works by nearly 500 authors', listed in Dessoir's exhaustive summary of published work on hypnotism, *Bibliographie des Modernen Hypnotismus*,[76] Milne Bramwell made the bold claim that he found 'little of value has been discovered which can justly be considered as supplementary to Braid's later work.'[77]

72 Podmore, *Mesmerism and Christian Science* (p. 153).

73 Podmore, *Mesmerism and Christian Science* (p. 143).

74 Bramwell, 'James Braid'.

75 Braid, *Neurypnology*; James Braid, *Magic, Witchcraft and Animal Magnetism, Hypnotism and Electro-Biology*, 3rd ed. (London: J. Churchill, 1853); James Braid, *The Physiology of Fascination and the Critics Criticized* (Manchester: Grant, 1855).

76 Max Dessoir, *Bibliographie des Modernen Hypnotismus* (Berlin: Carl Duncker, 1888).

77 John Milne Bramwell, 'On the Evolution of Hypnotic Theory', *Brain* (1896) 459–568 (p. 459).

In this chapter, I have considered the significance of historiography in the story of British hypnotism. I have focussed on the way that the New Hypnotists retold and reinterpreted trance healing practices and the lives of Elliotson and Braid to present a reassuring, scientific Anglocentric lineage. However, modern versions of the story of mesmerism and hypnosis can reveal just as much about the viewpoints and purposes of their authors. The social historian Alison Winter's academically dominant orthodox history of mid-century Victorian mesmerism provided an excellent cultural context to sympathetically understand Elliotson's life and work and his radical agenda. However, her concluding chapter describes the slow dissipation of mesmerism and the eclipse of medical mesmerism by chemical anaesthesia and Freudian psychotherapy which ignores the medical hypnotic revival of the century's end and New Hypnotist's important role in this.[78] This omission will be rectified in the following chapters.

Bibliography

Anon. 1833. 'Lancet Gallery of Medical Portraits: John Elliotson, M.D.', *Lancet* (8 June): 341–44.

Anon. 1838. 'Animal Magnetism', *Times* (6 September): 2.

Anon. 1838. 'Progress of Animal Magnetism', *Times* (15 September 1838): 3.

Anon. 1838. 'Chit-Chat', *The Satirist; or the Censor of the Times* (9 September): 285.

Anon. 1838. 'Animal Magnetism', *Medico-Chirurgical Review* (1 October): 636.

Anon. 1839. 'The Humbug called "Mesmerism"', *Times* (7 January): 6.

Anon. 1845. 'Pencillings of Eminent Men', *Medical Times* (1 February): 392.

Anon. 1860. 'Obituary: James Braid'. *Lancet* (31 March): 335.

Blumenbach, Johann. 1787. *Institutiones Physiologicae.* Gottingae: Jo. Christ. Dieterich.

Blumenbach, Johann. 1817. *The Institutes of Physiology,* 2nd ed., trans. by John Elliotson. London: Bensley.

Braid, James. Satanic Agency and Mesmerism Reviewed, In A Letter To The Reverend H. Mc. Neile, A.M., of Liverpool, in *Reply to a Sermon Preached by Him in St. Jude's Church, Liverpool, on Sunday, 10 April 1842.* Manchester: Simms and Dinham; Galt and Anderson.

Braid, James. 1843. *Neurypnology or the Rationale of Nervous Sleep.* London: J. Churchill.

[78] Winter, 'Conclusion: The Day after the Feast', in *Mesmerized* (pp. 345–54).

Braid, James. 1853. *Magic, Witchcraft and Animal Magnetism, Hypnotism and Electro-Biology*, 3rd ed. London: J. Churchill.

Braid, James. 1855. *The Physiology of Fascination and the Critics Criticized*. Manchester: Grant.

Braid, James. 2013. *The Discovery of Hypnosis: The Complete Writings of James Braid, the Father of Hypnotherapy*. ed. by Donald Robertson. Raleigh: Lulu.com.

Bramwell, John Milne. 1896. 'James Braid: Surgeon and Hypnotist', *Brain*, 19: 90–116.

Bramwell, John Milne. 1896. 'On the Evolution of Hypnotic Theory', *Brain*: 459–568.

Bramwell, John Milne. 1903. *Hypnotism: It's History, Practice and Theory*, 1st ed. London: Grant Richards. 37.

Brock, W. H. 1965. 'The Life and Work of William Prout', *Medical History*, 9: 101–26.

Bulwer-Lytton, Edward. 1842. *Zanoni*. London: Saunders and Otley.

Bulwer-Lytton, Edward. 1861–1862. *A Strange Story*. Leipzig: Tauchnitz.

Bulwer-Lytton, Edward. 1871. *The Coming Race*. London: William Blackwood and Sons.

Clarke, James Fernandez. 1874. *Autobiographical Recollections of the Medical Profession*. London: J. and A. Churchill.

Colquhoun, John Campbell. 1833. *Report of the Experiments on Animal Magnetism Made By a Committee of the Medical Section of the French Royal Academy of Sciences*. Edinburgh: Robert Cadell.

Darnton, Robert. 1970. 'Mesmerism and Popular Science', in *Mesmerism and the End of the Enlightenment in France*. New York: Schocken Books. 2–45.

Dessoir, Max. 1888. *Bibliographie des Modernen Hypnotismus*. Berlin: Carl Duncker.

Dickson, Melissa. 2019. 'Hats, Cloaks, and Stethoscopes: The Symbolic Fashions of the Nineteenth-Century Medical Practitioner'. *Fashion and Material Culture in Victorian Fiction and Periodicals*, ed. by Nickianne Moody and Janine Hatter. Brighton: Edward Everett Root. 105–20.

'Elliotson, John' in *Dictionary of National Biography*, Vol 17 (1885–1900). ed. by Robert Hunt. London: Smith and Elder.

Elliotson, John. 1829. 'Addendum', *London Medical and Physical Journal*, 62: 315–24.

Elliotson, John. 1838. 'John Elliotson's Letter', *London Medical Gazette* (23 March): 951.

Elliotson, John. 1840. *Human Physiology*, 5th ed. London: Longman, Orme, Brown, Green and Longmans.

Elliotson, John. 1844. 'Lecture Mania', *Zoist*, 1: 99.

Elliotson, John and Engledue, William. 1844. 'Prospectus', *Zoist*, 1: 2.

Elliotson, John. 1846. *The Harveian Oration*. London: H. Baillière.
Felkin, Robert. 1890. *Hypnotism or Psycho-Therapeutics*. Edinburgh: Y. J. Pentland.
Gauld, Alan. 1992. *A History of Hypnotism*. Cambridge: Cambridge University Press.
Gravitz, Melvin and Gerton, Manuel. 1984. 'Freud and Hypnosis: Report of Post-rejection Use', *Journal of the History of the Behavioral Sciences*, 17: 68–74.
Hawthorne, Nathaniel. 1850. *The Scarlet Letter*. Boston: Ticknor, Reed and Fields.
Hawthorne, Nathaniel. 1851. *The House of the Seven Gables*. Boston: Ticknor, Reed and Fields.
Hughes, William. 2015. *That Devil's Trick: Hypnotism and the Victorian Popular Imagination*. Manchester: Manchester University Press.
Kaplan, Fred. 1975. *Dickens and Mesmerism: The Hidden Springs of Fiction*. Princeton: Princeton University Press.
Kingsbury, George. 1891. *The Practice of Hypnotic Suggestion, Being and Elementary Handbook for the Use of the Medical Profession*. Bristol: John Wright.
Martineau, Harriet. 1845. *Life in the Sickroom: Essays by an Invalid*, 2nd ed. London: Edward Moxon.
Mayo, Herbert. 1838. '"Animal Magnetism"; or, "Mesmerism"', *Lancet* (1 September): 805–14.
Moore, Wendy. 2017. *The Mesmerist, the Society Doctor who held Victorian London Spellbound*. London: Weidenfield and Nicholson.
Nadis, Fred. 2005. *Wonder Shows: Performing Science, Magic, and Religion in America*. New Brunswick: Rutgers University Press. 108.
Preyer, William. 1881. *Die Entdeckung des Hypnotismus*. Berlin: Gebruder Paetel.
Podmore, Frank. 1909. *Mesmerism and Christian Science: A Short History of Mental Healing*. Philadelphia, George Jacobs.
Porter, Roy and Micale, Mark. 1994. 'Introduction: Reflections on Psychiatry and Its Histories', in *History of Psychiatry*. eds. by Mark Micale and Roy Porter. Oxford, Oxford University Press. 3–26.
Thackeray, William. 1986. *The History of Pendennis*. London, Penguin Books.
Tuckey, Charles Lloyd. 1907. *Psycho-Therapeutics: or Treatment by Hypnotism and Suggestion*, 5th ed. London: Baillière, Tindall and Cox. 128.
Wakley, Thomas. 1829. 'The Medical and Physical Journal', *Lancet* (13 June): 341–5.
Wakley, Thomas. 1830. 'Editorial', *Lancet* (17 April): 86.
Wakley, Thomas. 1838. 'University College Hospital: Animal Magnetism', *Lancet* (26 May): 282–7.
Wakley, Thomas. 1838. 'Editorial', *Lancet* (15 September): 873–7.

Wakley, Thomas. 1838. 'The Virtues of Animal Magnetism', *Lancet* (8 December): 413.
Wakley, Thomas. 1839. 'University College and Hospital', *Lancet* (5 January): 561–2.
Waterfield, Robin. 2004. *Hidden Depths: The Story of Hypnosis.* London: Pan.
Winter, Alison. 1998. *Mesmerized: Powers of Mind in Victorian Britain.* Chicago and London: University of Chicago Press. 131.

CHAPTER 6

The Medical Contest for Hypnotism in the 1890s

The battle for hypnotism took place over the 1890s between the New Hypnotists and their professional colleagues for credibility and with the general public for acceptability. This chapter focuses on the medical battle. The improved scientific credibility of therapeutic hypnotism came in part from the development of the new explanatory model for hypnotism. The tipping point came as the theoretical mode of action shifted from imagination to suggestion. While the doctrine of imagination had lost favour in the rest of medicine over the latter half of the nineteenth century, the transition to suggestion, as a model for hypnotism, occurred gradually over the course of the late 1880s and 1890s. The new British lineage and history of hypnotism combined with the books and scientific articles of the New Hypnotists helped to change medical as well as public opinion which were separate but overlapping spheres. Although the prevailing opinion of any group is notoriously hard to evaluate there were several events and developments that demonstrate that among the medical profession opinion was changing fast in the 1890s.

The first event was the creation of a committee by the British Medical Association to examine the therapeutic potential of hypnotism, which is covered in the first part of this chapter. There was an inevitable reactionary response to hypnotism from the medical establishment who shelved the positive report. The subject of the second section is the conflict in print

G. D. L. Bates, *The Uncanny Rise of Medical Hypnotism, 1888–1914*, Mental Health in Historical Perspective,
https://doi.org/10.1007/978-3-031-42725-1_6

between the New Hypnotists and the medical institutions personified by the *BMJ* editor Ernest Hart. Another aspect of the medical response was the result of the emerging internationalism of medicine at this time. The growing connections through journals, conferences and reliable correspondence between the physicians of Britain, Europe and America meant that there was international support for the British physicians trying to use hypnotism and suggestion in their clinical practice. This wider international interest also meant that it was harder for orthodox British medicine to ignore medical hypnotism.

Hypnotism and the BMA Committee of Inquiry

The idea of a struggle between the New Hypnotists and the establishment is not just my modern framing. In July of 1890 Charles Lloyd Tuckey wrote to his Dutch friend and colleague van Eeden asking for help with evidence for a debate: 'There is to be a great battle about hypnotism at the meeting of the British Medical Association next week at Birmingham and I am appointed to answer Dr Norman Kerr's contention that the practice should be forbidden.'[1] Tuckey revealed in his letter that he had contacted all of his European hypnotism colleagues. The establishment figure Norman Kerr was a friend of Ernest Hart and was known for his previous work with the British Temperance movement and his conviction that alcoholism or 'narcomania' was an illness.

The relatively newly founded Section of Psychology was convening as a part of the programme for the 58th BMA annual national conference. The Section of Psychology of the BMA had been established in 1870. At this time the BMA included more than 13,000 members or two thirds of all medical practitioners and the regular meetings helped to establish shared professional values as much as provide education about new medical innovations and discoveries.[2]

Psychology and the care of the mentally ill were not considered to be a prestigious or well-regarded branch of medicine but the *Times*, reporting

[1] Charles Lloyd Tuckey, letter to Frederik van Eeden, 14 July, 1890. In *Frederik Van Eeden Collection* (Amsterdam: Allard Pierson, University of Amsterdam).

[2] Anon, 'British Medical Association', *Times* (30 July 1890) (p. 9).

daily on the entire congress, unusually suggested that public interest 'centred chiefly on the psychological division' that year.[3] Before the debate format, Tuckey and Kingsbury both made presentations about the practice of hypnotism and then gave demonstrations of the technique on two medical subjects in front of an audience of 200 medical men.

One volunteer was well known to dislike public speaking but was told under hypnosis that he was the parliamentary candidate for Birmingham and the audience wanted to hear his address. He was then able to speak freely and clearly. The other subject was made to adopt a sitting posture without any support to his body, and he remained in that 'most uncomfortable attitude' for several minutes.[4] He was also made to imagine great pain in his thumb, paralysis of the left leg and an inability to move his arm. The medical reporter for the *BMJ* recorded that:

> The manner in which these demonstrations were carried out seemed to produce a strong impression on the minds of many of the speakers in the discussion that followed, who, admitting the spirit of scepticism with which they had come to the meeting, stated that they would leave it impressed with the necessity of having the subject thoroughly investigated.[5]

The resemblance to any Victorian mesmeric 'lecture' of the previous fifty years is unmistakeable but without irony, the conclusion of the assembly was that public performances should be banned and hypnotism should be restricted to medical practitioners. The discussion that followed appears to have been quite heated in that the following day George Kingsbury was commended for his equanimity in the face of 'the heckling and harsh cross-examination of members.'[6]

Norman Kerr, one of the most vocal critics had given the opening address of the debate and provided the standard criticisms of the day of hypnotism: that it weakened the will and reduced energy levels and its production of automatic obedience was too dangerous. Like Charcot, he also suggested that a susceptibility to hypnotism represented a neurosis of itself. But he had perhaps misjudged his audience with his reported

[3] Anon, 'British Medical Association', *Times* (2 August 1890) (p. 10).

[4] Anon, 'British Medical Association', *Times* (1 August 1890) (p. 13).

[5] Anon, 'Hypnotism as a Therapeutic Agent', *British Medical Journal* (23 August 1890) (p. 465).

[6] Anon, 'BMA' (2 August) (p. 10).

polemic: 'Each seance might bring the hypnotee [sic] more under the control of the hypnotist, ending often in the complete submission of the former to the will of the latter. A jellyfish slavery, without mental or moral backbone, was infinitely worse than days of pain and nights of agony.'[7] Kerr was either unable or did not try to provide any evidence for his claims and Kingsbury asked him whether he really meant that he preferred to 'have a man remain a drunkard than be cured by hypnotism.' Kingsbury went on to suggest that 'Such a statement was not only injurious, but positively wicked.'[8] This led to vocal support from the floor.

The end result of the meeting was unanimous agreement that the section should 'not allow the matter to rest' and that a committee should be appointed to 'investigate the subject, and to endeavour to ascertain the true phenomena of hypnotism and the value of its use in the treatment of disease.'[9] The ten man committee and secretary included an academic, several asylum superintendents, general practitioners and both Hack Tuke and George Kingsbury.

The cautious, reactionary medical profession was starting to take hypnotism seriously. This represented a major advance for the technique and easily surpassed the institutional medical reception that Elliotson had achieved in his lifetime. This was also very different from the response to the lecture of Salpêtrière physician Auguste Voisin only the previous year to the same group. He had given a paper to the Psychology Section on 'The Treatment of Mental Disease by Hypnotic Suggestion' and was met with incredulity.[10] Though for accuracy, it should be noted that Voisin had claimed the efficacy of hypnotism for an impossibly wide range of conditions from idiocy to mania and masturbation.

The establishment of a Committee of Inquiry to investigate hypnotism and provide a consensus statement was subsequently approved by the main board of the BMA. The group first met in December 1890.[11] Their first act was to vote the asylum superintendent Frederick Needham,

[7] Norman Kerr qtd. In Anon, 'BMA', *Times* (3 August 1890) (p. 13).

[8] Anon, 'BMA' (2 August) (p. 10).

[9] Anon, 'A Discussion on Hypnotism in Therapeutics', *British Medical Journal* (23 August 1890) 442–9 (p. 446).

[10] Anon, 'The Section of Psychology', *British Medical Journal* (21 September 1889) 646–51 (p. 649).

[11] Anon, 'The Committee on Hypnotism', *British Medical Journal* (13 December 1890) (p. 1389).

the president of the Section of Psychology, as their chair. They then drew up specific areas for their investigation: the nature of hypnotism and its nervous and mental relations; its general or limited applicability as a therapeutic agent in different classes of disease; the degree and mode of its influence on morbid conditions; and its dangers and the necessary safeguards. As a result of his experience and his talent for hypnotic induction, Kingsbury agreed to the onerous task of visiting the various committee members at their hospitals and asylums to assist them with their experiments.

In 1891, the committee reported to the BMA council at their annual congress that they had not completed their investigation. The following year in Nottingham, they presented their first report declaring that they had satisfied themselves of the genuineness of the hypnotic state but rejected animal magnetism as a credible theory. They had found that hypnotism was frequently effective in 'relieving pain, procuring sleep and alleviating many functional ailments' while the evidence in the treatment of alcohol dependency (drunkenness in the language of the day) was 'encouraging but not conclusive.'[12] They made a number of recommendations that later Kingsbury would claim to have instigated but which can be traced back to Tuckey's initial article 'Faith Healing' and *Psycho-Therapeutics*. These included the restriction of therapeutic hypnotism to medical practitioners, the presence of same-sex chaperones for women during treatment and a call for a ban on public exhibitions of hypnotic phenomena.

The BMA council elected to refer it back for 'further examination and report.' Essentially, this meant that the leaders of the BMA did not like the conclusions of the report and wanted changes. The committee duly obliged and resubmitted the document the following year at the AGM in Newcastle, adding further documentary evidence in the form of extensive appendices. However, the main summary of the report was left unaltered which presented a serious problem to the BMA leadership. By 1893, as a result of the efforts of Ernest Hart and other cultural developments, the societal backdrop had changed and hypnotism was not a trivial medical matter. As I will describe it had developed a significant public profile

[12] Frederick Needham and Thomas Outterson Wood, 'Report of the Committee Appointed to Investigate the Nature of the Phenomena of Hypnotism; Its Value as a Therapeutic Agent; and the Propriety of Using It', *British Medical Journal* (23 July 1892) 190–1 (p. 190).

and fictional representations of hypnotism merged with those of fictional mesmerism, generating significant anxiety among the general public.

Despite being viewed by some members within the hypnotism committee and the hypnotism lobby as 'too cautious and not sufficiently dogmatic,' the final report from the upstart Section of Psychology was seen by the BMA council as potentially damaging to public relations and medical reputations.[13] One of the council members, the surgeon and editor of the *Medical Times*, George Brown was especially hostile, asking:

> What was hypnotism? Could it be weighed in the balance? Was it a thing that could be administered in disease in a liquid, solid, or any other form? The whole thing was imaginary from beginning to end. They must know as professors of physical science that mental influence could not cure disease. It might cure imaginary disease, and doubtless did so. They knew the action of fear and many other things, but it was another thing to pledge the Association to hypnotism as a thing to cure disease.[14]

These comments clearly demonstrate the highly materialist nature of orthodox medical thinking and the fact that the origins of 'diseases of the imagination' had been forgotten, becoming instead imaginary or 'made up' diseases. Additionally, other factors were at play. As the cultural historian Mary Leighton has argued: 'the figure of the hypnotist *was* fraught with popular culture connotations that rendered it a risky position for medical men to assume in the mid-1890s.'[15] The treatment might have been effective but what did it look like for a professional, scientific doctor to adopt the instrument of spiritualists, magicians and fraudsters?

The BMA council took the decision to shelve the report. George Kingsbury summarised the affair, somewhat bitterly, five years later: 'The Committee, consisting of eleven eminent physicians and myself,' officially appointed by the association, investigated the subject of hypnotism as a therapeutic agency and reported favourably. The Association's leadership, represented at Newcastle in 1893 by a 'handful of gentlemen not having

[13] Anon, 'BMA Annual Meeting', *British Medical Journal* (5 August 1893) 321–9 (p. 324).

[14] Anon, 'BMA Annual Meeting' (1893) (p. 324).

[15] Mary Leighton, '"Hypnosis Redivivus": Ernest Hart, "The British Medical Journal" and the Hypnotism Controversy"', *Victorian Periodicals Review*, 34 (2001) 104–27 (p. 105).

investigated the subject,' felt that it was wiser for them to 'receive' the Committee's report with thanks rather than to formally 'adopt' it.[16]

Notwithstanding the above, Tuckey and John Milne Bramwell both mentioned the importance of the committee's investigation and their report in their subsequent books. Tuckey included the committee's entire findings in the appendix of several subsequent editions of *Psycho-Therapeutics* and portrayed the development in positive terms within the main text:

> The most important recent event connected with the progress of hypnotism in this country was the appointment of a commission by the British Medical Association as a result of the important discussion at the annual meeting held at Birmingham in 1890. [...] It is hoped that the result will be increased interest in the subject by medical men and the prohibition of its use by showmen and idlers.[17]

The council's policy of accepting but ignoring the report could be seen as short term and politically motivated. The issue of the legitimacy of therapeutic hypnotism would not go away and eventually the BMA passed a formal resolution approving it and recommending its instruction to medical students. However, this would not to be until 1955.[18] From a historical standpoint, the BMA's 1893 decision certainly did not represent either the British medical profession's wholesale rejection or acceptance of the technique in the 1890s as it has been sometimes portrayed.

Medical Internationalism and the Growth of Medical Hypnotism

In the medical battle for legitimacy, one of the advantages for the New Hypnotists which John Elliotson did not share, was the improvement in international communication and networks. The medical historian

[16] The original committee was of 11 men but as a result of the death of Dr. Ross led to his replacement by Mr. Langley, a Cambridge physiology lecturer, meaning that Kingsbury had 11 colleagues on the committee; George Kingsbury, 'Correspondence: The BMA and Hypnotism', *BMJ* (26 February 1898) (pp. 591–2).

[17] Charles Lloyd Tuckey, *Psycho-Therapeutics: or Treatment by Hypnotism and Suggestion*, 4th ed. (London: Baillière, Tindall and Cox, 1900) (pp. 6–7).

[18] British Medical Association, Psychological Medicine Group Sub-committee, 'The Medical Use of Hypnotism', *Supplement* to the *BMJ* (23 April 1955) (pp. 190–3).

William Bynum has identified the idea of a late nineteenth-century 'international medical community'.[19] Previously quite isolated and insular, British medicine had become much more outward-looking. A global viewpoint was manifest in the awareness of foreign scientific developments found in the weekly medical journals.

Another manifestation of this change was the arrival of the international medical congress. Although the trend had started in Paris, the centre of scientific medicine, by 1881 London had hosted its first major medical and scientific meeting, the Seventh International Medical Congress. All of the medical specialties were to take up this innovation as an opportunity to meet colleagues, exchange ideas and hear speeches which proclaimed, 'the capacity of objective scientific knowledge to transcend the divisiveness of multiple languages and the competitiveness of nations.'[20]

Medical hypnotism was no exception to this medical internationalism. The New Hypnotists had learned about the technique from Ambrose Liébeault in Nancy and from the Amsterdam hypnotic clinic run by Frederik van Eeden and Albert van Renterghem. Tuckey made clear his European debt in the introduction of every edition of his book *Psycho-Therapeutics*. Tuckey and Kingsbury went to see Dr. Luys's work at La Charité in Paris, in 1891.[21] It appears that it was not just the techniques that were important to Tuckey but also the relationships with his continental colleagues. He was responsible for initiating a testimonial gift for Liébeault when he retired in 1890. He also kept a lifelong friendship and correspondence with Edgar Bérillon and van Eeden, whom would stay with him when in London.[22]

Bérillon was the editor in chief of *La Revue de l'Hypnotisme* throughout its publication from 1887 to 1910. He oversaw the change of title to *Revue de psychothérapie et de psychologie appliquée* and the broadening of its scope. He invited Tuckey on to the editorial board of the journal. As an excellent linguist, he was able to write for the journal as

[19] William Bynum, *Science and the Practice of Medicine in the Nineteenth Century* (Cambridge: Cambridge University Press, 1994) (pp. 142–6).

[20] Bynum, *Science* (p. 142).

[21] Charles Lloyd Tuckey, 'A New Hypnotism: A Reply to Mr. E Hart's "The Revival of Witchcraft"', *Contemporary Review*, 63, 416–419 (p. 416).

[22] Charles Lloyd Tuckey, letter to Frederik van Eeden, 14 May, 1900. In *Frederik Van Eeden Collection* (Amsterdam: Allard Pierson, University of Amsterdam).

well as follow the European developments.[23] Tuckey certainly saw himself as part of an international group of medical hypnotists. He travelled to France after Liébeault's death and gave an address at the memorial service and inauguration of a bust in his honour in Paris in 1906. The bust had originally been proposed by van Renterghem and was funded largely by subscriptions from the Paris-based, 'La Société d'hypnologie,' publishers of *La Revue de l'Hypnotisme*. Tuckey suggested both the medical acceptance and the power of the medical internationalism in his memorial speech. He gave credit to Liébeault for the fact that 'in England, there are now, in almost every city, physicians who have specialised in the practice of hypnotism. This is all the more surprising since the English people are essentially attached to their age-old traditions and only welcome new developments with extreme distrust.'[24]

Bramwell too acknowledged the impact in Britain of the widespread acceptance of medical hypnotism in Europe. 'In most European countries hypnotism now plays an important part, while many of those who practise it are well known by their contributions to other departments of medicine.' He noted that in Europe, hypnotism has also found its way into 'university classrooms, and has occupied a prominent place at numerous medical congresses.'[25]

The medical hypnotists like other medical specialists organised and attended international conferences. The largest specialist event for medical and academic hypnotists was the Congress of Experimental and Therapeutic Hypnotism. The first of these took place in 1889, during the Universal Exhibition in Paris. There were 171 attendees in all. There were representatives from Germany, Poland and Italy including the physician Albert Schrenck-Notzing, the philosopher Julian Ochorowicz and the psychiatrist Cesare Lombroso. Francis Galton was on the organising committee and Edmund Gurney and Frederic Myers from the SPR were

[23] Charles Lloyd Tuckey, 'Perversion Sexuelle Guérie par l'Hypnotisme', *Revue de l'Hypnotisme et de la Psychologie Physiologique*, 20 (1906) (pp. 91–3).

[24] This pamphlet lists the international delegates and the eulogies delivered at the memorial. There is an English translation of Lloyd Tuckey's speech in the appendix. Edgar Bérillon, *L'Oeuvre Psychologique du Dr. Liébeault* (Paris: Aux bureaux de La Revue de l'Hypnotisme, 1906) 18–9 (p. 18). https://archive.org/details/Loeuvrepsycholog00br/page/n4/mode/2up [accessed 19 April 2020].

[25] John Milne Bramwell, *Hypnotism: History, Practice and Theory* (London: Rider and co, 1921) (p. 34).

invited from the UK and contributed. Although Jean-Martin Charcot himself could not attend, the majority of the speakers were French and the Salpêtrière and Nancy schools were well represented. Inevitably the battle between the two camps was quite prominent, with Joseph Babinski's paper openly critical of Hippolyte Bernheim.[26] Otherwise, the papers covered a variety of topics from the definition of terms and the exclusion of animal magnetism as a mechanism, to the therapeutic uses of hypnotism and its enhancement of human potential.

Hypnotism was also a regular feature of the international meetings of the new discipline of psychology, at least until 1905. The Congress of Psychology came to the UK in 1892 for only its second meeting. Here it was organised by James Sully and Frederic Myers and Henry Sidgwick of the Society for Psychical Research as there was no university-based psychology department. James Sully was a philosopher turned psychologist, who went on to set up the British Psychology Society.[27] Later that year, he became Britain's first professor of psychology at University College London. He, Myers and Sidgwick invited many of the leading names in hypnotism research who were mostly medically trained. They included Bernheim, Jules Liégeois, Bérillon, van Eeden and Janet. The published proceedings did not include a list of registrants but it seems most likely that Tuckey was in attendance. There were over 300 delegates, including nearly a hundred foreign visitors, from all parts of Europe, from America and Australia.[28] The significance of this event was threefold. Firstly, it helped to kickstart the discipline of academic psychology in the UK. The congress' chair Henry Sidgwick was a Cambridge philosophy professor and in his inaugural speech he bemoaned the absence of any properly equipped psychology labs in the UK compared with France,

[26] Carlos Alvardo, 'Nineteenth-Century Suggestion and Magnetism: Hypnosis at the International Congress of Physiological Psychology (1889)', *Contemporary Hypnosis,* 27 (2010) (pp. 48–60).

[27] Sully was also interested in dual consciousness and as a friend of Robert Louis Stephenson, is believed to have influenced *The Strange Case of Dr. Jekyll and Mr. Hyde.* Ed Block, 'James Sully, Evolutionist Psychology, and Late Victorian Gothic Fiction', *Victorian Studies*, 25 (1982) (pp. 443–67).

[28] Conference Archives found at Psychology Resources around the World: https://psychology-resources.org/conferences-events/conference-archives/international-congress-of-psychology-1889-present/1892-ii-international-congress-of-psychology [accessed 19 April 2020].

Germany and the United States.[29] Secondly, the programme shows that the majority of the delegates were interested in the therapeutic possibilities of hypnotism above all else. Thirdly, the conference marked the rise of the Nancy school of suggestion and the downfall of the Salpêtrière concept of hypnosis as an abnormal pathological phenomenon.[30]

Eleven years were to elapse between the first and second congresses of International Hypnotism which was held in Paris once more. By 1900, the landscape had changed completely. The death of Charcot had decisively ended the Salpêtrière-Nancy debate in favour of Nancy. The organising committee was entirely French, but according to Alan Gauld, by this time the intellectual momentum had shifted away from France to Germany.[31] Contrary to the rapid decline of hypnotism described by Pierre Janet and historian Henri Ellenberger, there were actually more delegates at the second meeting than at the first, with 211 attendees compared to 171. Therapeutic hypnotism remained a major theme though there were papers on physiology, applications in education and medicolegal aspects. Tuckey was an invited speaker, one of six from the UK.[32] Tuckey gave a presentation on the treatment of alcoholism with hypnotism and suggestion. Bramwell spoke on the use of hypnotism in general practice which gives a good indicator of the direction of British medical hypnotism at this time.

This is not to say that the New Hypnotists ignored the local national medical context in the 1890s. Tuckey and Bramwell contributed regular papers to a variety of medical journals including the *Lancet* and *Brain* which became more sympathetic over time.[33] The hostility of the editor Ernest Hart meant they could get nothing except letters published in

[29] It was not until 1898 that Sully opened the first psychology labs at University College, London.

[30] Mark Rosenzweig and others, *History of the International Union of Psychological Science* (Hove: Psychology Press, 2000) (pp. 31–5).

[31] Alan Gauld, 'The Decline of Hypnotism', Ch. 25 in *Hypnotism* (Cambridge: Cambridge University Press, 1992) 559–74 (p. 560).

[32] The other British delegates were Frederic Myers, William Crookes, Francis Cruise, James Sully and John Milne Bramwell, 'The Second Congress of International Hypnotism', *Journal of the Society for Psychical Research*, 9 (1900) (pp. 261–5).

[33] John Milne Bramwell, 'On the Evolution of Hypnotic Theory', *Brain* (1896) 459–568 (p. 459); John Milne Bramwell, 'James Braid: Surgeon and Hypnotist', *Brain*, 19 (1896) (pp. 90–116); Charles Lloyd Tuckey, 'Critical Digest of Hypnotism', *Brain*, 16 (1891) (pp. 539–56); Charles Lloyd Tuckey, 'Cases Treated by Hypnotism and Suggestion', *Lancet*, 134 (1889) (pp. 365–7).

the *BMJ*. They took the opportunity to promote hypnotism and suggestion directly to their British fellow professionals, too. They were invited to lecture and give demonstrations of hypnotism by general hospitals across the country, as well as local BMA branch committees. The *BMJ* records Tuckey's demonstrations of hypnotism at branch meetings of the BMA in Norwich and Southend.[34] In Ireland, Kingsbury presented on the medicolegal aspects of hypnotism to the Dublin Royal Academy of Medicine.[35]

The Battle for Legitimacy with Ernest Hart and the *BMJ*

The surge in the medical and public prominence of medical hypnotism was potentially destabilising to the British medical institutions and demanded a response. That challenge was taken up by Ernest Abraham Hart, the pugnacious editor of the *BMJ* from January 1876 until his death in January 1898. Not quite its longest-serving editor, he has been described as its most 'controversial, powerful and influential' (Figs. 6.1 and 6.2).[36]

Surprisingly, Hart has never been the subject of a full biography and his life variously dubbed as an 'enigma' and 'shadowy.' Some of this controversy stems from some shady financial dealings with the journal's money for which he was temporarily suspended from office; his advertising his own mineral water in the journal and his involvement by omission or design in the death by poisoning of his first wife Rosetta Levy, when he was just 22.[37] His wife had died from an overdose of the tincture of

34 Anon, 'Branch News—East Anglia Branch: Norfolk District', *British Medical Journal* (28 June 1890) (p. 923); Anon, 'Branch News—East Anglia Branch: Essex District', *BMJ* (18 October 1890) (p. 937).

35 George Kingsbury, 'Should We Give Hypnotism a Trial? *Dublin Journal of Medical Science* (May 1891), 396–406 (p. 896).

36 Peter Bartrip, Ch. 4 and 5, 'A Gigantic National Institution' and 'Campaigns and controversies', *Mirror of Medicine: A History of the British Medical Journal* (Oxford: British Medical Journal and Clarendon Press, 1990) 63–92 and 93–120 (p. 63).

37 Bartrip, *Mirror of Medicine* (p. 63); Leighton, '"Hypnosis Redivivus"'; David Ryde, 'Ernest Hart—A Forgotten Man', *Journal of the College of General Practice*, 12 (1966) (pp. 345–57).

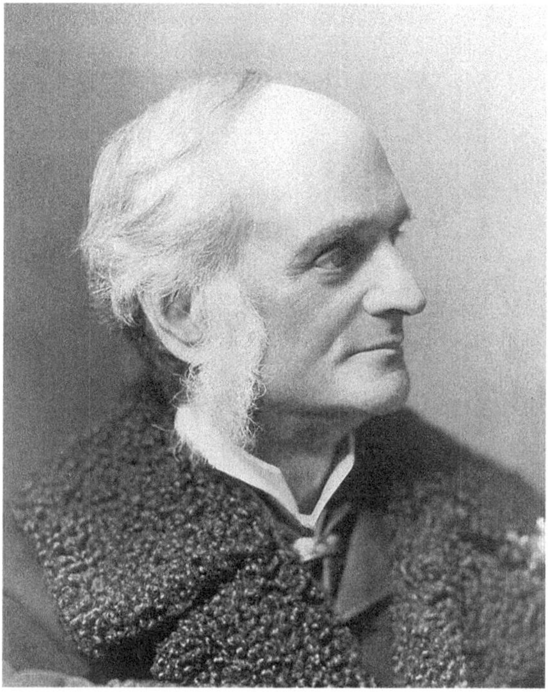

Fig. 6.1 Ernest Abraham Hart, Unknown artist. https://en.wikipedia.org/wiki/Ernest_Hart_%28medical_journalist%29#/media/File:Ernest_Abraham_Hart2.jpg

aconite that he had prescribed. The malicious rumours even inspired a contemporary novel, *Dr Phillips: A Maida Vale Idyll* (1887).[38]

Hart's medical background was in ophthalmic surgery, being the first to describe the nervous network that sits above the iris and to introduce medicated gelatine discs into routine ophthalmic practice.[39] However, he is best known for his achievements as a medical journalist. He was a precocious talent. While attending the City of London school, the only public school of merit that accepted boys from Jewish backgrounds, he submitted articles to periodicals for publication. He continued to pick up

[38] Frank Danby, *Dr. Phillips: A Maida Vale Idyll* (London: Keynes Press, 1989).

[39] Ryde, 'Ernest Hart' (p. 346).

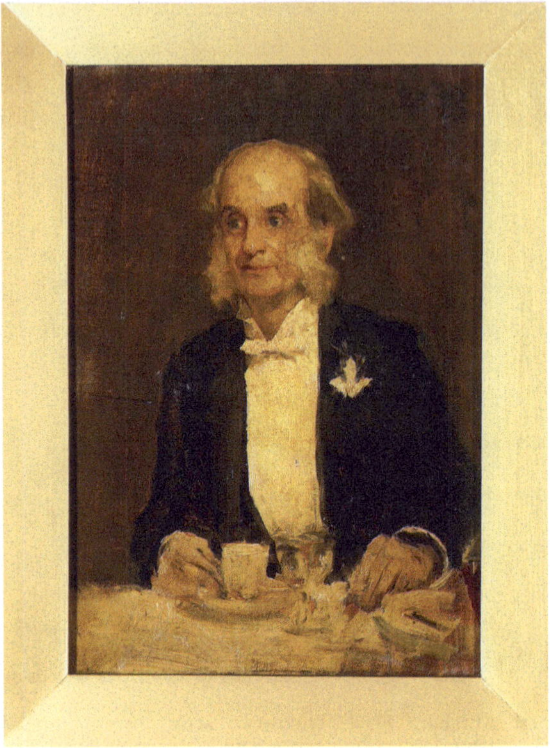

Fig. 6.2 Solomon Joseph Solomon (1860–1927). Ernest Abraham Hart (1835–1898), Editor of the British Medical Journal (Courtesy of the Wellcome Collection)

academic prizes and publish outside of medicine as a medical student at St. George's Medical school. He was promoted to junior consultant by the age of 22 and became the Dean of St. Mary's medical school at the age of 28.

Hart honed his writing skills while training as an ophthalmic surgeon by joining the staff at the *Lancet* in 1858. He worked under the editor James Wakley (the son of Elliotson's friend and unlikely nemesis, Thomas) with whom he fell out when he refused to make him co-editor. In August 1866, at the age of 31, he was appointed to the editorship of the *BMJ*. Over the course of the next 32 years, he secured the finances of both the journal and the BMA, by increasing its subscription tenfold.[40] In the process, he had turned the *BMJ* into a 'gigantic national institution,' in the words of the obituarist from the *Practitioner*, a rival medical journal.[41]

Under Hart's leadership, the *BMJ* moved away from being merely the newsletter of the association. Previously, it had narrowly represented the professional and business matters of the British Medical Association (the BMA remains the joint trade and professional body of all medical doctors). With Hart as editor, the *BMJ* started publishing high quality scientific papers and clinical material and developing a more international outlook. Hart's editorials in particular, offered a consistent, authoritative and independent voice. The *BMJ* and other contemporary medical journals like the *Lancet* also had a subtler social role in helping to establish the reputation of medicine as a socially responsible, beneficent and reputable professional enterprise with members who held shared values.

One particular aspect that marked out Hart's tenure as editor, was his engagement with social and political issues. He was described by the *Medical Magazine* as 'unquestionably the foremost public man of his day [...] in the modern science of preventative medicine.'[42] He campaigned for improvements in municipal sanitation, clean milk, air quality in cities and compulsory vaccination. He drew considerable criticism outside the medical profession for his views in favour of medical vivisection but also turned his pen against the lucrative business of baby-farming (the practice of purchasing the custody of infants or children from the poor), as well as against the working conditions in factories and the learning environment of pauper schools.[43] His editorials could be highly combative and he was responsible for destroying individual careers as well as a number of important public health campaigns which were highly effective.

Another general area of Hart's lobbying was for improvements in the life and prestige of medical doctors.[44] He ensured that physicians in the armed forces were given an officer's rank and treated that way. He

[40] Bartrip, *Mirror of Medicine* (p. 7).

[41] Anon, 'Obituary – Ernest Hart', *Practitioner*, 60 (1898) 117–8 (p. 117).

[42] Anon, 'Obituary', *Medical Magazine* (Januarry 1898) 34–5 (p. 34).

[43] Anon, 'Obituary: Ernest Hart', *British Medical Journal* (15 January 1898) (pp. 175–86).

[44] Ryde, 'Ernest Hart' (p. 346).

established a library for the BMA, donating his own book collection. He fought for proprietary medicines to show their ingredients on their label and for prosecutions against patent compounds containing poisons.[45] The Medical Act of 1858 had already enshrined in law that it was 'expedient that Persons requiring Medical Aid should be enabled to distinguish qualified from unqualified Practitioners.'[46] This legislation had effectively separated physicians trained through the universities and medical schools from other unlicensed healers. Hart used the pages of the *BMJ* and high-circulation national newspapers to rail against the harm done to the public by unqualified and unregistered quacks (and so promote the business of registered physicians).[47] He encouraged editors and newspaper owners to refuse advertising space to unlicensed practitioners and patent remedies.[48] In similar fashion to the *Lancet* under Thomas Wakley, an important role of the *BMJ* was to clearly demarcate trustworthy orthodox medicine from untrustworthy quackery. Such boundary work between science and non-science becomes more important when status, identity and mercenary factors are at stake.[49]

All of Hart's obituaries make mention of the enemies that he had made during his career. The *BMJ* historian, Peter Bartrip suggests that this was the result of a combination of his driving ambition, pushiness and plain antisemitism. Hart himself was not distressed by his developing enemies and saw it as a mark of good journalism and editorship. In an address to the American Medical Editors association in 1893 he said that 'An editor needs and must have many enemies; he cannot do without them. Woe be unto the journalist of whom all men say good things.'[50]

[45] Bartrip, *Mirror of Medicine* (pp. 190–1).

[46] Preamble from The Medical Act of 1858 (21 and 22 Vict. Cap. 90) (passed 2 August 1858).

[47] Ernest Hart, 'The Practice of Quacks. Collective Investigation', *British Medical Journal* (21 July 1894) (p. 153).

[48] Ernest Hart, 'The Press, The Quacks and the Public', *British Medical Journal* (27 January 1894) (p. 208).

[49] Thomas Gieryn, 'Boundary-Work and the Demarcation of Science from Non-Science: Strains and Interests in Professional Ideologies of Scientists', *American Sociological Review*, 48, 6 (December 1983) (pp. 781–95).

[50] Ernest Hart, 'American Editors Association', *British Medical Journal* (1 July 1893) 19–20 (p. 20).

This bellicose quality becomes important because one of Hart's battles was against hypnotism. Over the 1890s and right up until his death in 1898, he became increasingly hostile towards the topic and vindictive towards those physicians who were using it. He was particularly abusive and personal towards Charcot's colleague, Dr Jules Luys for his credulousness towards more bizarre aspects of hypnotism.[51] Hart's abrasive style meant that those that tried to oppose him could expect rough treatment in the pages of the *BMJ*. As editor he could also choose what to publish and what not to publish. In response the New Hypnotists were forced to promote medical hypnotism in the lay journals and periodicals, away from the medical journals. He used the *BMJ* to snipe at his opponents: 'Dr. Tuckey would do well to submit to impartial medical observation and criticism the cases upon which he bases his claims.'[52]

When Tuckey did write in reply to the criticisms, Hart did not deign to publish his letter instead criticising him for providing his personal records of cases rather than external validation of his cures.[53] This fractious debate with the medical hypnotists was neglected at the time by his obituarists and there is no space for the argument in the Bartrip chapters devoted to Hart's time at the *BMJ* (the closest we have to a contemporary biography). Fortunately, it has been examined more recently by the historians Mary Leighton and Teri Chettiar.[54] However, they have attempted to simplify Hart's attitude to hypnotism to a consistent hostile opposition.

Hart's personal and theoretical position was more complex and evolved significantly over time. He had enough of an interest in hypnotism to go personally to visit Charcot and the hypnotism demonstrations at the Salpêtrière as part of a trip to Paris in 1888. Hart was fully aware of Charcot's reputation and his initial reports of 'Medical Paris of To-Day'

[51] Ernest Hart, *Mesmerism and the New Witchcraft* (London: Smith and Elder, 1893). His articles on hypnotism were collected and republished in Ernest Hart, *Hypnotism, Mesmerism and the New Witchcraft*, enlarged ed. (London: Smith and Elder, 1896).

[52] Ernest Hart, 'Literary Intelligence', *British Medical Journal* (4 March 1893) (p. 483).

[53] Ernest Hart, 'Letters, Notes and Answers to Correspondents', *British Medical Journal* (18 March 1893) (p. 618).

[54] Leighton, '"Hypnosis Redivivus"; Teri Chettiar, '"Looking as Little Like Patients as Persons Well Could": Hypnotism, Medicine and the Problem of the Suggestible Subject in Late Nineteenth-Century Britain', *Medical History*, 56 (2012) (pp. 335–54).

in the *BMJ* were respectful and broadly favourable.[55] Based on the notes he had made at the time, Hart's series, which covered a range of Parisian medical developments that included hypnotism, ran from December 1888 to May 1889. He described Charcot as the 'master' and credited him with delineating at least a third of known neurological disorders. He also praised his work on hypnotism: 'The hypnotics of the Salpêtrière and the elaborate and admirable studies which have been made of them by M. Charcot are well known to all European physicians, and constitute the chief basis of our present knowledge of hypnotism.'[56]

Over five years after the first publication of Bernheim's book, *de la Suggestion* and three years after the Nancy visits and the subsequent publications of Tuckey, Kingsbury, Felkin and Bramwell, Hart reported in the *BMJ* on the ideas of the Nancy school for the first time.[57] It is unclear, but seems unlikely, whether he had actually attended the 1891 International Congress of Hypnotism held in Paris that year, but he quoted from its published addresses. In his report, he described the principal differences between the Nancy school of Liébeault and Bernheim and those of the Salpêtrière and Charcot. The article attempted to separate the key concepts of the two doctrines.[58]

It is apparent that Hart was still respectful of 'the master' (Charcot) who had raised the status of hypnotism to a subject worthy of scientific study. He favoured Charcot's views of three distinct hypnotic stages over those of the Nancy ideas that hypnotism represents a state of heightened suggestibility to the physician's curative instructions. Hart accepted the idea that suggestion played a role in hypnotic phenomena but argued against the Nancy school's belief in universal suggestibility, ultimately believing hypnotism to be a pathological state and that those who could be hypnotised must have an underlying pathological neurosis or hysteria. He was highly sceptical of the possibility of heightened sensory perceptions during trance, such as telepathy and clairvoyancy and scorned the public excitement this was causing.

[55] Ernest Hart, 'Special Correspondence Section: Medical Paris of To-Day', *British Medical Journal* (2 February 1889) (pp. 266–8).

[56] Hart, 'Special Correspondence' (p. 267).

[57] Hippolyte Bernheim, *De la Suggestion et de ses applications a la therapeutique*, (Paris: Doin, 1886).

[58] Ernest Hart, 'Schools and Doctrines of Hypnotism', *British Medical Journal* (28 March 1891) (pp. 721–3).

Despite his previous promotion of Charcot's work on hypnotism which explored the boundaries between hypnotism and hysteria, he started to show a more critical perspective towards therapeutic hypnotism. He referred it as mostly ineffective and potentially harmful. He felt that it had not lived up to its early promise and that there was insufficient evidence of usefulness.

> The hopes which the therapeutic hypnotist aroused have not been realised, and any expectations of producing by hypnotic methods any desirable moral or mental effect rest upon a totally inadequate basis of fact, and are far from being promising.[59]

Hart did not restrict his condemnations of therapeutic hypnotism to the journal which he edited. Like his opponents, he was happy to prosecute the battle in public view and to court public approval within the national newspapers and general journals. It was surely no coincidence that when he came to publish his first essay on hypnotism for a general audience in 1892, it was in the *Nineteenth Century*, the same journal that had published Tuckey's 'Faith-Healing' in 1888. The tone of the essay was scathing as can be gathered from its title, 'Hypnotism and Humbug,' reprising the Okey and Elliotson incident headline from the *Times* from fifty years before.[60]

The article was derived from a presentation that Hart had given to a non-medical audience at the Toynbee Hall in December 1891, as part of his philanthropic work.[61] The Hall had been established as a base for graduates of Oxford and Cambridge to support the poor, by Hart's sister-in-law and her husband, the social reformers, Henrietta and Samuel Barnett. It was located in Whitechapel, one of the poorer parts of East London, as a part of the reformist Settlement movement. As well as providing food, shelter and musical entertainment for the poor, it had links to the University and offered basic and higher education. Hart's talk was therefore part of a broader purpose of the intellectual improvement of the poor.

[59] Hart, 'Schools and Doctrines' (p. 723).

[60] Ernest Hart, 'Hypnotism and Humbug', *Nineteenth Century,* 31 (January 1892) (pp. 24–37).

[61] Anon, 'Mr. Ernest Hart on Hypnotism', *St. James Gazette* (7 December 1891) (p. 5).

In spite of the critical title, Hart makes some surprising revelations. We learn that Hart has some direct early experience of hypnotism, witnessing a relative with severe arthritis gain the ease of sleep following the intervention of John Elliotson. Hart claimed that as a result of this early exposure he had himself investigated and experimented with hypnotism. He disclosed that he had nearly lost his job as a house surgeon, when some friends had persuaded him to hypnotise a young woman in his rooms at a London hospital. She was spotted leaving his rooms unsteadily when she could not be fully roused following Hart's demonstration of hypnotism to his fellows. This incident Hart claimed taught him the danger of meddling. If these revelations are designed to give Hart a platform for his views by demonstrating his knowledge and experience then they appear limited grounds for expertise.

However, Hart's main conclusions were relevant and logically consistent. He proposed that as the means of hypnotic induction and influence were so many and varied, that it was likely that the hypnotised subject was more important than the hypnotist for the observed phenomena. Like Charcot and Henry Maudsley, Hart continued to view suggestibility or susceptibility to hypnosis as evidence of mental pathology. Also, like these two he had fixed, deterministic and organic views of mental illness and could not contemplate the kind of dynamic psychiatry that suggestion offered.

The features of the hypnotised were just as relevant to the public acceptance of therapeutic hypnotism as the qualities of the hypnotist. Susceptibility to fictional hypnotism was already associated with a variety of other characteristics: weak will, female gender or femininity, creativity, mental illness and South European or Celtic heritage. These qualities reflected in the early hypnotic fictions had to be challenged if therapeutic hypnotism was to gain acceptability with the general public. The New Hypnotists did attempt to develop a counter-narrative, demonstrating in their clinical work and experiments at the SPR that labourers, athletes, military men and university students (who were all male at this time) were the most suitable for hypnosis.[62]

[62] Charles Lloyd Tuckey, 'Faith Healing as a Medical Treatment', *Nineteenth Century*, 21 (1888) (p. 842); Charles Lloyd Tuckey, 'Some Phases of Hypnotism', *Occult Review*, 1 (1905) 51–7 (p. 54); John Milne Bramwell, 'Susceptibility to Hypnotism and the causes that Influence it', Ch 4 in *Hypnotism Its History, Practice and Theory*, 3rd ed. (London, William Rider & Son, 1921) (pp. 57–73); George Kingsbury, 'Who are Susceptible?', Ch

In his 'Humbug' essay, Hart uses the older language of the doctrine of imagination, noting that 'we can contrive to influence the *imagination* [my emphasis] or affect the physical condition of the subject by any of a great number of contrivances.'[63] However, he later calls upon the new language of suggestion to explain the effects of hypnotism when performed by Charcot, Albert Moll, Bernheim and Jules Dejerine: 'honest and capable men' (by which he means physicians of repute).[64] We can see that even a sceptic like Hart finds the idioms of suggestion more useful for explaining hypnotic phenomena than the romantically and mystically influenced doctrine of imagination. Hart rejects stage entertainments as trickery and the clairvoyance, telepathy and other special powers investigated by the SPR as 'imposture.' He concludes the essay in a rhetorical polemic fashion:

> these delusions, this miracle-mongering, these disordered visions and hysteric hallucinations, this exploitation of the love of the mysterious, these pseudo-magnetic attractions, these sham scientific floatings in the air or fixations of the body, these thought-readings and foretellings, these vain pronouncements concerning unseen worlds and invisible planes of being, these playings on the fears, the hopes, the feeble senses, the eager imaginations, and the ill-balanced reason of the masses, are as old as, nay, apparently older than history. Sometimes in this, as in other things, we are tempted to ask, 'Does the World make any progress?[65]

At the end of the same year, Hart picked up where he left off in looking at the history of trance states in healing in another article for the *BMJ* entitled 'Hypnotism, Animal magnetism and Hysteria.'[66] Once again it was based on a platform speech, this time one given at Sheffield Philosophical Institute. It was an odd and inconsistent paper with sections that claimed British ownership for the theory of the technique for healing but other sections that were highly critical. He still followed the Charcot

4 in *The Practice of Hypnotic Suggestion, Being and Elementary Handbook for the Use of the Medical Profession* (Bristol: John Wright, 1891) (pp. 59–66).

[63] Hart, *New Witchcraft* (1896) (p. 13).

[64] Hart, *New Witchcraft* (1896) (p. 23).

[65] Hart, *New Witchcraft* (1896) (p. 28).

[66] Ernest Hart, 'Hypnotism, Animal Magnetism and Hysteria', *British Medical Journal* (3 December 1892) (pp. 1215–20); Also collected in *New Witchcraft* (1896) (pp. 30–71).

school that hysteria and susceptibility to hypnotism were related morbid mental states. He expanded on his view that hypnotism depended entirely on the subject for its effects: that is, that the trance state was voluntary and the subject would only act in the way that they wished to. This was a marked change from his earlier views on automatic automatons.

For a medical audience, he went over similar ground to the 'Humbug' paper, covering the history of magnetism from Paracelsus to Mesmer but suggested that the accounts could be reinterpreted and explained in the light of modern knowledge. He credited James Braid, the Englishman, with the responsibility for the theory of hypnotism, favouring his more prosaic physiological explanation and his British heritage. He finished the article hostile to therapeutic hypnotism by supporting the Salpêtrière physicians (Charcot, and his pupils Paul Richer, Babinski and Dejerine) in their view that 'hypnotism is very rarely useful, generally entirely useless and often injurious.'[67] However, the uneven tone continues with a final paragraph which proposed that hypnotism should be limited to qualified medical doctors and banned from platform performances and private entertainment altogether. Hart went on to make the bold and damaging but unsubstantiated claim, that 'a confirmed and trained hypnotic subject is a maimed individual in mind and body, and likely at any time to be dangerous to himself and to society.'[68] The medical hypnotists could agree with the ban on hypnotic entertainments, even if they did not accept or recognise Hart's underlying rationale.

The Wimpole Street Sting

Hart's next attempt to discredit medical hypnotism was more brash and unethical. He wanted to show stage hypnotism to be a sham and more provocatively to expose the British hypnotism lobby to be the victim of a calculated deceit and therefore credulous fools. He described his carefully designed piece of subterfuge in an article for a journal with a wider, more general audience, named the *Century Illustrated Magazine*.[69] In 'The Eternal Gullible,' he shared the experiences of 'L,' a professional

[67] Hart, *New Witchcraft* (1896) (p. 70).

[68] Hart, *New Witchcraft* (1896) (pp. 70–1).

[69] Ernest Hart, 'The Eternal Gullible', *Century Illustrated Magazine,* 48 (1894) (pp. 833–9).

hypnotic subject whom he had met the previous year through another journal editor. He explained that L had wanted money as he had lost his commercial value through his overuse in hypnotic entertainments. Tragically for his career, the audience had started to recognise him.

L described the intensive and unpleasant training required to tolerate the foul tastes and smells and the passage of needles through his cheeks that characterised a magic mesmerism act. He also learned to swallow paraffin and had to develop his musculature to tolerate 'doing catalepsy' in order to perform at the Royal Aquarium for eight months and thereafter at other venues.[70] In addition to a permanent display of fish, the Royal Aquarium used to contain an art gallery, an ice rink and a theatre where L appeared as part of a magic shows featuring hypnotism and clairvoyancy. He told Hart that he earned £1 and 5 shillings a week for the work which Hart reflected was inadequate for the suffering entailed. L also revealed that he had regular work as a subject for a physiology lecturer at a London medical school who was unaware of his duplicity.

The second part of the article gave an account of a demonstration that Hart had arranged at his London house on Wimpole Street with L and two of his show business colleagues. Hart had invited many who had participated in the recent BMA section of psychology hypnotism committee like Hack Tuke, Thomas Outterson Wood and Surgeon-Colonel J. B Hamilton. He also invited John Milne Bramwell and Hugh Wingfield.[71] Apart from Tuckey and George Kingsbury, Hart had invited all of the major names of British medical hypnotism. One of the doctors was asked to hypnotise L, who acting as a stooge for Hart, disconcertingly kept 'waking up' from his hypnotic state. When eventually 'hypnotised,' he was then able to demonstrate that he was impervious to pain. Hart wrote that L made no reaction to any painful stimuli but accused him of over-acting badly at other times. He then mocked the doctors for their gullibility and for seeing only what they wanted to see: 'The impression left on my mind by L's performance was mainly a feeling of wonder that

[70] Tuckey had written to the *Lancet* complaining about hypnotic seances there in 1891; Charles Lloyd Tuckey, 'Correspondence', *Lancet* (31 October 1891) (p. 1024). In 1896, a Walter Johnson was put into a hypnotic trance and left there for 3 weeks drinking only occasional milk and Bovril; Anon, 'The Hypnotic Trance at the Royal Aquarium', *British Medical Journal* (15 February 1896) (p. 422).

[71] Hart, 'The Eternal Gullible' (p. 837).

so vulgar and transparent apiece of trickery should ever have imposed on anyone.'[72]

The above incident does seem a shabby if not unethical trick to play on one's colleagues and perhaps shows the desperate measures to which Hart would resort to discredit hypnotism. When republished in the *BMJ*, the first part of the 'Eternal Gullible' is reprinted but not the second part concerning the deception played on Kingsbury and friends.[73] I considered whether or not Hart had subsequently regretted the trickery but the entire *Century* article was included as an extra chapter when his *Mesmerism and Witchcraft* book went for its next edition in 1896.[74] I have found no record of the response of the deceived doctors and little mention in the press or medical press at the time.

His *New Witchcraft* book and a review of the hypnotic fiction *Trilby* were to be Hart's last counterblasts against hypnotism. He had been diagnosed with diabetes in 1883 and suffered from bouts of pneumonia and depression in the 1880s and 1890s which neither his work rate nor his foreign convalescences helped. He was in poor health when he moved out of London to Hertfordshire in 1896. He developed diabetic ulcers and then gangrene, requiring amputation of his leg in September 1897. While he continued to contribute to the *BMJ*, more and more of the work of the journal was done by Dawson Williams. He requested a leave of absence from the journal in late 1897 to go to Madeira for his health. He never made the trip and died in early 1898.

Hart's impact on the *BMJ* and the British medical profession was substantial and with his journal and role on the parliamentary committee of the BMA, he achieved many public health advances. However, it is clear that Hart was a figure who provoked mixed feelings: the obituarist from the *Practitioner* opined that he was a 'man who with a nobler ambition and a loftier ideal might have left the whole world his debtor for ever. He preferred a cheaper glory and he had his reward.'[75] Certainly, Hart's censure of hypnotism made it more difficult for the New Hypnotists. Hart would not publish their papers, negatively reviewed their books and actively attempted to discredit both the technique and the doctors

[72] Hart, 'The Eternal Gullible' (p. 839).

[73] Anon, 'Literary Intelligence' (p. 817).

[74] Hart, *Hypnotism, Mesmerism* (1896).

[75] Anon, 'Obituary', *Practitioner* (p. 118).

involved. After his death, Dawson Williams his successor took a more impartial view and the book reviews at least became more positive.

While Ernest Hart's position as a figurehead for the anti-hypnotism lobby has been acknowledged and is well-described by Mary Leighton, the response of the New Hypnotists, particularly Tuckey and Bramwell have not been previously described. I have examined how both parties made use of lectures, demonstrations, medical journals, gentleman's periodicals and their own public standing as a platform to advocate their view.

The American sociologist, Terry Parsinnen has argued that the reason for the failure of mesmerism in the 1840s compared to the success of the New Hypnotism in the 1890s was the increased standing and security of the medical profession at this time. He proposed that what had changed was not so much the theory or even the practice of hypnotism but rather the professional community that received it. By the 1890s, the British Medical profession was in a much stronger position with its legal foundation rather than struggling for acceptance. In his view, hypnotism was not associated with a dangerous popular culture phenomenon, as mesmerism had been. He concluded 'etiology and therapeutics were not areas of contention that they had been, and the profession was not beset by such fundamental challenges as it had been in the 1840s.'[76]

While I agree with Parsinnen's view that hypnotism did eventually find favour at the fin de siècle, I believe his thesis to be an oversimplification. There were other reasons for its success over and above the change in the fortunes of the profession. I also disagree with some of his central contentions. Firstly, inasmuch as the journals can be seen to represent medical culture, under Hart the *BMJ*, like other medical journals, remained staunchly orthodox and regularly called out quackery which in Parsinnen's view indicated continuing professional insecurity. Second, the improved standing of the medical profession at this time may have made some physicians more willing to promote some of the more fringe practices but the reception given to homoeopathy at the time (as illustrated by the Margaret Street Infirmary incident) demonstrates that acceptance and legitimacy were by no means guaranteed and the professional punishment for transgression remained severe. Finally, as

[76] Terry Parsinnen, 'Professional Deviants and the History of Medicine: Medical Mesmerists in Victorian Britain', *Sociological Review*, 27, Supplement 1 (1979) 103–20 (p. 117).

the next chapters will investigate, in the 1890s hypnotism was very much 'a popular culture phenomenon,' even if some of the belief systems and dangerous connotations differed to those of the 1840s.

Not all physicians accepted the efficacy of medical hypnotism and had either not followed or not accepted the transition of hypnotism's mode of action from the doctrine of medical imagination to that of suggestion. For this group, the public opinion of hypnotism and confusion with mesmerism was highly concerning. The action of the BMA's council confirms this.

I should stress that legitimacy and the acceptability of medical treatments are not the same thing and depend as much upon local cultural contingencies as medical opinion. Legitimacy is more of a professional concern which is linked to scientific proof of efficacy and low rates of tolerable side effects as well as an adequate explanation for action. As Geiryn has suggested, in interdisciplinary disputes, legitimacy may be portrayed and argued as scientific authenticity which may then be claimed by both sides.

What is deemed a legitimate treatment to the medical profession is not always acceptable to the general public. One recent example would be electroconvulsive therapy or ECT, a treatment for severe depression in which therapeutic seizures are induced by externally applied electrical current to the brain. ECT may have been shown in many studies to be medically effective with mostly tolerable side effects but it still generates significant anxiety for patients and families. In the face of such anxiety about a treatment it can be difficult for a new therapy to gain acceptance.

These anxieties may be traced to fictional as well as factual lay discourse. In the same way that the film *One Flew Over the Cuckoo's Nest* both generated and represented significant public unease about ECT, a number of books and plays did the same thing for hypnotism in the 1890s. While medical culture often views itself as objective, scientific and separate there are inevitably interactions between medical and popular culture over time which will help to establish or to reject any treatment. This topic is the subject of the next chapters.

Bibliography

1858. *The Medical Act*. 21 and 22 Vict. Cap. 90. UK.

Alvardo, Carlos. 2010. 'Nineteenth-Century Suggestion and Magnetism: Hypnosis at the International Congress of Physiological Psychology (1889)', *Contemporary Hypnosis*, 27: 48–60.

Anon. 1889. 'The Section of Psychology', *British Medical Journal* (21 September): 646–51.

Anon. 1890. 'Branch News—East Anglia Branch: Norfolk District', *British Medical Journal* (28 June): 923.

Anon. 1890. 'British Medical Association', *Times* (30 July): 9.

Anon, 1890. 'British Medical Association', *Times* (1 August): 13.

Anon. 1890. 'British Medical Association', *Times* (2 August): 10.

Anon. 1890. 'BMA', *Times* (3 August): 13.

Anon. 1890. 'A Discussion on Hypnotism in Therapeutics', *British Medical Journal* (23 August): 442–9.

Anon. 1890. 'Hypnotism as a Therapeutic Agent', *British Medical Journal* (23 August): 465.

Anon. 1890. 'Branch News—East Anglia Branch: Essex District', *British Medical Journal* (18 October): 937.

Anon. 1890. 'The Committee on Hypnotism', *British Medical Journal* (13 December): 1389.

Anon. 1891. 'Mr Ernest Hart on Hypnotism', *St. James Gazette* (7 December): 5.

Anon. 1893. 'BMA Annual Meeting', *British Medical Journal* (5 August): 321–9.

Anon. 1896. 'The Hypnotic Trance at the Royal Aquarium', *British Medical Journal* (15 February): 422.

Anon. 1898. 'Obituary—Ernest Hart', *Practitioner*, 60: 117–8.

Anon. 1898. 'Obituary', *Medical Magazine* (January): 34–5.

Anon, 1898. 'Obituary: Ernest Hart', *British Medical Journal* (January 15): 175–86.

Anon. 1900. 'The Second Congress of International Hypnotism', *Journal of the Society for Psychical Research*, 9: 261–5.

Anon. 'International Congress of Psychology 1892', Conference archives retrieved 19 April, 2020, from https://psychology-resources.org/conferences-events/conference-archives/international-congress-of-psychology-1889-present/1892-ii-international-congress-of-psychology.

Bartrip, Peter. 1990. *Mirror of Medicine: A History of the British Medical Journal.* Oxford: British Medical Journal and Clarendon Press.

Bérillon, Edgar. 1906. *L'Oeuvre Psychologique du Dr. Liébeault*. Paris: Aux bureaux de La Revue de l'Hypnotisme. 18–9. https://archive.org/details/Loeuvrepsycholog00br/page/n4/mode/2up [accessed 19 April 2020].

Bernheim, Hippolyte. 1886. *De la suggestion et de ses applications a la therapeutique*. Paris: Doin.

Block, Ed. 1982. 'James Sully, Evolutionist Psychology, and Late Victorian Gothic Fiction', *Victorian Studies*, 25: 443–67.
Bramwell, John Milne. 1896. 'James Braid: Surgeon and Hypnotist', *Brain*, 19: 90–116.
Bramwell, John Milne. 1896. 'On the Evolution of Hypnotic Theory', *Brain*, 19: 459–568.
Bramwell, John Milne. 1921. *Hypnotism: History, Practice and Theory.* London: Rider and co. 34.
British Medical Association, Psychological Medicine Group Sub-committee. 1955. 'The Medical Use of Hypnotism', *Supplement to the British Medical Journal* (23 April): 190–3.
Bynum, William. 1994. *Science and the Practice of Medicine in the Nineteenth Century.* Cambridge, Cambridge University Press.
Chettiar, Teri. 2012. '"Looking as Little Like Patients as Persons Well Could": Hypnotism, Medicine and the Problem of the Suggestible Subject in Late Nineteenth-Century Britain', *Medical History*, 56: 335–54.
Danby, Frank. 1989. *Dr Phillips: A Maida Vale Idyll.* London: Keynes Press.
Gauld, Alan. 1992. *A History of Hypnotism.* Cambridge: Cambridge University Press.
Gieryn, Thomas. 1983. 'Boundary-Work and the Demarcation of Science from Non-Science: Strains and Interests in Professional Ideologies of Scientists', *American Sociological Review*, 48, 6: 781–95.
Hart, Ernest. 1889. 'Special Correspondence Section: Medical Paris of To-Day', *British Medical Journal* (2 February): 266–8.
Hart, Ernest. 1891. 'Schools and Doctrines of Hypnotism', *British Medical Journal* (28 March): 721–3.
Hart, Ernest. 1892. 'Hypnotism and Humbug', *Nineteenth Century,* 31 (January): 24–37.
Hart, Ernest. 1892. 'Hypnotism, Animal Magnetism and Hysteria', *British Medical Journal* (3 December): 1215–20.
Hart, Ernest. 1893. 'Literary Intelligence', *British Medical Journal* (4 March): 483.
Hart, Ernest. 1893. 'Letters, Notes and Answers to Correspondents', *British Medical Journal* (18 March): 618.
Hart, Ernest. 1893. 'American Editors Association', *British Medical Journal* (1 July): 19–20.
Hart, Ernest. 1893. *Mesmerism and the New Witchcraft*. London: Smith and Elder.
Hart, Ernest. 1894. 'The Press, the Quacks and the Public', *British Medical Journal* (27 January): 208.
Hart, Ernest. 1894. 'The Practice of Quacks. Collective Investigation', *British Medical Journal* (21 July): 153.

Hart, Ernest. 1894. 'The Eternal Gullible', *Century Illustrated Magazine*, 48: 833–9.

Hart, Ernest. 1896. *Hypnotism, Mesmerism and the New Witchcraft*, enlarged ed. London: Smith and Elder.

Kingsbury, George. 1891. *The Practice of Hypnotic Suggestion, Being and Elementary Handbook for the Use of the Medical Profession*. John Wright.

Kingsbury, George. 1891. 'Should We Give Hypnotism a Trial?', *Dublin Journal of Medical Science* (May): 396–406.

Kingsbury, George. 1898. 'Correspondence: The BMA and Hypnotism', *British Medical Journal* (26 February): 591–2.

Leighton, Mary. 2001. '"Hypnosis Redivivus": Ernest Hart, "The British Medical Journal" and the Hypnotism Controversy', *Victorian Periodicals Review*, 34: 104–127.

Needham, Frederick and Wood, Thomas Outterson. 1892. 'Report of the Committee Appointed to Investigate the Nature of the Phenomena of Hypnotism; Its Value as a Therapeutic Agent; and the Propriety of Using It', *British Medical Journal* (23 July): 190–1.

Parsinnen, Terry. 1979. 'Professional Deviants and the History of Medicine: Medical Mesmerists in Victorian Britain', *Sociological Review*, 27, Supplement 1: 103–20.

Ryde, David. 1966. 'Ernest Hart—A Forgotten Man', *Journal of the College of General Practice*, 12: 345–57.

Rosenzweig, Mark and others. 2000. *History of the International Union of Psychological Science*. Psychology Press. 31–5.

Tuckey, Charles Lloyd. 1888. 'Faith Healing as a Medical Treatment', *Nineteenth Century*, 21: 839–50.

Tuckey, Charles Lloyd. 1889. 'Cases Treated by Hypnotism and Suggestion', *Lancet*, 134: 365–7.

Tuckey, Charles Lloyd. 1890. Correspondence to van Eeden, 14 July, 1890. In *Van Eeden Collection*. Amsterdam, Allard Pierson, University of Amsterdam.

Tuckey, Charles Lloyd. 1891. 'Correspondence', *Lancet* (31 October): 1024.

Tuckey, Charles Lloyd. 1891. 'Critical Digest of Hypnotism', *Brain*, 16: 539–56.

Tuckey, Charles Lloyd. 1893. 'A New Hypnotism: A Reply to Mr. E Hart's "The Revival of Witchcraft"', *Contemporary Review*, 63: 416–9.

Tuckey, Charles Lloyd. 1900. Correspondence to van Eeden, 14 May, 1900. In *Van Eeden Collection*. Amsterdam, Allard Pierson, University of Amsterdam.

Tuckey, Charles Lloyd. 1900. *Treatment by Hypnotism and Suggestion; or, Psychotherapeutics*. London: Baillière, Tindall and Cox.

Tuckey, Charles Lloyd.1905. 'Some Phases of Hypnotism', *Occult Review*, 1: 51–7

Tuckey, Charles Lloyd. 1906. 'Perversion Sexuelle Guérie par l'Hypnotisme' In *Revue de l'Hypnotisme et de la Psychologie Physiologique*. Paris. 20: 91–3.

CHAPTER 7

Hypnotism in the Public Sphere

A Scandal in Paris

In January 1893, a group of three distinguished Victorian gentlemen joined forces to condemn a new French enthusiasm in a British national newspaper. The forces of conservative orthodoxy were the editor of the *Times*, an eminent psychiatrist and Ernest Hart, the campaigning president of the *British Medical Journal (BMJ)*. The unlikely object of their outrage and Francophobic scorn was the newly fashionable subject of medical hypnotism. In a leading article for the *Times*, the editor George Buckle thundered:

> The new mesmerism, as our Correspondent shows to-day, is not really new at all. It has changed its jargon to some extent, and has been baptized with a new name, but it is in every essential respect the old mesmerism that our fathers and grandfathers used to argue about. It has exactly the same substratum of fact, and exactly the same huge superstructure of imposture, quackery, and downright fraud.[1]

[1] George Buckle, 'Leading Article: The New Mesmerism', *Times,* 11 January, 1893, p. 9.

G. D. L. Bates, *The Uncanny Rise of Medical Hypnotism, 1888–1914*, Mental Health in Historical Perspective,
https://doi.org/10.1007/978-3-031-42725-1_7

At the end of 1892, an unknown physician had visited the Charité clinic of the French neurologist Jules Luys and had written three anonymous, highly critical *Times* articles. Originally attributed in the *Times* to a 'Special Correspondent,' one of the medical authors of the subsequently published letters of response revealed the author to be John Bucknill.[2] His eminence and expertise were indisputable, Bucknill was an alienist, mental health reformer and originally the medical superintendent of the Devon County asylum. He had founded the journals *Brain* and *Mental Science* and wrote one of the first psychiatry textbooks with Daniel Hack Tuke.[3] He had been elected a fellow of the Royal College of Physicians in 1859. He was a man at the heart of the British establishment and medical orthodoxy.

Luys, whom Bucknill had exposed, was a celebrated physician in his own right. He had published the first photographic atlas of neuroanatomy in 1873 and launched the neurology journal, *L'Encéphale*. He was also the first to describe the subthalamic nucleus, part of the basal ganglia and a brain region critical for movement. However, in Bucknill's series of articles, like the disgraced physician John Elliotson before him, Luys was portrayed as a credulous fool and his patients as 'cunning hysterics.' Some of the doctors at Charcot's Salpêtrière had returned to the pseudoscience of Mesmer's original work, investigating the effects of iron magnets in hypnotism. Luys at the Charité had taken the mesmeric aspects further still, describing 'externalisation of the senses' (using a digit to see) and 'magnetic transference' (passing on the symptoms of one patient to another by direct contact). He returned to the dramatic theatricality of mesmerism and the theory of animal magnetism by making passes with magnetic bars over the affected body regions of his patients. Luys had his patients spectacularly 'transfer' the outward signs of their illness from one to another in sequence: an old man with a hand contracture passed this on to a young man with vertigo whose symptoms were then passed on to a child with St. Vitus dance (a movement disorder).[4]

Bucknill may not have been responsible for the title of his articles ('The New Mesmerism') but within the accounts he deliberately conflated

[2] George Kingsbury, 'Correspondence: The New Mesmerism', *Times*, 9 January 1893, p. 7.

[3] John Bucknill and Daniel Hack Tuke, *A Manual of Psychological Medicine* (London: John Churchill, 1858).

[4] John Bucknill, 'The New Mesmerism II', *Times,* 5 January, 1893, p. 6.

mesmerism and hypnotism. It seems likely that Bucknill did come with pre-formed ideas about Luys' mesmeric practice and he was very critical. By a strange chance, he had worked fifty years before as the house doctor for the surgeon Robert Liston at UCH at the same time that John Elliotson was there. Liston had headed the hospital consultants' efforts to prevent Elliotson from using or demonstrating mesmerism at the hospital.

Bucknill was unambiguous in his reaction to the healing events that he witnessed at the Charité:

> I have no words within the limits of politeness strong enough to condemn them, and I am at a loss to conceive why such reckless tampering with a human brain and a human intelligence [...] should be permitted to continue. Would any man allow his own daughter to be subjected to it?[5]

By coincidence, Hart had been in Paris at the time of the Bucknill's first publication, attending the Jubilee celebrations of physician and father of microbiology, Louis Pasteur. Like any good journalist, he had taken advantage of the good timing to pay a visit to Luys at the Charité. Hart already had medical hypnotism in his sights as a threat to medical professionalism and had started to criticise the practice in the *BMJ* as previously described. He claimed that he had visited Luys' patients to prevent medicine from returning to the 'old practices and conclusions of the mystics and sorcerers of the Middle Ages.' He witnessed exactly the same range of phenomena that Bucknill had been shown. The patients and their clinicians were apparently unaware of the articles in the British newspapers. However, in front of several observers, Hart had switched one of the magnets for a sham magnet and demonstrated that the remarkable events like 'externalization of the senses' would still occur. In a letter to the *Times*, he said that what he had seen was:

> only [with] another chapter of human folly, misled by fraud, a reproduction of the old frauds of Mesmer, of the self-deceptions of Reichenbach, and the malpractices of sham magicians of the Middle Ages who have still their ingenious imitators. These impostures and this self-deception mask themselves now under a new nomenclature, and avail themselves

[5] John Bucknill 'The New Mesmerism III', *Times*, 11 January, 1893, p. 8.

> of recent developments of psychological investigation in order to assume more plausible shapes and a pseudo-scientific character.[6]

There was an immediate response to the *Times exposé* and editorial, *in the letters' column of the newspaper*. The New Hypnotists had to counter these attacks in a national newspaper. George Kingsbury wrote to the *Times* because he and Tuckey had visited Luys in 1891.[7] A letter from Frederic Myers, representing the Society for Psychical Research, was also published.[8] The SPR valued hypnotism highly as a tool for investigating nonmaterialist phenomena like telepathy and communicating with the dead. Myers and Gurney from the SPR had visited Charcot and Luys and observed their demonstrations. Both Kingsbury and Myers took the position that while Dr. Luys was a thoroughly honest man who was eager to display his hypnotic work, his enthusiasm had led to his deception and his beliefs and practice were in no way representative of modern hypnotism.

The letters were necessarily brief for inclusion and could only counter some of the accusations. The job of writing a longer response fell to the leaders of the New Hypnotists Charles Lloyd Tuckey and John Milne Bramwell, who both published articles in separate journals. Tuckey argued that Hart had 'confounded medical hypnotism with matters totally unconnected with it,' and commented that 'nothing is harder to contend against than a half-truth, and Mr. Hart's articles are full of half-truths and of false deductions drawn therefrom.'[9]

On the face of it, it seems obvious why a senior psychiatrist and a medical editor might wish to expose quackery and charlatanry, even that occurring in another country. From a public health perspective, publicising the fraud of the fringe practice might help to protect the health and pockets of the unwary and credulous in the UK. It would also serve to bolster the scientific credibility of British medical professionals in

[6] Ernest Hart, 'Correspondence: The New Mesmerism', *Times,* 10 January, 1893, p. 8.

[7] George Kingsbury (1891) *The Practice of Hypnotic Suggestion*. Bristol, J. Wright p. 29; George Kingsbury, 'Correspondence: The New Mesmerism', *Times*, 9 January 1893, p. 7.

[8] Frederick Myers, 'Correspondence: The New Mesmerism', *Times*, 14 January 1893, p. 3.

[9] Charles Lloyd Tuckey (1893) 'A New Hypnotism: A Reply to Mr E Hart's "The Revival of Witchcraft".' *The Contemporary Review* (1893) 63: 416–9.

the process known as boundary-work.[10] However, the major puzzle for today's readers would be why the general readership of the Times newspaper might be interested in a technical medical matter about therapeutic hypnotism and a dispute about its name. The peaking public interest in hypnotism, at around this time, is the subject of this chapter.

Educating the Public

Despite the fact that the general public had routine exposure to mesmerism/hypnotism in the form of platform mesmerists, stage magicians and spiritualists, in the 1890s, the public appetite for information about medical hypnotism was insatiable. In an era before radio and television and other forms of mass communication, the main source of facts about new scientific developments was the printed word. The increased literacy that followed changes in Victorian education policy meant that the reading public was considerable and there were a large number of periodicals and journals, in addition to daily newspapers, which catered to them. Most of the gentleman's journals included scientific articles alongside short stories, news, opinion and poems.

Physicians were among the scientists who provided essays in the gentleman's journals, aimed primarily for a lay audience. The extent of the late Victorian interest in hypnotism is demonstrated by the sheer number of these articles in the general journals over and above the longer theoretical works and practical manuals that were published at this time. *Poole's Index* was developed by the American librarian William Poole as the first systematic attempt to catalogue and index Victorian journals. Examining the entries between 1887 and 1896, reveals a total of 64 relevant items under the subject heading of 'hypnotism'.[11]

When Tuckey's third edition of *Psycho-Therapeutics* was published in 1892 it was reviewed for the lay readership of the periodicals not just the medical journals. The critic for the *Spectator*, a weekly journal covering

[10] Thomas Geiryn, 'Boundary-Work and the Demarcation of Science from Non-Science: Strains and Interests in Professional Ideologies of Scientists', *American Sociological Review*, 48 (1983) (pp. 781–95).

[11] The American librarian William Poole developed the first systematic attempt to catalogue and index Victorian journals. Hypnotism entry in *Poole's Index to Periodical Literature 1887–92 (2nd Supplement)*, (Gloucester, US: Peter Smith, 1963) (p. 206); *Poole's Index to Periodical Literature 1892–97 (3rd Supplement)* (Gloucester, US: Peter Smith, 1963) (p. 271).

current affairs, politics and the arts declared that *Psycho-Therapeutics* was, 'a book of which the interest is by no means exclusively or principally professional. It will be found to have the highest possible interest or even fascination for the general reader, with even a superficial knowledge of medical science.'[12]

There was a real eagerness for factual information about the new technology and there was no shortage of medical experts prepared to write books. I have already mentioned the longer works of Robert Felkin, Bramwell and George Kingsbury which along with Tuckey's books did much to promote medical hypnotism.[13] There were also pamphlets and books from other physicians which were antithetic. Norman Kerr, who had participated in the Hypnotism debate at the 1890 BMA conference in Birmingham. His letters to journals and newspapers and his book clearly articulated the dangers of hypnotism to both patients and doctors and cast doubt on its efficacy.[14]

There were a variety of accounts from physicians which were both for and against the New Hypnotism.[15] Although written for the lay public they went into considerable detail about the subtle differences between the views at the Salpêtrière and the Nancy school. They did not always represent the complexities accurately. For example, the British psychiatrist, Theodore Ewart took the title of his article for the *Nineteenth Century* from the theoretical model of the Nancy school, 'The Power of Suggestion' but went on to describe the key beliefs of the doctors at the Salpêtrière.[16] Such was the reputation of Jean-Martin Charcot that translations of his essays and those of his colleagues like Jules Luys (before his

[12] Anon, 'Dr Tuckey on Hypnotism', *Spectator*, 68 (1892) 55–6 (p. 55).

[13] Robert Felkin, *Hypnotism or Psycho-Therapeutics* (*Edinburgh:* Y. J. Pentland, 1890); John Milne Bramwell, *Successful Treatment of Dipsomania, Insomnia,* etc., *and Various Diseases by Hypnotic Suggestion* (London: n.p.) (1890–92) I have only found a partial reference to this book from the early 1890s and have not been able to locate a copy; Kingsbury, *Hypnotic Suggestion.*

[14] Norman Kerr, *Should Hypnotism Have a Recognised Place in Ordinary Therapeutics?* (London: H.K. Lewis, 1890).

[15] *Inter alia* St. Clair Thomson, 'The Dangers of Hypnotism', *Westminster Review*, July 1890 (pp. 624–31).

[16] C. Theodore Ewart, 'The Power of Suggestion', *Nineteenth Century,* 28 (1890) (pp. 252–9).

disgrace) could be published directly in translation in many Anglophone journals.[17]

Hypnotism and Medicolegal Cases

Occasionally there are high-profile court cases which put the complexities of medical debate and in this era early psychological thinking into the spotlight. Criminal cases, in particular, have long fascinated the public and the historian Judith Flanders has argued that the Victorians revelled in murder and as a result created modern crime and its reporting.[18] In the early 1890s, there were two European high-profile murder cases that involved hypnotism which was closely followed and commented on in the UK. These were the French Eyraud-Bompard case of 1890 and the lesser-known Dutch De Jong murders of 1893.

Eyraud-Bompard Case: Hypnotism and Criminal Responsibility

The Eyraud-Bompard case seized the public imagination and put hypnotism back in the public eye both in France and Britain. It was reported in the *Times* that over 5000 people applied for the 80 available tickets to witness the hearing in Paris.[19] The previous year, Gabrielle Bompard had lured a wealthy Parisian bailiff named Alexandre-Toussaint Gouffé to her bedroom with promises of sex. While Gouffé was preoccupied, the waiting petty criminal Eyraud had strangled him with Bompard's silk belt (Fig. 7.1). The amateur scheme quickly unravelled when the couple discovered only a few Francs on Gouffé's person and realised they had to get rid of the body. They eventually dumped the corpse in an oilskin bag in woods outside Lyon, many miles from Paris. When the body was found and the police successfully identified the body, the pair fled the country. The case stayed in the newspapers for many months because, in an early triumph for the police and forensic procedure, the victim was successfully

[17] Jean-Martin Charcot, 'Magnetism and Hypnotism', *Forum*, 8 (1890) (pp. 566–77); Jean-Martin Charcot, 'Hypnotism and Crime', *Forum*, 9 (1890) (pp. 159–68); Jules Luys, 'The Latest Discoveries in Hypnotism I', *Fortnightly Review*, 47 (1890) (pp. 896–921); Jules Luys, 'The Latest Discoveries in Hypnotism II', *Fortnightly Review*, 48 (1890) (pp. 168–83).

[18] Judith Flanders, *The Invention of Murder* (London: Harper Press, 2011).

[19] Anon, 'The Gouffé Murder', *Times*, 17 December, 1890, p. 5.

identified and a trunk that had contained the bag and a boot linking the couple to the body were found near the crime scene. The couple fled to the United States and Cuba and, in another exciting scoop for the newspapers, were made subject to the first Interpol (international police) order and were tracked down and extradited for trial.

The infamous court case was closely covered by both the English and French press between December 1890 and February 1891 and has been subsequently reviewed by historians of law and psychology.[20] Gabrielle Bompard was only 22 years old and faced a death penalty for murder. Her defence claimed that she could not be held responsible because 'she had acted under a post-hypnotic suggestion implanted by her former lover.'[21] Several psychiatrists examined her and decided that while she was mildly hysterical, she was perfectly capable of knowing what she was doing. Jules Liégeois, a law professor who identified with the Nancy school, gave lengthy testimony to the effect that as Bompard had been hypnotised and was no more than an automaton. This testimony while damaging for the public confidence in medical hypnotism was apparently ignored by the court. Eyraud went to the guillotine while Bompard was imprisoned for 20 years. Her lesser sentence reflected the fact she had separated from Eyraud and had given herself up in the United States, rather than the success of the arguments of Liégeois.

The issue of criminal responsibility and the hypnotic state was discussed at length in the British daily press and periodicals. The Scottish solicitor and church historian Alexander Taylor Innes had written an essay on just that subject for the *Contemporary Review* the previous year.[22] Taylor Innes had observed that the 'scientific discussion of hypnotism/

[20] Robert van Plas, 'Hysteria, Hypnosis, and Moral Sense in French 19th-century Forensic Psychiatry. The Eyraud-Bompard case', *International Journal of Law and Psychiatry*, 21 (1998) (pp. 397–407); Steven Levingston, *Little Demon in the City of Light* (New York: Doubleday, 2014); Dorothy Hoobler and Thomas Hoobler, *The Crimes of Paris: A True Story of Murder, Theft, and Detection* (Lincoln, NE: Bison, 2010).

[21] Ruth Harris, 'Murder Under Hypnosis in the Case of Gabrielle Bompard: Psychiatry in the Courtroom in Belle Époque Paris' Ch 10 in *The Anatomy of Madness: Essays in the History of Psychiatry* II, ed. by William Bynum, Roy Porter and Michael Shepherd (London: Tavistock, 1987) (pp. 197–241).

[22] These are a fraction of the publications: 'The Gouffé Murder', *Times*; Charcot, 'Hypnotism and Crime'; A. Taylor Innes, 'Hypnotism in Relation to Crime and the Medical Faculty', *The Contemporary Review*, 58 (1890) (pp. 555–66); George Kingsbury, 'Hypnotism, Crime and Doctors', *Nineteenth Century*, 29 (1891) (pp. 145–53).

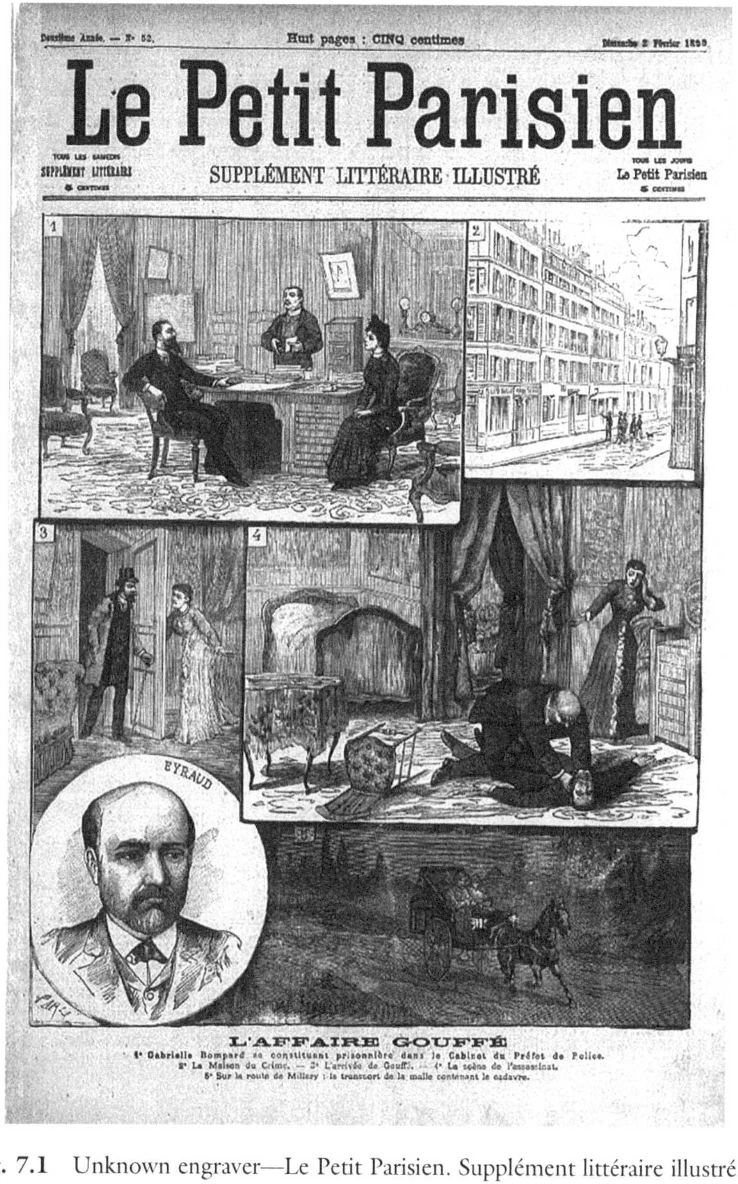
Deuxième Année. — N° 52. Hunt pages : CINQ centimes Dimanche 2 Février 1890

Le Petit Parisien

SUPPLÉMENT LITTÉRAIRE ILLUSTRÉ

L'AFFAIRE GOUFFÉ

1° Gabrielle Bompard se constituant prisonnière dans le Cabinet du Préfet de Police.
2° La Maison du Crime. — 3° L'arrivée de Gouffé. — 4° La scène de l'assassinat.
5° Sur la route de Millery : le transport de la malle contenant le cadavre.

Fig. 7.1 Unknown engraver—Le Petit Parisien. Supplément littéraire illustré, 2 février 1890, p. 1

mesmerism' had finally reached the UK and offered a legal viewpoint. He claimed that '[undoubtedly] hypnotism opens many possibilities of crime'.[23] He described hypnotic sleep as both passive and active proposing that the activity of somnambulism was of the imaginative not the rational faculty. This was portrayed negatively and shows that the associations with the doctrine of the imagination would not help the acceptance of hypnotism. He described several cases of automatic obedience and of post-hypnotic amnesia from his own experience and reflected how problematic this would be for both the victim and the 'witness box.' He chided the British medical profession for their previous reluctance to research the phenomena and wondered where the medical expert witnesses on the subject would come from. He finished by rejecting any legal restrictions on public hypnotism entertainments which the German medical profession had achieved.

Kingsbury's response to Taylor Innes was published in the sympathetic journal, the *Nineteenth Century*. Though written before the Eyraud-Bompard case, it was not published until January 1891 coinciding with the public interest in the case. Kingsbury had presciently predicted that there would be a case of murder with the defence of hypnotism 'at no distant date.' He took issue with Taylor Innes basic ideas of sleepwalking and automatic obedience under hypnosis. He agreed that there should be more research into hypnotism but reflected that some of the blame was down to the views of the general public and the 'alarmist writers who caused the public to look askance at any medical man who dared to identify himself with the "uncanny" thing.'[24] He described the links in the public mind to sorcery, witchcraft and the devil. He suggested that hypnotic entertainments should be banned but on the grounds of taste, the proofs of entrancement in stage hypnotism being cruel and degrading: stitching tongues and eating potatoes for apples.

Liegeois' assertion at the trial, that hypnotism caused automatic obedience may have contributed to a belief in the potency of hypnotism but it also became problematic for the Nancy school and its British adherents. Particularly so when they also made the claim that everyone was susceptible to hypnotism. The helpless automation image would continue to be used by hypnotism's detractors and would need to be regularly rebuffed.

[23] Taylor Innes, 'Hypnotism', p. 555.

[24] Kingsbury, 'Hypnotism, Crime', p. 148.

The De Jong Murders: Hypnotism in Forced Confessions

A few years later, a less famous European murder made headlines in the British press and led to further discussion of the power of hypnotism. The unsolved cases of the potential serial killer have been recently rediscovered and reviewed by the Dutch historians Jan Bondeson and Bart Droog.[25] In 1893, at least one Dutch newspaper had proposed the use of hypnotism to force a confession from the prime suspect Hendrik de Jong and to ascertain the whereabouts of his two missing wives. This was quickly picked up by the UK press, in part because one of his victims was English (Fig. 7.2).[26]

De Jong was a handsome confidence trickster well known to the Dutch police for preying on rich women. In June of 1893, the Dutch national

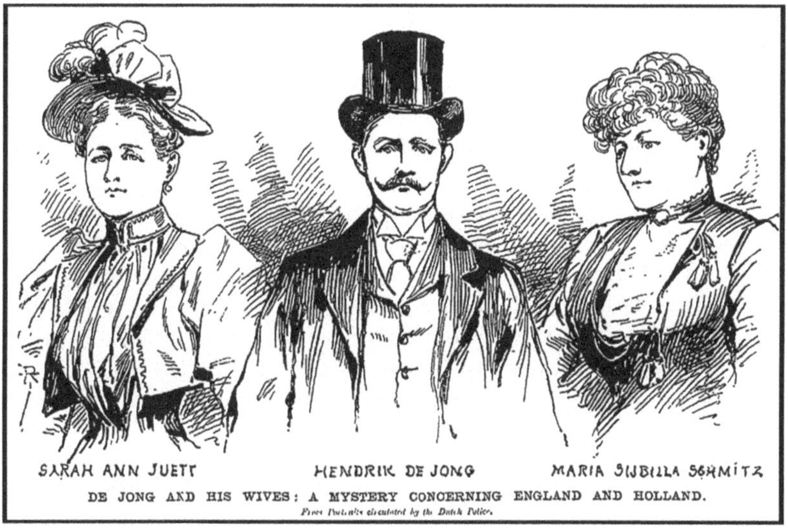
SARAH ANN JUETT
HENDRIK DE JONG
MARIA SIJBILLA SCHMITZ
DE JONG AND HIS WIVES: A MYSTERY CONCERNING ENGLAND AND HOLLAND.
From Portraits circulated by the Dutch Police.

Fig. 7.2 'The De Jong Case' (1893), unknown engraver in the Penny Illustrated Paper (London: Henry Taylor)

[25] Jan Bondeson and Bart Droog, 'The Dutch Jack the Ripper: New Light on Hendrik De Jong, "The Continental Suspect"' *Ripperologist, The Journal of Jack the Ripper, East End and Victorian Studies,* 159 (December 2017/ January 2018) (pp. 2–25).

[26] Anon, 'De Zaak-De Jong' *De Tijd*, 7 October, 1893 p. 4.

had married an English nurse named Sarah Ann Juett in Maidenhead, England. They had returned to the Netherlands where Sarah mysteriously vanished and de Jong then wasted no time in marrying a wealthy Dutchwoman, Maria Schmitz in the August. Before his proposal to Sarah Ann, he had claimed to the Juett family that he was a wealthy hotel proprietor who had studied medicine. He had told Maria Schmitz that he was a military surgeon from the Dutch East Indies. The truth was more prosaic: he was born to a peasant family and despite two periods in the Dutch army stationed in Batavia, he had been discharged as unfit for military service.

The Juett family was convinced that de Jong was a fraudster and probably a murderer. They made contact with the Dutch police who had arrested de Jong following the disappearance of Maria. The evidence against de Jong was suspicious but only circumstantial. Screams and moans had been heard in Laren's Camp, just outside Amsterdam, on the night of Maria's disappearance and a spade had been found inside one of de Jong's cases. Despite the involvement of over forty constables and volunteers the bodies of his wives were never found.

Juett's brother travelled to Amsterdam and interviewed de Jong and identified two dresses and a gold necklace found in a local pawn shop as belonging to Sarah Anne. The Dutch papers were convinced of his guilt but de Jong appeared unflappable in police custody and repeated his view that both women would soon reappear. Even when Juett's father came to see him begging for an admission of guilt, de Jong showed no remorse stating 'I shall be free. I shall walk out of here. You cannot keep me.'[27] The case started to attract more attention in the UK when Tom Fielders, the Amsterdam correspondent of the *Pall Mall Gazette* repeated the growing speculation in the Dutch press about De Jong's probable previous murders and the possibility that he might even be Jack the Ripper.[28] De Jong never confessed to the crimes and was eventually tried for fraud in April 1894 and imprisoned for three years.[29]

These hypnotic criminal cases also led to ideas around criminal responsibility and the moral limits of hypnotic control being played out within fiction. The early fictions of mesmerism had mostly centred on fears

[27] Anon, 'The De Jong Case', *New York Herald,* 1 November, 1893.

[28] Tom Fielders, 'The Maidenhead Mystery. De Jong's antecedents. Is he "Jack the Ripper"?', *Pall Mall Gazette*, 2 October, 1893, p. 3.

[29] Anon, 'The De Jong Case', *Times*, 13 April 1894, p. 5.

of romantic infatuation and loss of virtue and reputation. These were linked to the prevalent views about increased female susceptibility and the intimacy of mesmeric passes and rapport. However, by the end of the nineteenth century, the societal fears about hypnotism had moved on to include the consequences of loss of will and the fearsome power of the evil hypnotist if automatic obedience was correct.

In keeping with his growing national profile, Tuckey was soon identified as the leading English expert on hypnotism. In October 1893, a reporter for the *Illustrated London News* stated that 'One would certainly like to hear what Dr. Lloyd Tuckey would say about the proposal to hypnotise de Jong.'[30] However Tuckey chose to wait a few months to give his view. He accepted an interview about his opinion towards the possible use of hypnotism to extract a confession in the De Jong case for *The Sketch* in February 1894.[31] The *Sketch* was a weekly journal that had been established the previous year. It was primarily a society magazine which had regular features on the aristocracy and royalty, theatre and literature. It is significant that the journalist, T.H. claims that he went to see his 'friend' Tuckey, reporting the interview over a page of the journal:

> Such knowledge of modern hypnotism as we have arrived at in this country – from the scientific and medical standpoints – is owing mainly to Dr Tuckey, who was the first West-End physician of repute courageous enough to give the treatment a fair trial and whose treatise on the subject, "Psycho-Therapeutics", is the clearest and ablest exposition of it that may be read in English.

Tuckey told T.H. that he had been in contact with his friend, the Netherlands' premier medical hypnotist Frederik van Eeden whose clinic he had previously visited in 1888. Despite the Dutch newspapers' claims, Tuckey had clarified by letter that the police had not made any contact with either van Eeden or his physician colleague de Jong [same surname] about a possible hypnotic interview with the suspect de Jong.[32] The interviewer asked whether or not he believed in the possibility of the 'famous scene in *The Bells* where Mathias, under the influence of a mesmerist,

[30] Anon, 'De Jong Case', *Illustrated London News*, 14 October, 1893, p. 4.

[31] T.H., 'Hypnotism in Criminal Investigation', *Sketch*, 4, (1894) p. 244.

[32] Charles Lloyd Tuckey to van Eeden correspondence, 14 October 1893. *Van Eeden Collection*. Amsterdam, Allard Pierson, University of Amsterdam.

shows how he murdered the Polish Jew.' *The Bells* was a popular play written by Leopold Lewis in 1871, earlier than the 1890s flowering of hypnotic fiction. It had run intermittently for several decades in the West End as a vehicle for the great actor-manager Henry Irving. As a marker of the enduring popularity of hypnotic-themed work in late Victorian Britain, Irving revived it on many occasions, playing the role of the Polish Jew Mathias right up until the night before his own death in 1905. Tuckey replied to the reporter that it was very unreal. 'A person who had never before been mesmerised, could not suddenly be taken in hand and compelled to betray himself in this way.'[33]

He maintained that a hypnotic subject could not be hypnotised against their will which limited its possible role both for the police and criminal parties: 'Where there is not only an absence of sympathy but vehement opposition, then hypnotism can accomplish very little.'[34] He was pushed as to whether crimes might be commissioned or induced by hypnotism. He said there was little cause for alarm as only the weak-minded and morally lax might be persuaded so the numbers would be small.

There are several details in the article which provide an interesting subtext. The journal, the *Sketch* was aimed at the gentry and affluent middle class. The journalist's description of Tuckey as a 'friend' and 'West-End physician' suggests that he would expect his readership to be already familiar with his name. It also repeats the view that some bravery was required to advocate and experiment with hypnotism, demonstrating that the impact of Elliotson's fall was felt even in the lay community over fifty years later.

The high-profile cases on the continent sparked further British interest in hypnotism and therapeutic hypnotism and the New Hypnotists became the experts, significantly raising their profile. The belief that hypnotism was fake and therefore ineffective was challenged by the antithetic idea that it was very real and too dangerous to use. These mutually exclusive views were both held by the public.

[33] T.H., 'Criminal Investigation'.

[34] T.H., 'Criminal Investigation'.

Hypnotic Fictions and Trilby Madness

The cultural prominence of hypnotism in the 1890s was inescapable. By 1895, the poet, novelist and literary critic, *Q* or Arthur Quiller-Couch had had enough. He had written a critical notice for the British journal *The Speaker*, a popular, liberal-leaning magazine that reviewed the week's literature, science and politics. The object of his exasperation was the contemporary popularity but what Q perceived to be the literary limitations of what he termed 'hypnotic fiction'.[35] Q saw George du Maurier's *Trilby* as one of the better examples of a rather hackneyed, well-worn storyline, which he had identified and could not abide. He was scornful of the genre as a whole but grudgingly complimentary about du Maurier's 'charming' original novel which had been published in instalments in *Harper's Monthly*, the year before (Fig. 7.3).[36]

Q drew attention to the recurring themes of hypnotiser and his subject, a good and beautiful woman, who is induced by the nefarious, foreign beast to 'commit any excesses that his beastliness may suggest'.[37] He complained that the plot device of hypnotism, by removing free will, removed any sense of a personal struggle against immoral behaviour. He worried that this lack of realism diminished the human drama and in the hands of authors with 'less tact' than du Maurier could lead to fictions that were more 'brutish,' for which I read sexually explicit.

There were, of course, several pornographic novels already published that utilised hypnotism or mesmerism as the central plot device for exactly this brutish, narrative end. One of the anonymous underground pornographic books that survive from this period is *The Power of Mesmerism—A Highly Erotic Narrative of Voluptuous Facts and Fancies*. In this titillating book, Frank Etheridge dabbles for a summer with mesmerism and sex with his entire family. In so doing, he repeatedly breaks the oldest taboo of all, that of incest.[38]

[35] Arthur Quiller Couch, 'A Literary Causerie: Hypnotic Fiction', *Speaker* (14 September 1895) (p. 316).

[36] George du Maurier, *Trilby*, (Peterborough, Canada: Broadview Press, 2003).

[37] Couch, 'Hypnotic fictions' (p. 316).

[38] Anon, *The Power of Mesmerism* (Moscow: For the Nihilists, 1891).

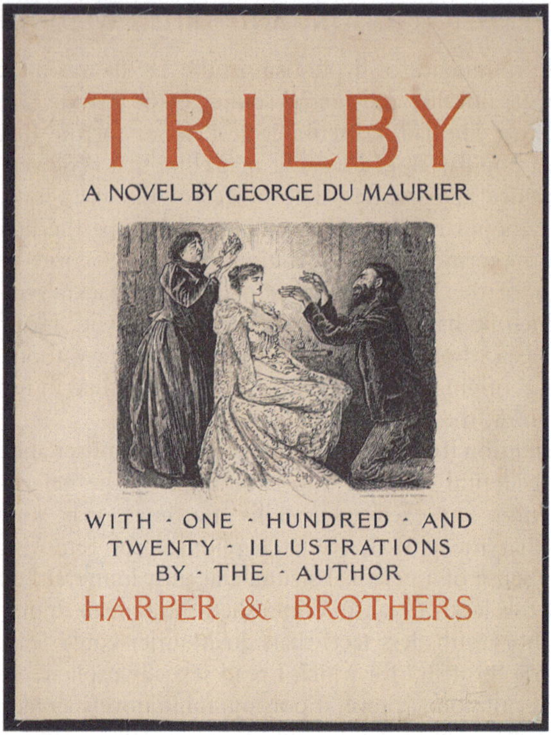

Fig. 7.3 Du Maurier, George, Artist. *Trilby, a novel by George Du Maurier.*, 1894. [New York: Harper & Brothers] Photograph. https://www.loc.gov/item/2014649141/

Mary Leighton, the cultural historian, has confirmed both the accuracy and quantity of publications in Q's newly described genre and narrative stereotype.[39] Though mesmerism had been a small aspect of many mid-Victorian novels, from the mid-1880s to the mid-1890s there was a sudden outburst of published fictions, mostly short stories for the literary journals but also dozens of full-length novels, which corresponded to his

[39] Mary Leighton, 'Under the Influence: Crime and Hypnotic Fictions of the Fin de Siècle', Ch. 10 in *Victorian Literary Mesmerism*, ed. by Martin Willis and Catherine Wynne. (Amsterdam: Rodolphi, 2006) pp. 203–26.

description.[40] The librarian and anthologist, Donald Hartman collected and published a bibliography of over 60 English language novels featuring mesmerism and hypnotism themes between 1885 and 1898.[41]

While crazes and fads were not new, with the hypnotic fiction *Trilby*, the 1890s saw some of the first examples of genuine modern mass culture. Primarily writing about the North American context, several writers have explored the publishing, printing and advertising framework which created the positive feedback loop that led to the cultural phenomenon that was 'Trilbyana' or 'Trilbymania'.[42] These aspects still held true in Britain. Even at the time the mass obsession was so unprecedented that there were books written reflecting on the story's reach and ubiquity.[43] *It has been described* as the first great example of how the 'machinery of promotion, distribution, secondary rights, and social hoopla would work.'[44]

The remarkable success of the novel *Trilby* and its subsequent dramatisation marked the high-water mark for 'hypnotic fictions' (no longer mesmeric).[45] *Trilby* was the zenith if not artistically, at least culturally and by the sheer scale of books sold. It sold so many copies of the one volume edition, that it is acknowledged as one of the first ever bestsellers. It sold 200,000 copies in the United States alone and is believed to be among the highest selling novels of the nineteenth century.[46] To capitalise on

[40] Walter Besant, *Herr Paulus: His Rise, His Greatness and His Fall* (London: Chatto and Windus, 1888); Robert Buchanan and Henry Murray, *The Charlatan* (London: Chatto and Windus, 1895); Ernest Clark Oliphant, *The Mesmerist* (London: Eden Remington, 1890).

[41] Donald Hartman, 'Hypnotic and Mesmeric Themes and Motifs in Selected English-Language Novels, Short Stories, Plays and Poems, 1820–1983', *Bulletin of Bibliography,* 44 (1987) (pp. 156–66).

[42] Emily Jenkins, 'Trilby: Fads, Photographers, and "Over-Perfect Feet"', *Book History*, 1 (1998) pp. 221–67 (p. 221); Edward Purcell, '*Trilby* and Trilbymania: The Beginning of the Best-Seller System', *Journal of Popular Culture,* 11 (1977) (pp. 62–76); *Joanna Levin, Bohemia in America, 1858–1920* (Stanford: Stanford University Press, 2009) (p. 193).

[43] J.B. Gilder and J.D. Gilder, *Trilbyana: The Rise and Progress of a Popular Novel* (New York: The Critic, 1895).

[44] L. Edward Purcell, qtd in Emily Jenkins, 'Trilby: Fads, Photographers, and "Over-Perfect Feet"', *Book History*, 1 (1998) pp. 221–67 (p. 221).

[45] Couch, 'Hypnotic Fiction' (p. 316).

[46] Gilder, Preface in '*Trilbyana*'.

the trend, American manufacturers produced *Trilby*-branded merchandise: perfumes, cigars, waltzes, corsets, cocktail sausages, hair styles and even foot-shaped ice-creams. Trilby's foot became an unlikely commoditization of the girl in both the book and the play and symbolised her widespread popularity. In a strange example of life imitating art, representations of her image and particularly her foot were sold because her celebrated voice was ephemeral.[47]

The magazine serialisation of *Trilby* may have been first published in the UK but the cultural obsession of Trilbymania had started in the United States. By the autumn of 1895, London too, had 'lost its head'.[48] The drama was so popular that the play ran for 254 performances at the West End theatre, the *Haymarket* from October 1895. It then went on to tour the provinces and crossed the Atlantic to tour the States, where several previous US productions had already been successful. It made so much money for its actor-manager, Herbert Tree that he was then able to rebuild and become a lessee of *Her Majesty's Theatre*.[49] Even the new style of short-brimmed hat worn by the women attending the *Trilby* matinee shows, became known by the name of the play.

The *Trilby* story itself was set in mid-nineteenth-century Bohemian Paris. Starting as a love story, it chronicles the life of the artists' model, Trilby O'Ferrall and her relationship with four men: three struggling British artists and a Jewish musician. She turns down the offer of marriage to one of the artists to protect his societal standing. She is then taken in by the musician, Svengali who hypnotises her, initially to cure her headache. However, he discovers her beautiful singing voice while in trance and keeps her in his hypnotic thrall. She becomes a music-hall diva as a result of her newfound range and exquisite tone before Svengali dies dramatically mid-concert, leaving her as she was: without talent. There is a brief reunion with her artist lover but Trilby fades and dies soon after.

The reasons for the enduring popular appeal of the various iterations of *Trilby* appear to transcend the original, mawkish novel concerning the life and loves of a tone-deaf laundress, living with British artists in 1850s Paris and transformed into a singing superstar by her hypnotist manager. The

[47] Emily Jenkins, 'Trilby: Fads' (p. 250).

[48] Daniel Pick, *Svengali's Web: The Alien Enchanter in Modern Culture* (New Haven: Yale University Press, 2000) (p. 22).

[49] Tracy Davis, *The Economics of the British Stage, 1800–1914* (Cambridge: Cambridge University Press, 2000) (p. 225).

characters and depictions of power are far more resonant than the details and style of the story. From the first dramatic production onwards, the focus was shifted away from the innocent girl and the romantic aspects, to the unequal relationship between Trilby and the Jewish mesmeric manipulator, Svengali. The story made an easy transition from stage to screen and thence to other European nations. The first silent cinematic version was released as early as 1896 and by 1915, there had been 10 cinematic versions. However, after this the films were usually named after the villain of the piece, *Svengali*.

The historian and psychotherapist, Daniel Pick has written extensively about *Trilby* and its cultural implications and consequences, particularly focussing on the sinister Jewish foreigner stereotype.[50] He has identified four aspects which might have led to its overwhelming popularity at the turn of the last century: its 'complicity with anti-Semitism, the charm of its picture of Bohemia, its fascination with mesmerism, or the mournful and melancholic rendition of a lost Paris'.[51]

For the purposes of this book, it is the presentation of hypnotism which is most relevant. Clearly, the success of any book or play depends upon aspects of the story connecting and resonating with the general public, in the case of Trilby these are the hypnotic elements. One reviewer for *Harper's Weekly* observed 'Hypnotism and kindred psychological problems are immensely attractive to most of us and Du Maurier's use of mesmeric tools is masterly.'[52] Trilby displays two tropes that will recur and which reflected the contemporary views of hypnotism, that of automatic obedience and its use in uncovering latent artistic and creative ability. In the chapter after next I will look at other fictions to demonstrate the specific themes that hypnotic stories both reflected but also shaped in the cross-fertilisation between medical and popular culture.

Bibliography

Anon. 1890. 'The Gouffé Murder', *Times* (17 December) 5.

[50] Pick, Svengali's Web.

[51] Daniel Pick, 'Powers of Suggestion: Svengali and the Fin-de-Siècle', Ch. 6 in *Modernity, Culture and 'The Jew'* ed. by Bryan Cheyette and Laura Marcus (Cambridge: Polity Press, 1998) pp. 105–25 (p. 119).

[52] Margaret Sangster, '"Trilby" from a Woman's Point of View', *Harpers Weekly,* 38 (September 1894) (p. 883).

Anon. 1891. *The Power of Mesmerism*. Moscow: For the Nihilists.
Anon. 1892. 'Dr Tuckey on Hypnotism', *Spectator*, 68: 55–6.
Anon. 1893. 'De Zaak-De Jong' *De Tijd* (7 October) 4.
Anon. 1893. 'The De Jong Case', *New York Herald* (1 November).
Anon. 1893. 'De Jong Case', *Illustrated London News* (14 October) 4.
Anon. 1894. 'The De Jong Case', *Times* (13 April) 5.
Besant, Walter. 1888. *Herr Paulus: His Rise, His Greatness and His Fall*. London: Chatto and Windus.
Bondeson, Jan and Droog, Bart. 2017–8. 'The Dutch Jack the Ripper: New Light on Hendrik De Jong, "The Continental Suspect"' *Ripperologist, The Journal of Jack the Ripper, East End and Victorian Studies*, 159: 2–25.
Bramwell, John Milne. 1890–2. *Successful Treatment of Dipsomania, Insomnia, etc., and Various Diseases by Hypnotic Suggestion*. London: n.p.
Buchanan, Robert, and Henry Murray, Henry. 1895. *The Charlatan*. London: Chatto and Windus.
Buckle, George. 1893. 'Leading Article: The New Mesmerism', *Times* (11 January) 9.
Bucknill, John, and Tuke, Daniel Hack. 1858. *A Manual of Psychological Medicine*. London: John Churchill.
Bucknill, John. 1893. 'The New Mesmerism II', *Times* (5 January) 6.
Bucknill John. 1893. 'The New Mesmerism III', *Times* (11 January) 8.
Charcot, Jean-Martin. 1890. 'Magnetism and Hypnotism', *Forum*, 8: 566–77.
Charcot, Jean-Martin. 1890. 'Hypnotism and Crime', *Forum* 9: 159–68.
Ewart, C. Theodore. 1890. 'The Power of Suggestion', *Nineteenth Century* 28: 252–9.
Davis, Tracy. 2000. *The Economics of the British Stage, 1800–1914*. Cambridge: Cambridge University Press. 225.
du Maurier, George. 2003. *Trilby*. Peterborough, Canada, Broadview Press.
Felkin, Robert. 1890. *Hypnotism or Psycho-Therapeutics. Edinburgh:* Y. J. Pentland.
Fielders, Tom. 1893. 'The Maidenhead Mystery. De Jong's antecedents. Is he "Jack the Ripper"?', *Pall Mall Gazette* (2 October) 3.
Flanders, Judith. 2011. *The Invention of Murder*. London: Harper Press.
Gieryn, Thomas. 1983. 'Boundary-Work and the Demarcation of Science from Non-Science: Strains and Interests in Professional Ideologies of Scientists', *American Sociological Review* 48, 6: 781–795.
Gilder, J.B., and Gilder, J.D. *Trilbyana: The Rise and Progress of a Popular Novel*. New York: The Critic.
Hart, Ernest. 1893. 'Correspondence: The New Mesmerism', *Times* (10 January) 8.
Harris, Ruth. 1987. 'Murder Under Hypnosis in the Case of Gabrielle Bompard: Psychiatry in the Courtroom in Belle Époque Paris', Ch 10 in *The Anatomy*

of Madness: Essays in the History of Psychiatry II, ed. by William Bynum, Roy Porter and Michael Shephard. London: Tavistock. 197–241.

Hartman, Donald. 1987. 'Hypnotic and Mesmeric Themes and Motifs in Selected English-Language Novels, Short Stories, Plays and Poems, 1820–1983', *Bulletin of Bibliography,* 44: 156–66.

Hoobler, Dorothy, and Hoobler, Thomas. 2010. *The Crimes of Paris: A True Story of Murder, Theft, and Detection*. Lincoln, NE: Bison.

Innes, A. Taylor. 1890. 'Hypnotism in Relation to Crime and the Medical Faculty', *The Contemporary Review* 58: 555–66.

Jenkins, Emily. 1998. 'Trilby: Fads, Photographers, and "Over-Perfect Feet"' *Book History* 1: 221–267.

Kerr, Norman. 1890. *Should Hypnotism Have a Recognised Place in Ordinary Therapeutics?* London: H.K. Lewis.

Kingsbury, George. 1891. 'Hypnotism, Crime and the Doctors', *Nineteenth Century* 29, 167 (January): 145–153.

Kingsbury, George. 1891. *The Practice of Hypnotic Suggestion, Being and Elementary Handbook for the Use of the Medical Profession*. Bristol: John Wright.

Kingsbury, George. 1893. 'Correspondence: The New Mesmerism', *Times* (9 January 1893) 7.

Leighton, Mary. 2006. 'Under the Influence: Crime and Hypnotic Fictions of the Fin de Siècle', Ch 10 in *Victorian Literary Mesmerism,* ed. by Martin Willis and Catherine Wynne. Amsterdam: Rodolphi. 203–26.

Levin, Joanna. 2009. *Bohemia in America, 1858–1920.* Stanford: Stanford University Press. 193.

Levingston, Steven. 2013. *Little Demon in the City of Light.* New York: Doubleday.

Luys, Jules. 1890. 'The Latest Discoveries in Hypnotism I', *Fortnightly Review* 47: 896–921.

Luys. Jules. 1890. 'The Latest Discoveries in Hypnotism II', *Fortnightly Review* 48: 168–83.

Myers, Frederick. 1893. 'Correspondence: The New Mesmerism', *Times* (14 January) 3.

Oliphant, Ernest Clark.1890. *The Mesmerist.* London: Eden Remington.

Pick, Daniel.1998. 'Powers of Suggestion: Svengali and the Fin-de-Siècle', Ch. 6 in *Modernity, Culture and 'The Jew'* ed by Bryan Cheyette and Laura Marcus. Cambridge: Polity Press. 105–25.

Pick, Daniel. 2000. *Svengali's Web: The Alien Enchanter in Modern Culture.* New Haven: Yale University Press.

Poole, William. 1963. *Poole's Index to Periodical Literature 1887–92* (2nd Supplement). Gloucester, MA: Peter Smith.

Poole, William. 1963. *Poole's Index to Periodical Literature 1892–97* (3rd Supplement). Gloucester, MA: Peter Smith.
Purcell, Edward. 1977. '*Trilby* and Trilbymania: The Beginning of the Best-Seller System', *Journal of Popular Culture,* 11: 62–76.
Quiller-Couch, A. 1895. 'A Literary Causerie: Hypnotic Fiction.' *Speaker* (14 September).
Sangster, Margaret. 1894. '"Trilby" from a Woman's Point of View', *Harpers Weekly,* 38 (September) 883.
T.H. 1894. 'Hypnotism in Criminal Investigation', *Sketch* 4: 244.
Thomson, St. Clair. 1890. 'The Dangers of Hypnotism', *Westminster Review* (July) 624–31.
Tuckey, Charles Lloyd. 1893. Letter to van Eeden, October 24th, 1893. In *Van Eeden Collection.* Amsterdam, Allard Pierson, University of Amsterdam.
Tuckey, Charles Lloyd. 1893. 'A New Hypnotism: A reply to Mr E Hart's "The Revival of Witchcraft".' *Contemporary Review* 63: 416–419.
van Plas, Robert 1998. 'Hysteria, Hypnosis, and Moral Sense in French 19th-century Forensic Psychiatry. The Eyraud-Bompard case', *International Journal of Law and Psychiatry* 21: 397–407.

CHAPTER 8

Social Networks and Hypnotic Influences

Charles Lloyd Tuckey and the other New Hypnotists were all highly socially active. It could never harm a doctor's practice to be well-connected. These connections are particularly relevant because these clubs were sites of discussion, exploration and elaboration of hypnotic ideas. Tuckey in particular was a member of many different clubs, some of which were more predictable, traditional and conservative, like the Royal Institution which Tuckey visited for scientific lectures and the ritualistic, secretive, business-promoting Freemasons. In the late 1880s, Tuckey joined their 'Imperial Lodge 1694,' which held its meetings in Chelsea. He was elected as its Worshipful Master, serving from 1898 to 1899. This meant he was the most senior officer at the lodge and the one who presided over all the ceremonies.[1]

However, some of Tuckey and his colleagues' other non-medical clubs might appear surprising at first sight, they also joined societies for ceremonial magic, psychical research and educational reform. We know that John Milne Bramwell was a member of the Society for Psychical Research

[1] He subsequently kept his involvement to a modest level. He did not achieve any position in the national organization, the United Grand Lodge of England. Sue Young, 'Charles Tuckey', in *Work on the Hermetic Order of the Golden Dawn*. www.wrightanddavis.co.uk/GD/TUCKEYCHARLESL.htm [accessed 13 April 2023].

G. D. L. Bates, *The Uncanny Rise of Medical Hypnotism, 1888–1914*, Mental Health in Historical Perspective,
https://doi.org/10.1007/978-3-031-42725-1_8

(SPR) and that Robert Felkin became involved in Theosophy and then occultism. With their social links the New Hypnotists did not just teach others about hypnotic possibilities, they learned about other potential hypnotic futures from others' perspectives. Occultists, psychic researchers, theosophists and educationalists all rubbed shoulders and shared their own ideas about hypnotism and what they could achieve with it. Within the social networks, theories about hypnotic action and uses were freely discussed.

The Hermetic Order of the Golden Dawn

As was the standard procedure, Tuckey's membership of the Freemasons made him eligible to become a member of two other freemasonry groups: a lodge, and a 'lodge-like order.' He chose as his second lodge *Quatuor Coronati*, which was a forum for research into the history and rituals of freemasonry. His chosen lodge-like group was the *Societas Rosicruciana in Anglia* (*SRIA*), which was not identical to a freemasons' lodge but only freemasons could join. Like *Quatuor Coronati*, the *SRIA* focused on the esoteric side of freemasonry. The members were particularly interested in the contributions that Rosicrucian legends had made and could make to freemasonry.[2] Rosicrucianism was a seventeenth-century form of mysticism which claimed access to hidden truths which provided insight into nature, the physical world and the spiritual realm. There were close links between the Hermetic Order of the Golden Dawn (henceforth Golden Dawn) and the SRIA, both in membership and rituals. It seems likely that this was Tuckey's route for discovery and then entry into the Golden Dawn, itself.

At the fin de siècle the boundaries between science and magic were not so distinct and obvious as today. The idea of a physician becoming interested in the occult was not so strange and a club was the place to further those interests. The Golden Dawn was one of the most exclusive and influential of the occult groups. It was established by two freemason doctors, William Wescott and William Woodman and the Rosicrucian and talented linguist, Samuel Mathers. Drawing their complex tiered organisational structure of neophytes to adepts to magi, from British Freemasonry

[2] Sue Young, www.wrightanddavis.co.uk/GD/TUCKEYCHARLESL.htm [accessed 13 April 2023].

and their teachings primarily from the Jewish Kabbalah and Egyptian writings, together they founded their first temple, Isis-Urania in London in 1888.[3] Perhaps as a result of its emphasis on the role of the imagination in human development, writers and artists had a particular affinity with the Golden Dawn. Other famous members of the London branch included the authors and poets Arthur Machen, W. B. Yeats, Arnold Bennett and Edith Bland (better known as E. Nesbit).[4] The society also claimed the most prominent occultists of their day, though some would go on to follow their own separate mystic inquiries and establish their own orders: A. E Waite, Aleister Crowley and Dion Fortune.

The Golden Dawn had many physician members: there were a total of 14 physicians prior to 1900 in a total membership of only a few hundred.[5] Other doctors in the Golden Dawn who were likely to be known to Tuckey included the homoeopath, Edward Berridge and one of the London temple's most active members, Henry Pullen Burry.

In a letter to his colleague van Eeden written in 1894, Tuckey talks of his plans of 'going in seriously for a course of occultism and I expect to emerge from it more liberal minded and with extended sympathies. I find it so necessary to take up new lines of thought from time to time or I become petrified.'[6] The casual almost flippant nature of the comment in Tuckey's letter about taking a course makes it clear that Tuckey was simply interested in another source of knowledge that he did not view as either sinister or spurious or antithetic to scientific inquiry. This would be consistent with the view of occultism as a method of self-development rather than the amoralistic sexmagic with which it would become later associated. With his growing expertise in hypnotism, it seems likely that Tuckey wished to investigate all avenues of learning on the subject.

[3] Dennis Denisoff, 'The Hermetic Order of the Golden Dawn, 1888–1901', *BRANCH: Britain, Representation and Nineteenth-Century History*, ed. by Dino Franco Felluga. Extension of *Romanticism and Victorianism on the Net* [accessed 8 July 2019].

[4] R. A. Gilbert, *The Golden Dawn Companion: A Guide to the History, Structure and Workings of the Hermetic Order of the Golden Dawn* (Wellingborough: Aquarian Books, 1986) (pp. 125–75). Gilbert's book contains a membership list.

[5] Alex Owen, *The Place of Enchantment: British Occultism and the Culture of the Modern* (Chicago: University Press of Chicago, 2004) (p. 61).

[6] Charles Lloyd Tuckey to van Eeden correspondence (19 August 1894). *Van Eeden Collection* (Amsterdam: Allard Pierson, University of Amsterdam).

Tuckey was initiated into the outer order of the Golden Dawn at its Isis-Uranis temple in London on July 21, 1894.[7] The membership of the temple was deliberately small and exclusive. Only 29 people were nominated and accepted for membership that year including George Rowell, an anaesthetist at Guys Hospital. All neophytes would appear blindfolded in front of an altar decorated with a cross and triangle, a red rose and a red lamp. They would wear a black gown, red shoes and a sash and hold a rope. During the ceremony they would take on a new name to symbolise their rebirth and Tuckey chose the Latin motto, *Stant Robora Vires* or 'virtues stand like trees.'[8]

Robert Felkin also became a member at the Amen-Ra temple, another Golden Dawn centre, in Edinburgh later the same year before moving to London for a more senior role at Isis-Uranis. The historian Alex Owen has proposed that it was Felkin who helped to screen and then invited Conan Doyle to join the arcane order in 1898, during an apparently chance meeting with the medical author.[9] This is a clear demonstration of the unlikely proximity of hypnotism, medicine, spiritualism and the occult at this time. Conan Doyle recalled the unsettling incident in his autobiography more than 25 years later, describing the feeling that he was being interrogated from afar: 'I remain under the impression that I brushed against something strange, and something that I am not sorry that I avoided.'[10]

While Felkin played an important role in the history of British occultism, Tuckey's membership with the organisation was short-lived. We must assume that Tuckey took his training further than the initiation ritual though, since the letter to van Eeden was written after he had gone through that ceremony. It seems he took his studies no further than the basics, as he did not proceed to the inner order and formally resigned from the order in November 1895.

[7] Gilbert, 'Membership' (p. 153).

[8] Darcy Kuntz, *The Golden Source Book.* (Edmonds, WA: Holmes, 1996) (p. 216).

[9] Owen, *The Place of Enchantment* (p. 224).

[10] Arthur Conan Doyle, *Memories and Adventures* (Oxford: Oxford University Press, 1989) (p. 151).

Personal Development and the Will

The Golden Dawn's message of personal betterment through industry, private study and arcane teaching resonated powerfully with many middle-class professionals and was a powerful draw in the late Victorian period. Their teaching on personal will and hypnotism are also relevant to my argument. There was ongoing debate about automatic obedience and susceptibility to hypnotism being 'a battle of wills,' which found their way into fiction as well as medical debate. As part of the 'ceremony of admission' vows for neophytes, the novices must promise: 'I will not suffer myself to be hypnotized, or mesmerized, nor will I place myself in such a passive state that any uninitiated person, power, or being may cause me to lose control of my thoughts, words or actions.'[11]

Occultists were very wary of the possibility of being under attack by other malign magi or ethereal beings using hypnotism or their will which amounted to the same thing. The wiccan historian, Ronald Hutton highlights the importance of the Victorian magical societies in formalising earlier witchcraft practices. He summarises that the aim of any magical ritual is to move the practitioner 'closer to spiritual maturity and potency, by inflaming the imagination, providing access to altered states of consciousness, and strengthening and focusing will-power.'[12] We can see the ideas of hypnotism, the will and the imagination coalescing in esoteric thinking as well as in medical discourse.

Many magicians saw themselves in a constant battle of wills, attempting to keep their own personal agency and psychic integrity. Two occultists in particular, were preoccupied by the malign power of ill-will and saw it as an aspect of hypnotism: Dion Fortune (1890–1946) and Anna Kingsford (1846–1888). Having studied in Paris, Anna Kingsford was one of the UK's first female medical graduates. She was also a fervent anti-vivisectionist and the president of the London Lodge of the Theosophical Society from 1883 to 1884. In 1886, she claimed to further her occult studies with a notable expert, believed to be Samuel Mathers, who had yet to found the Golden Dawn.

In correspondence with Lady Caithness, Kingsford claimed that one of the reasons that she had pursued the practice of ceremonial magic was

[11] Gilbert, *Dawn Companion* (p. 45).

[12] Ronald Hutton, *The Triumph of the Moon* (Oxford: Oxford University Press, 1999) (p. 82).

so she could direct 'elemental forces' at vivisectors especially M. Pasteur, one of France's foremost physicians and advocates of animal experimentation in medicine.[13] If her diaries are to be believed, she had already caused the death of Claude Bernard, physiologist and medical doctor. While studying medicine in Paris, she heard him say how he had slowly baked live animals to death to study the physiological effect of body heat. Kingsford wrote that she was so overwhelmed with anger that she jumped up and denounced him as a murderer. After a further angry exchange of words, she marched out of the classroom. She was incensed by his cruelty and wanted to see him punished. She described feeling herself become 'a spiritual thunderbolt.' With all her might, she willed the doctor dead. And then she fainted. Shortly afterwards, Dr. Bernard suddenly fell very ill of a disease that no one could identify. Six weeks later, he died.

Some have speculated that some aspects of Kingsford's diary and letters may have been fictionalised before their release following her death by her partner, George Maitland.[14] This suspicion was raised by his burning all the originals before publication. However, they do read as if Kingsford genuinely believed that she had achieved the death of her vivisectionist enemies. After her occult training in London, she next targeted Paul Bert, the most notorious of the vivisectors who kept his neighbours awake with the sounds of the experimentation on animals at his Parisian house. Bert died in November 1886. Kingsford gloated: 'I have killed Paul Bert, as I killed Claude Bernard; as I will kill Louis Pasteur, and after him the whole tribe of vivisectors – it is a magnificent power to have, and one that transcends all vulgar methods of dealing out justice to tyrants.'[15]

After Bert, Kingsford next turned her lethal will to Louis Pasteur. Although seen today as a heroic figure who saved millions of lives through developing the science of microbiology and the heat treatment of milk, he routinely used animals for experimentation. Kingsford's husband, Maitland, wrote that she admitted to him that her projections against the doctors 'took from me my nervous force,' but she saw the ends as justifying the means. In November 1886, she was caught in a sudden storm

[13] Letter to Lady Caithness 12 May 1884, in *Anna Kingsford—Her Life, Letters, Diary and Works*, ed. by Edward Maitland, 2nd ed., 2 vols. (London: George Redway, 1896), vol. 2 (p. 168).

[14] Alan Pert, *Red Cactus, The Life of Anna Kingsford* (New South Wales: Books and Writers, 2007) (p. 2).

[15] Maitland, *Anna Kingsford* (p. 291).

while secretly visiting Pasteur's Parisian laboratory. She caught a chill and subsequently pneumonia which Maitland attributed to her weakened state. She went on to develop pulmonary tuberculosis which killed her four months later.

Although a slightly later historical figure, Dion Fortune, born Violet Firth (1890–1946), was both a Theosophist and ceremonial magician. She also connects to the later development of suggestive therapy, training in psychology and psychoanalysis at the University of London and Brunswick Square. She was so preoccupied by the possibility of magical willed attack that she wrote an entire book titled *Psychic Self-Defence* based on her own experiences.[16] She described the strong links between psychic attack and hypnotism, citing earlier work such as the Christian scientist, Mary Eddy's writing on malicious animal magnetism. She felt compelled to do it because 'I know for myself the peculiar horror of such an experience, its insidiousness, its potency, and its disastrous effects on mind and body.'[17]

Any publicity of Tuckey and Felkin's membership of the Golden Dawn would not have helped the cause of the New Hypnotists in the 1890s, at a time when the conflict seemed to be about scientific credibility with an agenda set by a very materialist medical perspective. The least evidence of mystical leanings would have been seized upon by their medical critics and 'looked on askance,' in the language of the day. It was not until the next century that many physicians felt confident enough to declare more esoteric ideas. Tuckey was to write for the *Occult Review*, an illustrated monthly magazine which was the pre-eminent English-language occult journal of the first quarter of the twentieth century. In 1905, its first year of publication, he declared that the 'revival of interest in hypnotism was one of the of the first signs of the reaction against crude materialism which marked the last quarter of the nineteenth century. Hypnotism may be considered as a connecting link between occultism and materialism, [...] demonstrating the truth of spiritualism [and] offering a rational explanation to apparently mysterious phenomena.'[18]

16 Dion Fortune, *Psychic Self-Defence* (London: Rider, 1930).

17 Dion Fortune, *Psychic Self-Defence* (London: Rider, 1930) (p. 3).

18 Charles Lloyd Tuckey, 'Some Phases of Hypnotism', *Occult Review*, 1 (1905) 51–57 (p. 51).

Tuckey and Felkin both saw hypnotism as a way towards understanding many of the aspects of medicine and the doctor-patient relationship that could not be explained by the crude materialism of the day. Their links to ceremonial magic led to a belief in the possibility of automatic obedience, the vulnerability of the public to malign hypnotists and an understanding of the hypnotic relationship as a battle of wills. This is seen most clearly in the foreword to Tuckey's fifth edition of *Psycho-Therapeutics* which was written by Dublin physician Francis Cruise: '*suggestion* [original emphasis] is the basis of your new departure. You must learn to dominate by your will-power, those whom you treat'.[19]

The Theosophy Society and Hypnotism

Like many other Britons, Robert Felkin was a devout Christian (he had previously worked as a medical missionary) but was dissatisfied. While working as a lecturer at Edinburgh medical school in the late 1880s, he was introduced to Theosophy, after showing interest in Hinduism at a bible discussion group. The Edinburgh section had only been established in 1884, following a visit by the society's president, Henry Olcott. Felkin was first drawn to Theosophy and thence to ceremonial magic.

Theosophy societies were also places where hypnotism was considered and discussed. Established in New York in 1875, the Theosophy Society was an influential international group which spread a partly religious and partly philosophical message drawn from many Eastern and Western sources, religious and esoteric. They appeared to offer an alternative middle way between the constrictions of a rigid and dogmatic religion and an overly materialist scientific world view. The Ukrainian émigré Helena Blavatsky had hosted the inaugural meeting and quickly rose to prominence in the organisation, which was run by Henry Olcott. In her first book *Isis Unveiled*[20] (1877) she outlined a complex 'theology,' based on wisdom from outside the traditional Christian church. There were commonalities with the beliefs of the Platonists, Kabbalists and Hermeticists. She presented these 'wisdoms' as the gifts of the Masters, clandestine, ageless adepts of the philosophy and practice. Magic

[19] Francis Cruise, 'Introductory Chapter', in Charles Lloyd Tuckey, *Psycho-Therapeutics*, 5th ed. (London: Baillière, Tindall and Cox, 1907) (p. xx).

[20] Helena Blavatsky, *Isis Unveiled*, 2 vols. (New York: Bouton, 1877).

and paranormal phenomena were described in depth and presented as a true science beyond the understanding of close-minded material scientists.

At over 1300 pages, *Isis Unveiled* remains a remarkable piece of work, seeking to refute Western materialist science with a combination of scientific and esoteric scholarship. In addition to equality for men and women, it also included beliefs like reincarnation and immortality which were highly attractive to Victorians who had lost their faith in a life after death in a Christian heaven. The society's founding coincided with a new religious scepticism in Britain which was the result of the publication of Darwin's *On the Origin of Species*.[21] The book had called into question the age of the earth and indirectly the historical accuracy of the Bible. This popular turn towards spiritualism which followed is described by Janet Oppenheim and Alex Owen and known as the occult revival (Janet Oppenheim 1985; Alex Owen 2004). Oppenheim makes the point that the public engagement with the occult was far greater than the numbers indicated by the membership lists of the Theosophy Society, the Rosicrucians or the Golden Dawn. The national obsession was better reflected by the numbers who participated in spiritualist parlour room seances, the interest in spirit writing, the mesmerism lecture circuit and the magicians using spiritualism themes in their acts.

After some faltering success in the US, in 1879 Blavatsky moved to India and made important converts there, among them Alfred Sinnett, a journalist who went on to write *The Occult World*, which was to be what introduced many British readers to the principles of Theosophy.[22] Blavatsky arrived in London in 1885, suggesting that she believed that the British general public might be particularly receptive to these kind of ideas at this time or that there might be rich patrons for her religion at the centre of the world's greatest empire.

Theosophy was initially quite positive about hypnotism as a spiritual practice. In various writings, Blavatsky and other Theosophists viewed it as a form of meditation and advocated self-hypnotism. They believed that hypnotism could help to unlock latent mental powers like telepathy and astral projection. However, as hypnotism was becoming the subject of more scientific scrutiny, Blavatsky rejected the prevailing medical theories

[21] Charles Darwin, *On the Origin of the Species* (London: John Murray, 1859).

[22] Alfred Sinnett, *The Occult World* (London: Trübner, 1881).

of hypnotism both as a pathological state and operating through suggestion. She returned to the mystical theories of animal magnetism and the imagination.[23] She viewed visually induced hypnotism as less potent than the passes of mesmerism. Another Theosophy founder, William Judge talked of the dangers of being hypnotised by another which he called subjugation which caused a separation between the 'soul man and the astral body.'[24] This disjunction might not be reunited with the result of long-term spiritual damage.

In *The Key to Theosophy*, Blavatsky's question and answer style introduction to Theosophy, she directly mocked the medical hypnotists of the day who would never be able to understand the phenomenon they researched, because they were not 'Masters' and so not granted with sufficient esoteric knowledge. Demonstrating her knowledge of the scientific literature, she disdainfully mentions several physicians by name including Hippolyte Bernheim, Frederik van Eeden and Tuckey.[25]

Like the physicians, Blavatsky wished to make a clear separation between hypnotism and mesmerism, but her purpose was quite different. They wished to embellish the scientific credentials of hypnotism while she wished to emphasise the esoteric and historical aspects. Blavatsky portrayed hypnotism as an unhealthy inert state of fatigue, in which the hypnotised becomes a passive agent of the will of the hypnotist. She differentiated it from therapeutic mesmerism by calling on the older theories of animal magnetism. She described the process in ways similar to the mesmerist Joseph Deleuze: 'The method of true mesmerism is entirely different [to hypnotism]. The mesmerizer throws out his own Auric Fluid... through the etheric double, on his patient; he may thus, in the case of sickness, regularize the irregular vibrations of the sufferer, or share with him his own life-force, thereby increasing his vitality.'

For Theosophists, hypnotism and trance were a potent means of self-development as well as healing. Like Frederic Myers of the SPR, they saw it as a way of accessing powerful internal resources. They saw it as an important part of an ancient and mystical tradition. They believed that its use should be regulated and that the study of Theosophy was the best way

[23] Helena Blavatsky, 'Hypnotism and Its Relations to Other Forms of Fascination', *Lucifer*, 7 (December 1890) (pp. 295–301).

[24] William Judge, 'Hypnotism', *Path*, 8 (February, 1894) 335–9 (p. 337).

[25] Helena Blavatsky, *The Key to Theosophy* (London: Theosophical Publishing Company, 1889) (p. 293).

of safely accessing and protecting oneself from that power. These beliefs were well-publicised within the Theosophy society but also in the wide range of occult journals which were popular at the time.

The Society for Psychical Research and Hypnotism

The SPR was the society which had the most significant impact on the thinking of the New Hypnotists. Both Bramwell and Tuckey remained active members of the SPR for over thirty years. Tuckey resigned only when forced by ill health in 1921. It is clear from his writing on hypnotism and other subjects that Tuckey was profoundly influenced by his membership of the group. This is true to a lesser extent for Bramwell, who stayed close to the ideas of James Braid throughout his writings. The scholarship of Myers and Edmund Gurney in particular can be seen in Bramwell and Tuckey's views and understanding of hypnotism: from dual consciousness to enhancing mental abilities and the 'subliminal self'.

The SPR remains the most well known and influential of all the British psychic research groups. It was founded in 1882 by a group of spiritualists and psychic investigators primarily for the purpose of providing scientific evidence of the existence of life after death. Spiritualists and mediums like William Stainton Moses were balanced by Cambridge academics Myers, Gurney and Henry Sidgwick. Their stated aims were: 'to approach these varied problems without prejudice or prepossession of any kind, and in the same spirit of exact and unimpassioned enquiry which has enabled science to solve so many problems, once not less obscure nor less hotly debated.'[26]

The SPR was interested in hypnotism from its foundation. They viewed hypnotism as an empirical practice which could be used to scientifically investigate a variety of psychic phenomena: 'No line of investigation seems to us more hopeful than this for our purposes if pursued in a serious and scientific manner.'[27] They established a specific committee to investigate the technology which was initially chaired by the brilliant Edmund Gurney.

[26] Edmund Gurney, Frederic Myers, and Frank Podmore, *Phantasms of the Living* (London: Trübner, 1886) (p. xxxvii).

[27] Anon. 'Mr Hansen's Hypnotic Demonstrations', *Journal of the Society for Psychical Research*, 4 (June 1889) (p. 86).

Gurney and the co-founder Frederic Myers and Myers' brother, the doctor Arthur, were among the first British scientists to travel to France to learn about hypnotism in Paris under Charcot and then in Nancy with Liébeault. Gurney edited the SPR journal *Proceedings* in which he reported experiments in mentally normal volunteers apparently revealing 'secondary selves' during trance and post-hypnotically. Gurney, Myers, and the American psychologist William James would use this as evidence for the non-pathological nature of hypnotism an important difference from Janet and Charcot's work which contended that hypnotism was only effective in the neurotic.

Such was his expertise that Gurney, who was not a physician, was invited to make a presentation on hypnotism at the BMA annual meeting in 1890. In the absence of a university base for the emerging discipline of experimental psychology, the SPR were the organisation to convene the second International Congress in London in 1892. Hypnotism was well-represented on the agenda. All of which demonstrate both the importance of the SPR for the British development of the discipline of psychology and the early importance of hypnotism for that discipline.

Critically, for the emerging field of psychology, the SPR's leading theorist, Frederic Myers used the observation of the phenomenon of post-hypnotic suggestion as a way of demonstrating the reality of dual or multiple consciousness, an important milestone in early psychological thinking:

> I suggest, then, that the stream of consciousness in which we habitually live is not the only consciousness which exists in connection with our organism. Our habitual or empirical consciousness may consist of a mere selection from our multitude of thoughts and sensations, of which some at least are equally conscious with those that we empirically know. I accord no primacy to my ordinary waking self, except that among my potential selves this one has shown itself the fittest to meet the needs of common life.[28]

As one of his supporting proofs, Myers described how it was possible to experimentally demonstrate that a man could carry out an action that had been planted while in trance and remain unconscious of the command and later believe that he was acting from his own choice and free-will.

[28] Frederic W.H. Myers, 'The Subliminal Consciousness: Chapter 1—General Characteristics of Subliminal Messages', *Proceedings for the SPR*, 7 (1891) 298–327 (p. 301).

Perhaps, Myers greatest legacy was his idea of the 'subliminal self,' the deepest, most creative aspect of human consciousness. He believed that only a fraction of the human personality, or soul, found expression through the ordinary mental processes, because the brain and body had not yet reached an adequate phase of evolution. He believed that much of the power of the soul remained hidden and untapped. He proposed that the subliminal self was connected to a reservoir of psychical energy, from which it drew forces that influence the physical body. He used this mechanism to explain the inspiration of genius, the amplification of the perceptive and intellectual faculties in hypnosis. Finally, psychic phenomena such as automatic writing and automatic talking, table turning and telepathy were caused by these internal psychical forces rather than by any external 'spirit' influences. Myers' and the SPRs major contributions to the development of psychology as a science in the UK and US are increasingly accepted, despite contemporary views about psychic powers.[29]

The Hypnotism Committee

Tuckey was one of the more active and influential members of the SPR. As a bibliophile, he sat on the library committee of the SPR from 1894 till 1918. He donated money and books and was involved in the growth of the collection, particularly the Edmund Gurney section on hypnotism. He regularly reviewed texts on hypnotism for the *Proceedings of the SPR*.[30] In 1894, he and Bramwell had joined the Hypnotism committee and Tuckey became its chairman the following year. Here he could explore the nonmaterialistic aspects of hypnotism using scientific methods. His appointment was an important step forward in the written aims of the SPR which as early as 1883 had included persuading the medical profession to admit the validity of hypnotism. Myers' biographer

[29] Andreas Sommer, 'Psychical Research and the Origins of American Psychology', *History of the Human Sciences*, 25 (2012) (pp. 23–44).

[30] *Inter alia* Charles Lloyd Tuckey, 'Reviews', *Proceedings of the Society for Psychical Research*, 14 (1898) (pp. 139–43); Charles Lloyd Tuckey, 'Reviews', *Proceedings of the SPR*, 16 (1901) (pp. 103–4).

Trevor Hamilton suggests that 'one of the [later] triumphs of the SPR was gradually to increase the medical profession's awareness of hypnosis.'[31]

The hypnotism committee met regularly. Over their busiest times, this was more than twice a month. They experimented with professional English clairvoyants like Maud Lancaster and George Smith in addition to famous hypnotic entertainers like the Dane, Carl Hansen. Hansen and the Belgian-born, Donato (Alfred Edouard D'Hont) had both had careers touring Europe between the late 1870s and 1880s. They were great self-publicists and often arranged to meet with local scientists and journalists to promote their travelling shows. Frequently performing in medical white coats, both offered a new spin on older mesmeric entertainments, blurring the distinctions between magic and science. The historian of hypnotism Alan Gauld credits Hansen with 'stirring the interest' of the German-speaking doctors Heidenhain, Kraft-Ebbing and Benedikt.[32] Donato is said to have inspired van Eeden and Renterghem.[33]

However, by the 1890s most of the work of the committee was more prosaic using young male volunteers obtained by newspaper advertisements. Tuckey gave updates on the results of their experiments. The most detail of these trials is given in the report for 1895. The members of the committee were particularly looking at telepathy or thought transference under hypnotism, combining Myers' ideas of with Puységur's much older beliefs of enhanced perception in the trance state. They undertook 61 experiments, in which the committee member was able to see a playing card but the hypnotised subject who was *en rapport* could not and had to guess the suit and number. A total of 817 cards were tried, out of which the subjects correctly told 214 suits, 79 pips [the number on the card] and 19 whole cards. They calculated that the most probable number of successes by chance would be 204, 63 and 16, respectively.[34]

[31] *Trevor Hamilton, Immortal Longings: F.W.H. Myers and the Victorian Search for Life after Death* (Exeter: Imprint Academic, 2009) (p. 124).

[32] Alan Gauld, *A History of Hypnotism* (Cambridge: Cambridge University Press, 1992) (pp. 302–6).

[33] Ilse Bulhof, 'From Psychotherapy to Psychoanalysis: Frederik van Eeden and Albert Willem van Renterghem', *Journal of the History of Behavioral Science*, 17 (1981) (pp. 209–21).

[34] Charles Lloyd Tuckey, 'Report of the Hypnotic Committee', *Proceedings of the Society for Psychical Research*, 11 (1895) 594–8 (pp. 594–5).

They investigated whether success rates improved with direct physical contact (which they did) and noticed that the subject sometimes guessed the preceding card. However, Tuckey concluded that the 'excess [of successes] was not very great, and the successes in every case fell short of the numbers required to prove some other cause than chance.'[35]

In a later report for the same committee, he writes more personally and less objectively 'we do not despair of finding subjects who will enable us to offer convincing evidence of their reality [advanced psychical phenomena, such as telepathy and clairvoyance].'[36] While all scientists hope for observations, data and evidence that will confirm their a priori hypotheses, this comment sums up the needy form of intellectual agnosticism that characterised the SPR. In their search for evidence of spiritualist manifestations they were examining the nature of consciousness and creating a very English school of psychology. They were investigating what Charles Richet called 'transcendental psychology.'

Tuckey was a significant if historically neglected member of the SPR. He sat on the main council from 1898 till his resignation through illness in 1921. He helped the society to navigate the existential crisis that followed the close deaths of Sidgwick in 1900 and Myers in 1901. Myers had been their president until his unexpected demise. The loss of two of their founding and most illustrious members in quick succession was a difficult blow for the SPR.

Both Tuckey and Bramwell held on to several important concepts of hypnotism that came from their SPR membership. They sided with the Nancy school over Charcot; they both saw hypnotism as an important therapeutic force and as a way of exploring mental functioning. They accepted post-hypnotic suggestion as a fact and therefore secondary consciousness. It appears that Tuckey was more open to the creative possibilities of the subliminal self, including telepathy. Bramwell remained sceptical of extraordinary mental powers throughout his writing.

[35] Tuckey, 'Report' (p. 597).

[36] Charles Lloyd Tuckey, 'The Hypnotic Committee', *Proceedings of the Society for Psychical Research*, 13 (1897) (p. 32).

The Sesame Club and Hypnosis in Education

In one of his letters from 1899, Tuckey invited van Eeden to address 'a club for men and women that I belong to' which is 'interested in new and educational ideas.'[37] The Sesame Club was a liberal and progressive society which was unusual for its time in accepting both male and female members. It had been formed by a 'group of friends' who had children of their own and who wished to study and discuss how best to educate them. Among those involved in the club were the Hebrew scholar and intellectual founder of Anglo-Liberal Judaism Claude Montefiore, the artist and educator Ebenezer Cooke and Lady Isabel Margesson, a eugenicist who was a relative by marriage to Emily Shirreff, the Victorian pioneer of women's higher education.

At first, the club was housed in what was described as a 'modest flat' in Victoria but in 1896 it had moved to 'a fine house in Piccadilly'.[38] By 1897, it had claimed membership of over nine hundred which included author and playwright George B. Shaw, biologist T.H. Huxley and the poet and critic Edith Sitwell. It was composed of those who used it purely as a social club and those parents and teachers who wished to pursue their interest in educational theories and practices. There were several members of the Froebel Society which meant that the ideas of the German educator Friedrich Froebel (1782–1852) were well-represented. He believed in the importance of play and the experience of nature in learning. In 1899, those members who were interested chiefly in the educational aspects of the club, formed the Sesame League and they announced their intention to establish a 'House for Home Life Training' modelled on the Pestalozzi-Froebel House. This institution, which was given the name of Sesame House, was opened by the Marchioness of Ripon at St Johns Wood in July 1899.[39]

Tuckey's membership of the Sesame Club might be seen as unusual for a bachelor. However, his previous writing demonstrated that he was interested in the medical needs of children. His earliest book was *Diseases*

[37] Charles Lloyd Tuckey to van Eeden correspondence (20 October 1899). *Van Eeden Collection* (Amsterdam: Allard Pierson, University of Amsterdam).

[38] Anon, 'Sesame Club Notes', *Child Life*, 1, 1 (1899) (pp. 53–5).

[39] Kevin Brehoney, 'The Sesame House for Home Training', in *The Froebel Movement and State Schooling 1880–1914: A Study in Educational Ideology* (PhD thesis, The Open University, 1987) (pp. 528–30).

of Children with Cases and Remarks presumably taking a homoeopathic approach.[40] He also refers to the effects of suggestion on young people from the third edition of *Psycho-Therapeutics* onwards.[41] His comparatively progressive views towards women are most clearly articulated in his 1914 article on marriage for the *Contemporary Review*.[42] In this article Tuckey advocates for matrimony but also supports economic independence, female doctors and scientific training for women. Apparently unironically he says, 'my suffragist friends assure me that the Kingdom of Woman is at hand, and that it will prove the Kingdom of God. I earnestly hope so.'[43]

Tuckey was not alone in sensing an important role for hypnotism within education. Many researchers from the United States and European centres had been able to prove by experiment an improvement in memory for volunteers in the hypnotic state.[44] This enhanced memory included the ability to memorise verse or musical melodies. The American physician Osgood Mason was enthusiastic about the value of hypnotism in education, devoting several chapters of his book to the subject, *Hypnotism and Suggestion in Therapeutics, Education and Reform*.[45] Tuckey describes a conversation with the head teacher of a British boys' school whose pupils found their sums 'came easier to them' than usual after suggestive treatment.[46]

However, for Tuckey and members of the Sesame club, education did not just mean academic training, it included moral education: the teaching of values and morality to young people. In the 1900 edition of *Psycho-Therapeutics* he writes that the beneficial and curative action of suggestion is not confined to bodily ailments. 'We are all acquainted with numerous examples where 'a word in season' i.e. a suggestion falling

[40] Charles Lloyd Tuckey, *Diseases of Children*. Cited but no copies extant.

[41] Charles Lloyd Tuckey, *Psycho-Therapeutics: Treatment by Hypnotism and Suggestion*, 3rd ed. (London: Baillière, Tindall and Cox, 1891).

[42] Charles Lloyd Tuckey, 'Some Thoughts on Marriage', *Contemporary Review*, 105 (1914) (pp. 366–75).

[43] Tuckey, 'Some Thoughts' (p. 370).

[44] John Milne Bramwell, 'Memory in Hypnosis', in *Hypnotism: Its history, Practice and Theory* (London: Grant Richards, 1903) (pp. 100–11).

[45] Rufus Osgood Mason, *Hypnotism and Suggestion in Therapeutics, Education and Reform* (London: Kegan Paul, Trench, Trübner, 1901).

[46] Tuckey, *Psycho-Therapeutics*, 5th ed. (1907) (p. 112).

on a receptive soil, has so influenced moral conduct that it has changed the entire life of the individual.'[47] Hypnotism offered the prospect of moral education which might counter some of the 1890s anxieties of rising criminality, moral decline and typified by physician Max Nordau's contemporary essay *Degeneration.*[48]

Physicians like Tuckey and Bramwell had already started to treat behavioural disorders like alcohol and drug dependency and the newly pathologized sexual disorders. Previously seen as moral problems, the Victorian doctors had begun to claim these behaviours as illness and amenable to medical treatment. Hypnotism and suggestive therapy were among the therapies to show promise in these areas. If these kinds of behaviours responded to hypnotism, it followed that anti-social behaviours might too. As children were more susceptible to hypnotism and the anti-social behaviours less engrained and habitual, they seemed a good place to start.

Tuckey had previously written two case reports on this topic for the *Edinburgh Medical Journal* and *Provincial Medical Journal.*[49] The first described a 13-year-old girl who was cured of repeatedly using scissors to cut up her own and other's clothes by a course of suggestive therapy. The second reported a 16-year-old boy with kleptomania who also responded to hypnotism. In *Psycho-Therapeutics,* he acknowledged that some would be reluctant to hypnotise their child for their behavioural problems, agreeing that he would rather a child naturally naughty than hypnotically good if by 'naturally' they meant 'the ordinary faults and shortcomings of free, happy, healthy childhood.' However, in the case of the parents of the 13-year-old girl described, he felt that in such severe circumstances most would employ the only available remedy.[50]

In *Hypnotism in Medicine*, Bramwell recorded his treatment of six children and adolescents who were 'vicious and degenerate' in the medical

[47] Charles Lloyd Tuckey, *Psycho-Therapeutics Treatment by Hypnotism and Suggestion*, 4th ed. (London: Baillière, Tindall and Cox, 1900) (p. 64).

[48] Max Nordau, *Degeneration* (London: Heinemann, 1895).

[49] Charles Lloyd Tuckey, 'Case of Mischievous Morbid Impulse in a Child, Treated by Hypnotism', *Edinburgh Medical Journal*, 1 (1897) (pp. 635–6); Charles Lloyd Tuckey, 'Case of Kleptomania Treated by Hypnotism', 13, *Provincial Medical Journal* (December 1894).

[50] Tuckey, *Psycho-Therapeutics*, 5th ed. (1907) (p. 116).

vocabulary of the day.[51] The majority were lower middle-class teenage girls who were deceitful and insolent, while two had a violent temper. He agreed with Berillon's conclusions on the treatment of such children presented at the 1889 International Congress of Hypnotism in Paris. He viewed suggestion as an excellent 'auxiliary' in their education, especially where there were habits of lying, cruelty, inveterate idleness or cowardice. 'Suggestion ought to be confined to cases where normal educational methods had failed and medical men alone should employ it.'[52]

Inasmuch as the British system of education of the time could be said to have a philosophy behind its practice of learning by rote and repetition, the ideas of the Johann Herbart (1776–1841), the German psychologist were most prominent. Herbart had created pedagogy, an academic approach and theory to teaching practice. He based his ideas on contemporary psychology and believed in the importance of the choice of the subject topics of instruction and in instilling character or moral judgement.

At the Sesame Club, as the new century dawned more liberal ideas about education were being discussed. As well as the progressive beliefs of Froebel, the new ideas of suggestion and the newly fashionable pedagogy of the Italian physician Maria Montessori were shared and distributed by the opinion-formers of the day. Tuckey was there to promote suggestive therapy and a medical role in future education.

In summary, it can be seen that the fact that these New Hypnotists held membership of these occult and quasi-scientific organisations does not represent some quaint or romantic leaning on their parts but suggests an attempt to engage with the complexity of modernity: contemporary, personal and spiritual. It also shows that at that time the boundaries between science and non-science were not so clearly dichotomised as they have become now. The borders were much more porous, and ideas from one discourse could freely move to another. The institutions also served to shape their respective ideas about suggestion and provided an important support network to develop therapeutic hypnotism and suggestion in the UK.

[51] Bramwell, 'Vicious and Degenerate Children', in *Hypnotism* (pp. 232–8).

[52] Bramwell, 'Vicious and Degenerate Children', in *Hypnotism* (p. 233).

Bibliography

Anon. 1889. 'Mr. Hansen's Hypnotic Demonstrations', *Journal of the Society for Psychical Research*, 4 (June): 86.

Anon. 1899. 'Sesame Club Notes', *Child Life*, 1: 53–5.

Blavatsky, Helena. 1877. *Isis Unveiled*, 2 vols. New York: Bouton.

Blavatsky, Helena. 1889. *The Key to Theosophy*. London: Theosophical Publishing Company.

Blavatsky, Helena. 1890. 'Hypnotism and Its Relations to Other Forms of Fascination', *Lucifer*, 7 (December): 295–301.

Bramwell, John Milne. 1903. *Hypnotism: It's History, Practice and Theory*, 1st ed. London: Grant Richards.

Brehoney, Kevin. 1987. 'The Sesame House for Home Training', in *The Froebel Movement and State Schooling 1880–1914: A Study in Educational Ideology* (unpublished PhD thesis). The Open University. 528–30.

Bulhof, Ilse. 1981. 'From Psychotherapy to Psychoanalysis: Frederik van Eeden and Albert Willem van Renterghem', *Journal of the History of Behavioral Science*, 17: 209–21.

Cruise, Francis. 1907. 'Introductory Chapter', in Charles Lloyd Tuckey. *Psycho-Therapeutics*, 5th ed. London: Baillière, Tindall and Cox. xx.

Darwin, Charles. 1859. *On the Origin of the Species*. London: John Murray.

Denisoff, Dennis. 'The Hermetic Order of the Golden Dawn, 1888–1901', in *BRANCH: Britain, Representation and Nineteenth-Century History*, ed. by Dino Franco Felluga. Extension of *Romanticism and Victorianism on the Net* [accessed 8 July 2019].

Doyle, Arthur Conan. 1989. *Memories and Adventures*. Oxford: Oxford University Press.

Fortune, Dion. 1930. *Psychic Self-Defence*. London: Rider.

Gauld, Alan. 1992. *A History of Hypnotism*. Cambridge: Cambridge University Press.

Gilbert, R.A. 1986. 'Membership List', *The Golden Dawn Companion: A Guide to the History, Structure and Workings of the Hermetic Order of the Golden Dawn*. Wellingborough: Aquarian Books. 125–75.

Gurney, Edmund, Myers, Frederic, and Podmore, Frank. 1886. *Phantasms of the Living*. London: Trübner.

Hamilton, Trevor. 2009. *Immortal Longings: F.W.H. Myers and the Victorian Search for Life After Death*. Exeter: Imprint Academic.

Hutton, Ronald. 1999. *The Triumph of the Moon*. Oxford: Oxford University Press.

Judge, William. 1894. 'Hypnotism', *Path*, 8 (February): 335–9.

Kingsford, Anna. 1896. 'Letter to Lady Caithness, 12 May 1884', in *Anna Kingsford—Her Life, Letters, Diary and Works*, ed. by Edward Maitland, 2nd ed., 2 vols. London: George Redway.

Kuntz, Darcy. 1996. *The Golden Source Book*. Edmonds, WA: Holmes.

Mason, Rufus Osgood. 1901. *Hypnotism and Suggestion in Therapeutics, Education and Reform*. London: Kegan Paul, Trench, Trübner.

Myers, Frederic W.H. 1891. 'The Subliminal Consciousness: Chapter 1—General Characteristics of Subliminal Messages', *Proceedings for the SPR*: 298–327.

Nordau, Max. 1895. *Degeneration*. London: Heinemann.

Oppenheim, Janet. 1985. *The Other World: Spiritualism and Psychic Research in England, 1850–1914*. Cambridge: Cambridge University Press.

Owen, Alex. 2004. *The Place of Enchantment: British Occultism and the Culture of the Modern*. Chicago: University Press of Chicago.

Pert, Alan. 2007. *Red Cactus, The Life of Anna Kingsford*. New South Wales: Books and Writers.

Sommer, Andreas. 2012. 'Psychical Research and the Origins of American Psychology', *History of the Human Sciences*, 25: 23–44.

Sinnett, Alfred. 1881. *The Occult World*. London: Trübner.

Tuckey, Charles Lloyd. 1891. *Psycho-Therapeutics: Treatment by Hypnotism and Suggestion*, 3rd ed. London: Baillière, Tindall and Cox.

Tuckey, Charles Lloyd. 1894a. 'Letter to van Eeden, 19 August 1894'. In *Van Eeden Collection*. Amsterdam: Allard Pierson, University of Amsterdam.

Tuckey, Charles Lloyd. 1894b. 'Case of Kleptomania Treated by Hypnotism', *Provincial Medical Journal* (December).

Tuckey, Charles Lloyd. 1895. 'Report of the Hypnotic Committee', *Proceedings of the Society for Psychical Research*, 11: 594–8.

Tuckey, Charles Lloyd. 1897a. 'Case of Mischievous Morbid Impulse in a Child, Treated by Hypnotism', *Edinburgh Medical Journal*, 1: 635–6.

Tuckey, Charles Lloyd. 1897b. 'The Hypnotic Committee', *Proceedings of the Society for Psychical Research*, 13: 32.

Tuckey, Charles Lloyd. 1898. 'Reviews', *Proceedings of the Society for Psychical Research*, 14: 139–43.

Tuckey, Charles Lloyd. 1899. 'Letter to van Eeden, 20 October 1899'. In *Van Eeden Collection*. Amsterdam: Allard Pierson, University of Amsterdam.

Tuckey, Charles Lloyd. 1900. *Psycho-Therapeutics: Treatment by Hypnotism and Suggestion*, 4th ed. London: Baillière, Tindall and Cox. xx.

Tuckey, Charles Lloyd. 1901. 'Reviews', *Proceedings of the Society for Psychical Research*, 16: 103–4.

Tuckey, Charles Lloyd. 1905. 'Some Phases of Hypnotism', *Occult Review*, 1: 51–7.

Tuckey, Charles Lloyd. 1907. *Psycho-Therapeutics: Treatment by Hypnotism and Suggestion*, 5th ed. London: Baillière, Tindall and Cox. xx.

Tuckey, Charles Lloyd. 1914. 'Some Thoughts on Marriage', *Contemporary Review*, 105: 366–75.

Young, Sue. 'Charles Tuckey', in *Work on the Hermetic Order of the Golden Dawn*. www.wrightanddavis.co.uk/GD/TUCKEYCHARLESL.htm [accessed 13 April 2023].

CHAPTER 9

Imaginary Hypnotism

Hypnotism and the trance state were not just a part of medical discourse and discussion. They had meanings well beyond scientific and medical culture. These ranged from historic ones (via mesmerism) to those of spiritualism, mysticism and entertainment. These alternative readings and connotations were both a curse and a boon to the New Hypnotists, who wished to portray hypnotism as safe, effective and credible. A later convert to medical hypnotism Albert Davis, described it vividly: 'The average man is repelled by the word hypnotism: he associates it with a grotesque stage character like Svengali, or with some mountebank who possesses a power that is dangerous and wicked.'[1]

Previously, I showed the ways that the various discourses were mixing in the 1890s as a result of the surprising social connections of Victorian cultural life and the efforts of the New Hypnotists. I have also demonstrated the prominence of hypnotism in wider British cultural life through the print media of newspapers and journals. This chapter describes the final important site of discourse for trance: that within fiction.

Many scholars have commented about the wide breadth of concerns of Victorian intellectual life. At this time, the distinct demarcations between

[1] Albert Davis, *Hypnotism and Treatment by Suggestion*, 2nd ed. (Liverpool: Liverpool Book Sellers, 1918) (p. 1).

G. D. L. Bates, *The Uncanny Rise of Medical Hypnotism, 1888–1914*, Mental Health in Historical Perspective,
https://doi.org/10.1007/978-3-031-42725-1_9

artistic culture and scientific culture were not yet fixed and an interest in both fields was expected as part of a normal healthy intellectual life. The notion that fictions and scientific theories could influence each other reciprocally is well-established idea within Victorian Studies. Psychological thinking in particular, has been well examined. Since the pioneering work of Sally Shuttleworth and Jenny Bourne Taylor in the 1980s, scholars have moved from Freudian readings of Victorian literature to those informed by the psychology of the time. Victorian psychology was broad, described by Bourne Taylor as a 'point of intersection between various fields of knowledge – philosophy, physiology, aesthetic and social theory'.[2] It was also accommodating enough to include fields that would now be considered to be pseudoscience such as mesmerism and supernatural psychic abilities.

The complex relationship between a fictional representation and the real-world object or idea is not unidirectional. Another critic Gillian Beer, mostly concerned with the Victorian period too, writes of the transformations and translations that occur when science is represented in art, 'Scientific and literary discourses overlap, but unstably.'[3] Beer uses the allegory of a field to represent a region in which different zones of influence play upon bodies or cultural moments, rather like iron filings in magnetic fields. Her terms of translation and transformation make us focus on the specific language used, but the concepts that the language represents can also be directly reflected, subtly distorted or shifted completely in the process.

Beer's own examples show the way that the scientific Darwinian ideas of order and natural selection find their way into late Victorian fiction in unexpected ways. Conversely, she also demonstrates the way that Victorian scientists use classical allusion to demonstrate authority and the way that they utilise novel comparisons during the attempt to say something new and original. Critically, she writes that 'Symbol and metaphor, as opposed to analysis, *can allow insight without consequences* because

[2] Jenny Bourne Taylor, *The Secret Theatre of Home: Wilkie Collins, Sensation Narrative and Nineteenth-Century Psychology* (New York: Routledge, 1988) (p. 19).

[3] Gillian Beer, 'Translation or Transformation? The Relations of Science and Literature', Ch. 8 in *Open Fields, Science in Cultural Encounter* (Oxford: Oxford University Press, 1996) 173–95 (p. 173).

perceptions are not stabilised and categorised.'[4] In other words, she draws attention to the power of allegory or story to enable scientists to conceptualise and communicate new ideas.

Beer also makes links between the contemporary fictions that were available within the culture for the scientists to draw upon, calling them 'the imaginative currency of the community.'[5] The New Hypnotists drew upon this imaginative currency in their writing and practice. Sometimes they used the fictional representations to help lay readers understand therapeutic hypnotism and sometimes they were forced to confront the anxieties which were represented in and sometimes generated by hypnotic fictions. In an 1894 interview with the journalist T.H., from the *Sketch*, about the de Jong murder cases, Charles Lloyd Tuckey was clearly conversant with the central plot of the play *The Bells*, as it was used as an example of hypnotism being used to induce a criminal confession.[6] *The Bells* was a popular play written by Leopold Lewis in 1871, which ran intermittently for several decades in the West End as a vehicle for the great actor-manager Henry Irving. As a further sign of the enduring fascination with hypnotic fictions in late Victorian Britain, Irving revived it on many occasions, playing the role of the Polish Jew Mathias right up until the night before his own death in 1905.

The New Hypnotists were well aware of the impact of imaginary hypnotism and complained that the cause of medical hypnotism was harmed, 'through the confusion existing in the popular mind between it and the hypnotism of shows and entertainments.'[7] However, not all fictional examples of hypnotism and mesmerism which were usually considered to be equivalent, were negative. One of the largest best-sellers of the time was Marie Corelli's *The Romance of Two Worlds* which imagined trance positively, as part of an ancient Eastern tradition of healing, spiritual and psychical development that was ripe for rediscovery.[8] Its

[4] Gillian Beer, *Darwin's Plots: Evolutionary Narrative in Darwin, George Elliot and Nineteenth-Century Fiction* (London: Routledge and Kegan Paul, 1983) (p. 14).

[5] Beer, *Open Fields* (p. 179).

[6] T.H., 'Hypnotism in Criminal Investigation', *Sketch*, 4 (1894) (p. 244).

[7] Charles Lloyd Tuckey, 'The Applications of Hypnotism', *Contemporary Review*, 60 (1891) 672–86 (p. 682).

[8] Marie Corelli, *A Romance of Two Worlds: Edinburgh Critical Editions of Nineteenth Century Texts*, ed. by Andrew Radford (Edinburgh: Edinburgh University Press, 2019).

success was based upon the growing interest in Theosophy and occultism with which it shared many themes.

I am suggesting that the fictions that individuals read were a part of a much wider shared social milieu which had the power not only to change people's attitude to trance but their beliefs of what trance could actually achieve. In other words, the fictions could be constitutive (creative and constructive), not just reflective (secondary, or degraded versions of the scientific 'truth'). I will discuss three themes that are encountered in the hypnotic fictions of the time: automatic obedience and the English will; gender and sexology; and medical professionalism.

Automatic Obedience and the English Will

The idea of will was a crucial Victorian concept. The possibility that one's will could be overridden by another was alarming and played out repeatedly in fiction. Its repetition marked it as more than just a useful plot device to cause jeopardy and change in the predictable respectable and moral behaviours of the heroes and heroines. The Victorians viewed their will as a self-evident entity. The mid-Victorian legal writer, James Stephen expressed it this way: 'Every human creature attaches to the words "to will", or their equivalents as vivid a meaning as every man with eyes attaches to the words "to see."'[9] To choose when to enact one's mental impulses and when not to, was fundamental.

The literary critic John Reed has usefully separated the three different aspects of will in the nineteenth century.[10] He separates out free will (as distinct from determinism), volition (the agency to initiate action) and strength of will (as a character trait of self-control and determination). The last two concepts are frequently blurred in mesmeric and hypnotic fictions, as one's strength of will reduces one's chances of losing volition and self-agency through hypnotism. There is the additional aspect of influencing the external world through the force of will which Reed touches on in his chapter which links Christian progress to the will. This idea of the mind directly influencing the material world resonates with the magical thinking and beliefs of the occultists and anti-materialists:

[9] James Stephen, *A General View of the Criminal Law of England* (London: Macmillan, 1863) (p. 73).

[10] John Reed, *Victorian Will* (Athens: Ohio University Press, 1989) (p. ix).

> Because Christian values continued to influence much thinking about progress, the familiar paradox of self-suppression as a means to self-fulfilment found expression in theories of progress as well. In England, a substantial body of opinion concluded that the modern Christian Englishman stood at the pinnacle of progress because he represented the highest development of will.[11]

Continuing on the theme of will and progress, the Victorian journalist and essayist, Walter Bagehot, wrote in his 1872 essay, 'Physics and Politics,' that the British were the most advanced nation because they had achieved power over nature and *themselves* [my emphasis] and were thus morally superior. This view finds expression in Rider Haggard's 1887 follow up novel to *King Solomon's Mines*, *Allan Quatermain* whose author and hero believe that 'the highest rank that can be reached upon this earth' is that of an English gentleman.[12] Bagehot also proposed that this high point of civilisation that had been reached was the result of a morality of self-restraint. It was the Englishman's ability to assert his will over his impulses and instincts that led him to his lofty position.[13] In other words, one of the reasons for the success of the British Empire was English willpower.

This perhaps explains the number of hypnotic narratives in the 1890s in which the hypnotist is foreign. The worries about the declining state of the British Empire become symbolised as a battle of wills between English men and women and foreign villains. Richard Marsh's villainous man/woman/insect in *The Beetle* (1897) was from Egypt and Svengali from *Trilby* (1894) was both Polish and Jewish. Perhaps most memorably, Bram Stoker's *Dracula* (1897) was Transylvanian, that is from Romania at the edge of Eastern Europe. Stoker was well-placed to write about hypnotism and mesmerism. He had friends in the Society for Psychical Research and Golden Dawn as well as two medical brothers.[14] He also wrote a

[11] Reed, *Victorian Will* (pp. 83–4).

[12] H. Rider Haggard, *King Solomon's Mines* (Oxford: Oxford University Press, 2016); H. Rider Haggard, *Allan Quatermain,* (London: Longman, Green's, 1887) (p. 276). See also the original introductory dedication to Rider Haggard's son.

[13] Walter Bagehot, 'Physics and Politics', Ch 14 in *The Works and Life of Walter Bagehot*, ed. by Mrs Russell Barrington (London: Longman's Green, 1915) (p. 52).

[14] Hans Corneel de Roos, *Bram Stoker's Hidden World: A Sociogram of London's Esoteric Circles* (E-book, Munich: Moonlake Editions, 2021).

chapter on Mesmer for his nonfiction book *Famous Impostors*.[15] There has been speculation that the character of Van Helsing was based on Tuckey himself or his Dutch friend van Renterghem.[16] The critic Steven Arata has described the fear of geopolitical decline represented as the empire's hub becoming invaded from beyond its periphery as 'reverse colonization'.[17] These fin de-siècle fears also surfaced in fictions of physical invasion like *War of the Worlds* and *The Yellow Danger* as well as the psychological thraldom of the hypnotic stories.[18]

If strength of will and self-control were linked to both English maleness and a successful empire, then the loss of will and self-mastery was associated with madness and femininity. Victorian clerics like Reverend John Barlow saw the exercise of self-control as fundamental to sanity. In his Royal Institution lecture of 1843, Barlow asserts than those who expressed all thoughts and feelings would be 'as wild as a madman.' However, 'the man of strong mind represses them, and seeks fresh impressions from without if he finds that aid needful: the man of weak mind yields to them and he is insane.'[19]

Writing over 30 years later, the eminent and influential psychiatrist, Henry Maudsley's views appear to draw from the same moral perspective of mental illness and they read very similarly. Although he is an organicist (that is the brain is the site of the mind), he views the loss of moral control as the first sign of mental illness: 'One of the first symptoms of insanity [...] is a deadening or complete perversion of the moral sense. In extreme cases it is observed that the modest man becomes presumptuous and exacting, the chaste man lewd and obscene.'[20]

Like the French neurologist, Jean-Martin Charcot and the *Salpêtrière* school, Maudsley believed that only hysterics and neurotics could be

[15] Bram Stoker, *Famous Impostors* (London: Sidgwick & Jackson, 1910).

[16] Hans Corneel de Roos, *Professor Abraham van Helsing: A Psychiatrist from Amsterdam? Hypnotism, Telepathy, Spiritualism and Magic in the Victorian Age* (Munich: Moonlake editions, 2012).

[17] Stephen Arata, 'The Occidental Tourist: "Dracula" and the Anxiety of Reverse Colonization', *Victorian Studies*, 33 (1990) 621–45 (p. 623).

[18] H.G. Wells, *War of the Worlds* (London: Heinemann, 1898); M.P. Shiel, *The Yellow Danger* (London: Grant Richards, 1898).

[19] John Barlow, *On Man's Power Over Himself to Prevent or Control Insanity* (London: William Pickering, 1843) (p. 44).

[20] Henry Maudsley, *Responsibility and Mental Disease* (London: King, 1874) (p. 67).

hypnotised. He devoted an entire chapter to hypnotism in his textbook of psychopathology, *Pathology of the Mind:* 'Were his [the subject's] will strong, the operator [mesmerist] could not succeed.'[21] He asserted that those with hysteria and neurosis were more susceptible to hypnotism because they had a hereditary predisposition to insanity. This tied in with his worry about degeneration, the belief that there was a rising rate of neurosis and hysteria among civilised city people which would lead to societal decline.[22] Maudsley's views influenced Max Nordau and his influential essay, *Degeneration*. The Austrian physician and writer used the term to convey both a specific form of mental illness and the decline of Western culture and civilisation. The concept has been taken up by critics of the late Victorian era to encapsulate a range of prevailing moral, social and scientific concerns.

This meant that in fiction those who were susceptible to hypnotism were generally depicted as morally or mentally weak. If this was generally believed to transfer to reality, this was not a good advertisement for the treatment and needed to be challenged by the New Hypnotists to be publicly acceptable. In his first article for the general public Tuckey emphasised the rude health of the rustic French peasants easily treated by Liébeault's hypnotism in an attempt to demonstrate their wholesome and undecadent qualities.[23] Within subsequent editions of *Psycho-Therapeutics*, Tuckey addressed the fear of automatic obedience more directly. He described it as a fiction which arose from attending magic shows and mesmeric lectures and recommended that a lighter hypnotic state be used for therapy: '[People's fear] rests very frequently upon the conception that loss of volition and amnesia are ordinary accompaniments of medical hypnotism. Such an idea arises from witnessing public performances, and it is difficult to eradicate. The physician who employs hypnotism as a remedial agent [does not] seek to obtain somnambulism (in which state alone the patient's memory and willpower are seriously

[21] Henry Maudsley, 'Hypnotism', in *Pathology of Mind* (London: Macmillan, 1867) 50–83 (p. 60).

[22] Max Nordau, *Degeneration* (London: William Heinemann, 1895).

[23] Charles Lloyd Tuckey, 'Faith Healing as a Medical Treatment', *Nineteenth Century*, 21 (1888) 839–50 (p. 842).

affected).'[24] This observation does not exclude the potential that a malicious physician could overpower their patient's will, if they so desired! In his interview with the *Sketch*, he was more definitive indicating that it would be impossible to hypnotise someone who did not wish to be.[25]

In 1895, W.L. Alden, the London-based, American-born literary critic of the *Idler* magazine confidently predicted the imminent demise of hypnotism fiction.[26] The *Idler* was another late Victorian monthly periodical catering to the newly literate middle-class offering mainly comic pieces and sensational fiction but also light poetry and travel-writing. 'The Book Hunter' column was idiosyncratic and quite personal: over several pages every month, Alden expressed his own fictional interests and pet peeves. He argued that although Conan Doyle's recent novelette, *The Parasite* which is covered in the next section was 'clever and interesting,' Doyle was 'just in time' with his story.[27] He proposed that outside of fiction, hypnotism could not compel people to do objectionable things and so the story form would become obsolete very soon. Alden was suggesting that the scientific developments in the understanding of hypnotism were leading to the debunking of myths such as automatic obedience and views of hypnotism as a kind of slavery. The New Hypnotists were succeeding in shifting opinion.

While Alden was wrong about the end of hypnotic fictions, they certainly did decline after 1895 and hypnotism was no longer the central part of the plot. For many writers, hypnotism had become a well-established trope and convenient plot device. Perhaps its literary characteristics had by then been fixed and there was no need for further fictional play. The hypnotists themselves became universally malign and their ability to influence others was a manifestation of their power, cunning and dangerousness.

[24] Charles Lloyd Tuckey, *Psycho-Therapeutics: Treatment by Hypnotism and Suggestion*, 3rd ed. (London: Baillière, Tindall and Cox, 1891) (p. 103).

[25] T.H., 'Hypnotism' (p. 244).

[26] W.L. Alden, 'The Book Hunter', *Idler*, 7 (May 1895) (p. 567).

[27] Arthur Conan Doyle, 'The Parasite', *The Parasite and The Watter's Mou*, ed. by Catherine Wynne (Kansas City: Valancourt Books, 2009) (pp. 3–47); Alden, 'Book Hunter' (p. 567).

Hypnotism, Gender and Sexology

Another view that Maudsley shared with Charcot was that women were highly suggestible since they were the weaker sex and so more biologically prone to neurosis and hysteria. This female susceptibility was a longstanding societal and medical view and the mesmeric fictions which predated the hypnotic ones commonly featured an evil male mesmeric protagonist and his female victim. As early as 1788, there had been a theatre production called *Animal Magnetism* in which two couples have to thwart the unwanted amorous advances of a physician who has one of Dr. Mystery's magnets to control the women.[28] Dr. Mystery was a thinly disguised caricature of Mesmer himself. The passes of animal magnetism invited a proximity between the male doctor and the usually female patients, which society frowned upon and provoked rumours and accusations of sexual impropriety.

Just as English masculine will was being questioned by the late Victorian gothic, so was the male gender role and the erotic aspect of masculinity. This is particularly obvious in two of Arthur Conan Doyle's hypnotic short stories, 'John Barrington Cowles' (1884) and *The Parasite* (1894).[29] In both tales, the typical gender roles of trance are deliberately inverted and there is a clear underlying erotic tension. The first was set among Edinburgh medical students who attend a Mesmeric stage show and the second among medical professors formally investigating hypnotism. In the ten year gap between the stories there has been a marked improvement in the scientific status of hypnotism.

Doyle was fascinated by mesmerism, hypnotism and the supernatural. His well-known spiritualist beliefs are usually attributed to the loss of his son Kingsley in the First World War but his autobiography makes it clear they began much earlier.[30] Significantly, he had trained in Edinburgh,

[28] Elizabeth Inchbald, *Animal Magnetism, A Farce of Three Acts* (Dublin: P. Byron, 1788).

[29] Arthur Conan Doyle, 'John Barrington Cowles', *Cassell's Saturday Journal*, 1 (12 and 19 April 1884); Arthur Conan Doyle, 'John Barrington Cowles', in *Arthur Conan Doyle Gothic Tales* (Oxford: Oxford University Press, 2016) (pp. 91–112). Arthur Conan Doyle, *The Parasite* (London: Constable, 1894).

[30] Arthur Conan Doyle, 'Pulling Up the Anchor', Ch. 9 in *Memories and Adventures* (Oxford: Oxford University Press, 1989) 82–93 (p. 82).

studied Theosophy and was a member of the SPR.[31] Doyle had received a personal invitation to join the group from Frederic Myers in 1887, as they needed doctors who were 'trained to assess evidence carefully'.[32] Doyle accepted but never assisted Bramwell and Tuckey on the hypnotism committee though he did investigate a haunted house for the society.[33] In 1930, Doyle left the society very publicly as he thought that they had become too sceptical of spiritual phenomena.

Doyle disliked *The Parasite* and 'John Barrington Cowles,' suppressing them later in his career. It was reprinted just twice while he lived and only once in the States. Doyle went so far as to remove from it his anthologies and even from the list of his previous publications in his later books. Some critics have speculated that this might relate to its negative handling of hypnotism which he came to re-evaluate as he became more interested in spiritualism though this ignores the fact that at the time of writing *The Parasite* he had already joined the SPR, specifically because of his interest in telepathy and hypnotism. It seems more likely that he was concerned by its thinly veiled sexual themes. The critic Anne Cranny-Francis first advanced this theory, interpreting the story as a demonstration of Doyle's sexual frustration.[34] Sexual relations between Doyle and his wife would have been forbidden after the diagnosis of tuberculosis which she had received in 1893.

Doyle subtitled *The Parasite*, 'a mesmeric and hypnotic mystery.'[35] His conflation of mesmerism and hypnotic was deliberate. His scientific and professional interest in hypnotism meant that he would have been well aware of the differences between mesmerism and hypnotism but he knew that the two practices were blurred in the public mind. In gothic stories the concepts of mesmerism and hypnotism are frequently merged: the

[31] Gordon Bates, 'The Fascinating Fictions of Arthur Conan Doyle', in *Re-examining Arthur Conan Doyle*, ed. by Nils Clausson (Newcastle: Cambridge Scholars, 2021) 59–74 (p. 61).

[32] Trevor Hamilton, *Immortal Longings: F.W.H. Myers and the Victorian Search for Life After Death* (Exeter: Imprint Academic, 2009) (p. 74).

[33] Gordon Bates, 'Arthur Conan Doyle in Mesmeric Edinburgh and Hypnotic London', *Victoriographies*, 11 (2021) (pp. 314–330).

[34] Anne Cranny-Francis, 'Arthur Conan Doyle's *The Parasite*: The Case of the Anguished Author', in *Nineteenth-Century Suspense from Poe to Conan Doyle*, ed. by Clive Bloom and others (Basingstoke: Macmillan, 1988) 93–106 (p. 105).

[35] Doyle, 'The Parasite' (2009).

modern aspects of hypnotism dragged back to the past by the mystical and sinister features of mesmerism (Fig.9.1.

Both 'John Barrington Cowles' and *The Parasite* are unorthodox hypnotic fictions, in featuring a dominant female mesmerist/hypnotist and a submissive male subject. However, to achieve this both protagonists John Cowles and Austin Gilroy are feminised in the narrative. Cowles is unusually intimate with the male narrator of the short story, confiding 'in a manner which is rare among men.' He is described as Mediterranean-looking: 'a tall slim young fellow, with an olive Velasquez-like [sic] face and dark tender eyes.'[36]

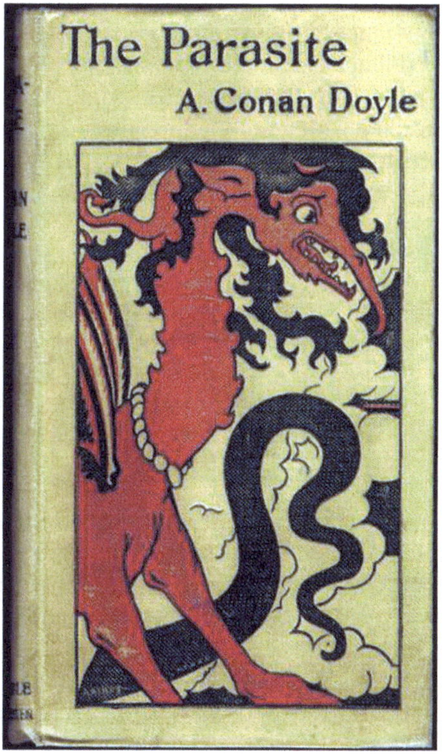

Fig. 9.1 Cover of the Constable Artist Series Edition (1898) of Arthur Conan Doyle's *The Parasite*

[36] Doyle, 'Cowles' (p. 91).

In 'The Parasite', Gilroy, writing in the first person, describes his appearance to be similar to Cowles: black hair and dark eyes, a thin olive face and tapering fingers. He also describes his change of temperament to be the result of his education, growing from a 'nervous sensitive boy, a dreamer, a somnambulist, full of impressions and intuitions' to a 'rank' materialist adult.[37] However, he makes it clear that his physical features and previous temperament mean that he is a 'highly psychic man' which carries both possible contemporary meanings of intellectualism and spiritual sensitivity. These features also mark him as susceptible to hypnotism as the northern Europeans physicians viewed the southern Europeans as highly suggestible.

Doyle slowly builds the humiliation and destruction of Gilroy as the consequence of his ambition. He is repeatedly tormented by Penelosa for meddling with forces that he does not understand. Particularly memorable is his first-person description of the youthful professor Gilroy recalling with a shudder his entranced amorous encounter with the elderly Penelosa, which resurrects the old fear that the intimacy of mesmeric rapport can be indistinguishable from erotic love:

> She smiled at me and pointed to a stool beside her. It was with her left hand that she pointed, and I, running eagerly forward, seized it – I loathe myself as I think of it – and pressed it passionately to my lips. [...] She lay quietly looking down at me with imperious eyes and her provocative smile. Once I remember that she passed her hand over my hair as one would caress a dog. And it gave me pleasure, the caress. I thrilled under it. I was her slave, body and soul, and for the moment I rejoiced in my slavery.[38]

Conventionally gothic, both Miss Penelosa and Kate Northcott use their mesmeric power for sinister ends. Like the gothic vampires, they are alien and other: both of them simultaneously attractive and repulsive in their alterity. While Northcott is young and breath-takingly beautiful, she is morally and sexually dangerous and has previous lovers who have taken their lives. Miss Penelosa, on the other hand is over forty, dark-skinned, small and frail and walks with a stick. This makes Gilroy's hypnotically

[37] Doyle, 'The Parasite' (2009) (p. 5).

[38] Doyle, 'The Parasite' (2009) (p. 31).

induced desire for her, all the more disturbing for him: 'She is far older than me, and a cripple'.[39]

Conventionally for mesmeric and hypnotic narratives, her striking eyes are described in detail. Penelosa's eyes are grey-green and 'furtive,' 'fierce' and 'feline'.[40] Doyle repeatedly uses animal similes. Gilroy is like a spaniel or terrier in his obedience. Later, as Gilroy comes to know of her attempts to possess him, mesmerically and in love, Penelosa is compared to a hermit crab that can pick up and drop shells at will. She is described as 'scarcely human' and as a 'loathsome parasite'[41] ('TP' 36). In another gender inversion from the conventional gothic, it is Gilroy who becomes weak, enervated and neurotic while he is under the thrall of the parasitic, psychic vampire. He complains about his nervous tension and even his fiancée recognises that he has become 'thinner and darker under the eyes' and 'pale and worn'.[42] The male physician has developed the symptoms of neurasthenia, the medical condition of the marginalised and impotent Victorian woman (Fig. 9.2).

Bramwell and the others tried to develop a counter-narrative demonstrating in their clinical work and experiments at the SPR that in contrast to fictional representations, women and the mentally ill were not easier subjects for hypnosis. Citing the widest European medical literature, Bramwell baldly states that 'sex has little or no influence on susceptibility.'[43] Instead, George Kingsbury and Tuckey claim that those from highly masculinised occupations like labourers, athletes, military men and university students (who were almost all male at this time) were those most suitable for hypnotic induction.[44]

There are echoes of the same gender inversion in *Dracula*. Throughout the story, there are many incidents of emasculated men and sexually predatory women. Gothic novels are traditionally subversive and

[39] Doyle, 'The Parasite' (2009) (p. 21).

[40] Doyle, 'The Parasite' (2009) (p. 7).

[41] Doyle, 'The Parasite' (2009) (p. 36).

[42] Doyle, 'The Parasite' (2009) (p. 27).

[43] John Milne Bramwell, 'Susceptibility to Hypnosis and the Causes That Influence It', Ch 4 in *Hypnotism*, 3rd ed. (London: Rider, 1921) (pp. 57–73).

[44] George Kingsbury, 'Who Are Susceptible?', Ch. 4 in *Hypnotic Suggestion: The Practice of Hypnotic Suggestion, Being and Elementary Handbook for the Use of the Medical Profession* (Bristol: John Wright, 1891) (pp. 59–66); Charles Lloyd Tuckey, 'Some Phases of Hypnotism', *Occult Review*, 1 (1905) (pp. 51–57).

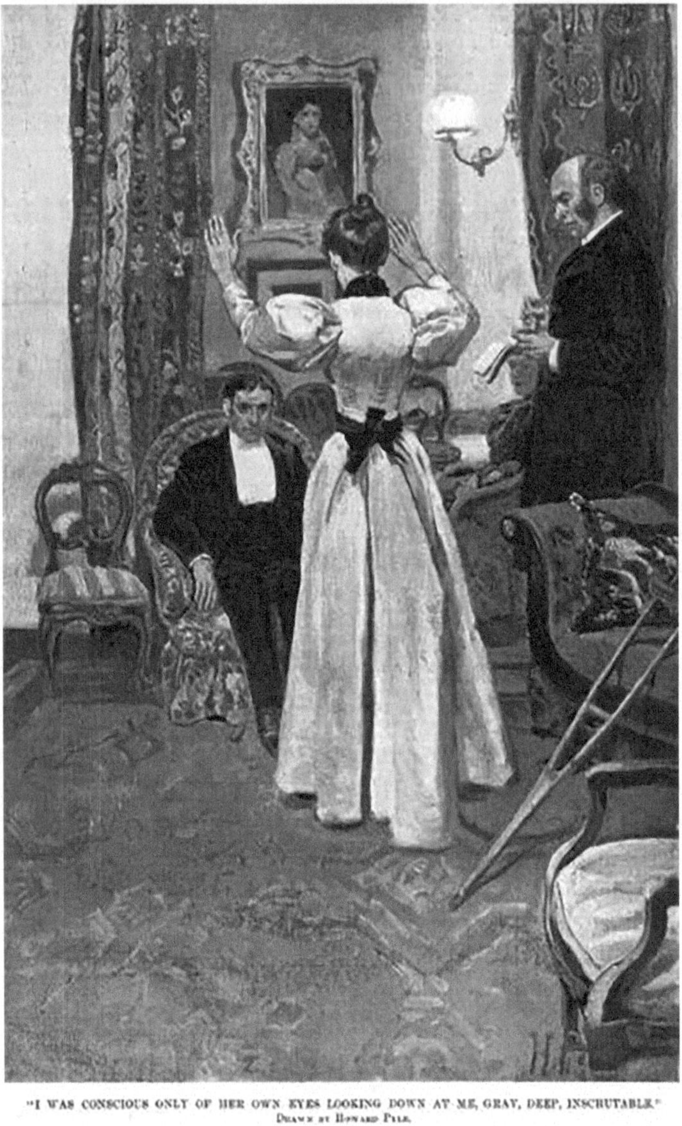

"I WAS CONSCIOUS ONLY OF HER OWN EYES LOOKING DOWN AT ME, GRAY, DEEP, INSCRUTABLE."
DRAWN BY HOWARD PYLE.

Fig. 9.2 'I was conscious only of her eyes…' illustration from 'The Parasite' (1894) by Howard Pyle for *Harpers Weekly* (New York, Harper and Brothers)

reactionary. Repeated challenges to the patriarchal orthodoxy are staged but do eventually resolve with the punishment or destruction of the transgressors and a return to the conservative status quo. Many critics have observed *Dracula's* confused and conflicted gender boundaries.

Soon after Jonathan Harker arrives at Castle Dracula, he is visited by three 'weird sisters,' female vampires who are either the Count's sisters or his wives or his lovers or all three. In a sexually charged scene, Harker feels 'in his heart a wicked, burning desire that they would kiss [him] with those red lips.' He describes their 'deliberate voluptuousness which was both thrilling and repulsive'. Despite his gender, he adopts the traditional Victorian female sexual passivity: 'I closed my eyes in a languorous ecstasy and waited – waited with a beating heart.'[45] This eroticism of control and submission implies a hypnotic component which we discover more clearly in Dracula's encounters with Lucy and Mina.

Some critics have considered this gender play within the book both as a response to the 'New Woman' and through the lens of queer theory.[46] The New Woman was a loose construct and stereotype that emerged at the end of the nineteenth century due to anxiety about the growing women's rights movement and suffragettism.[47] Portrayed in comic fiction or *Punch* cartoons, the New Woman was either overtly sexual or crudely manly, wearing trousers and smoking. The critic Christopher Craft was one of the earliest to offer a queer reading of *Dracula*.[48] The scene with the weird sisters climaxes without the penetration of the sister's teeth on Harker's neck but instead with Dracula's declaration, 'This man belongs to me.' This statement is even clarified in the text as an assertion of romantic love not just ownership.

As the trial of Oscar Wilde demonstrates, homosexuality provoked considerable public anxiety at the fin de siècle and was viewed as part of a wider problem of degeneration. The scientific interest in the behaviour led to the medicalisation of sexuality and the medical policing of these boundaries. Heike Bauer's recent collection has demonstrated that this

[45] Bram Stoker, *Dracula* (Oxford: Oxford University Press, 2011) (pp. 38–9).

[46] Carol Senf, 'Dracula and Women', *The Cambridge Companion to Dracula*, ed. Roger Luckhurst (Cambridge: Cambridge University Press, 2018) (pp. 114–22).

[47] The name was coined by Sarah Grand, 'The New Aspect of the Woman Question', *North American Review*, 158, 448 (1894) (pp. 270–6).

[48] Christopher Craft, '"Kiss Me with Those Red Lips": Gender and Inversion in *Dracula*', *Representations*, 8 (1984) (pp. 107–33).

new 'science' was also very much an international concern.[49] Richard Krafft-Ebbing among others, had started to define normality and abnormality using hundreds of case examples in his work, *Psychopathia Sexualis* (1886).[50] His new names were to come quickly into common parlance. Terms like sexual inversion (homosexuality), sadism and masochism were rapidly taken up beyond medical culture. These new distinctions and this novel approach moved sexual practices away from morality, the traditional domain of the priest and the church and towards doctors and medicine in the new discipline of 'sexology'.[51] Abnormality was viewed as evidence of degeneracy and the presence of mental illness which required medical treatment. However, the treatments of the new dynamic psychiatry were limited and hypnotism was one of those tried. After a decline in usage in the twentieth century, hypnotic treatment and suggestion were rediscovered in the 1960s as part of wider attempts to treat homosexuality as an illness at this time.[52]

The art historian and literary critic, John Addington Symonds (1840–1893) was homosexual and wrote a courageous autobiography of his own experiences.[53] He was married and had a family but chose to risk his reputation and prosperity by advocating male same-sex love. He worked with Britain's foremost medically trained expert on sexual inversion, Henry Havelock Ellis on his book *Sexual Inversion*, which did not characterise the subject as immoral, criminal or evidence of mental illness.[54] In 1893, he asked Havelock Ellis in a letter about the possible effectiveness of hypnotism and the usefulness of Charles Lloyd Tuckey's experience.

[49] Heike Bauer, ed. *Sexology and Translation: Cultural and Scientific Encounters Across the Modern World* (Philadelphia: Temple University Press, 2015).

[50] Richard Krafft-Ebbing, *Psychopathia Sexualis* (London: Staples, 1965).

[51] 'Sexology' was not coined until 1906. It derives from the German term *Sexualwissensschaft* first used by Iwan Bloch.

[52] Peter Roper, 'The Effects of Hypnotherapy on Homosexuality', *Canadian Medical Association Journal*, 96 (1967) (pp. 319–27).

[53] John Addington Symonds, *The Memoirs of John Addington Symonds: A Critical Edition*, ed. by Amber Regis (Basingstoke: Palgrave Macmillan, 2016).

[54] Havelock Ellis and John Addington Symonds, *Sexual Inversion: A Critical Edition*, ed. by Ivan Crozier (Basingstoke: Palgrave Macmillan, 2008).

Havelock Ellis was dismissive and did not think that hypnotism was helpful nor that Tuckey 'had any important contributions to make.'[55]

Despite this, Tuckey claimed to have treated 'a good number' of men troubled by their homosexuality as well as others with a range of sexual problems from masturbation to sterility.[56] He summarises his organic views of sexual problems in his 4th edition:

> If hypnotism had done nothing more for medical science than bring such melancholy cases as the above within the scope of curative treatment, it would have conferred a lasting benefit on humanity. In even worse cases of perverted sexual instinct it is frequently successful [...] Hypnotic suggestion seems to act by checking excessive functional irritability, and by developing and bringing into play the inhibitory action of the higher brain centres, which have either not developed or have undergone impairment.[57]

Bramwell confessed that he had had little experience of the 'grosser forms of sexual disorder' but some success with impotence and 'sexual inversion'.[58] He wondered if this was because they were rare in England or because those who suffered from them did not seek medical aid. He recommended the work of the Krafft-Ebbing and the German psychiatrist and psychic researcher, Albert Schrenck-Notzing who strongly advocated suggestion as the best treatment for all kinds of paraphilias, fetishes and homosexuality.[59]

The only such case history that Tuckey published outside of his books concerned paedophilia. He wrote it in 1906 for *Revue de l'hypnotisme*.[60] It is difficult to know whether this paper was written in French and

55 Havelock Ellis, 'Letter to John Addington Symonds, 19 February 1893', qtd in Sean Brady, *John Addington Symonds (1840–1893) and Homosexuality: A Critical Edition of Sources* (Basingstoke: Palgrave Macmillan, 2012) (p. 254).

56 Charles Lloyd Tuckey to van Eeden correspondence. 28 December 1888. *Van Eeden Collection* (Amsterdam: Allard Pierson, University of Amsterdam); Charles Lloyd Tuckey, 'Case 22 – Moral Breakdown', *Psycho-Therapeutics*, 4th ed. (London: Baillière, Tindall and Cox, 1900) (p. 308).

57 Tuckey, 'Sexual Perversion', *Psycho-Therapeutics*, 4th ed. (1900) (pp. 308–10).

58 Bramwell, *Hypnotism*, 3rd ed. (1921) (pp. 209–10).

59 Albert von Schrenck-Notzing, *Therapeutic Suggestion in Psychopathia Sexualis*, trans. by Gilbert Chaddock (Philadelphia: F.A. Davis, 1895).

60 Charles Lloyd Tuckey, 'Perversion Sexuelle Guérie par l'Hypnotisme', *Revue de l'Hypnotisme et de la Psychologie Physiologique*, 20 (1906) (pp. 91–3).

published in France due to prudishness or sensitivity on his part or on the part of the British journals. It concerned Tuckey's successful treatment of a 43-year-old American schoolteacher and professor of music whose life had been 'poisoned by his passion for [sexual] attacks on little girls' which he associated with his own 'corruption' at the age of six by a similarly aged girl. After hypnotic suggestive treatment the patient found himself 'very fond of little girls in a proper way.'[61] As evidence of both the cross-fertilisation between the nascent psychotherapies and the new medical internationalism, this case report was then discussed by Freud's Vienna Psychoanalytic Society early the following year.[62]

Medical Professionalism

It would be expected that the rise of medical hypnotism would result in fictions in which the hypnotists were medical practitioners. There were significant societal anxieties about the motivations and methods of the growing and increasingly influential profession at the end of the century. The decade gave rise to several unflattering tales of evil or misguided doctors. Among them, Arthur Machen's *The Great God Pan* (1894) and the H.G. Wells' *The Island of Doctor Moreau* (1896) both have driven, medical protagonists of the mad scientist archetype.[63] Machen and Wells seem to criticise their clinical objectivity and lack of empathy, as well as the clear anti-vivisection themes of *The Island of Doctor Moreau*.

However, there were surprisingly few instances of negative portrayals of medical hypnotism (discrete from hypnotism) or medical hypnotists. Margaret Brandon's *Hypnotized; or a Doctor's Confession* is one such, though it is more of a hypnotic romance than gothic in tone.[64] Dr. Digby Heblethwaite confesses to his faithful nurse, that his accidental hypnotic link to Blossom, the intimate friend of his fiancée Dora, has led to her tragic death in his care. He leaves the country for a few years out of grief

[61] Tuckey, 'Perversion sexuelle' (p. 92).

[62] Herman Nunberg and Ernest Federn, eds., '23 January 1907', in *Minutes of the Vienna Psychoanalytic Society. Vol. I: 1906–1908* (New York: International Universities Press, 1962) (p. 88).

[63] Arthur Machen, *The Great God Pan* (London: John Lane, 1894); H.G. Wells, *The Island of Doctor Moreau* (London: Heineman, 1896).

[64] Margaret Brandon, *Hypnotized; or a Doctor's Confession* (London: Hutchinson, 1891).

or remorse but at the end returns to England to be reunited with Dora, older and wiser.

It was much more common to have a heroic male doctor, often equipped with some knowledge of hypnotism to enable them to tackle the villain. In *Dracula*, Dr. van Helsing is the central member of the 'crew of light,' using his esoteric knowledge to fight against Dracula's evil special powers. Stoker depicts van Helsing as the embodiment of wisdom and virtue. He is an authority figure who presents a highly professional front. Van Helsing has read Charcot and uses an amalgam of 'metaphysical' mesmerism and modern medical hypnotism to combat Dracula's animal magnetism.

In Maclaren Cobben's *Master of His Fate* (1989), both the hero Dr. Lefevre and the psychic vampire Julius Courtney have been trained in hypnotism in Paris by Charbon [sic].[65] The charming Wilde-like Courtney is a gentleman bon-viveur who has no profession. His friend Lefevre is a hard-working neurologist who admits two young people to his hospital ward who are inexplicably unconscious. He discovers that Courtney has used hypnotism to drain their psychic energy to extend his own life. Lefevre is able to design a novel medical apparatus which revives his patients. The book was written by a clergyman who dedicated it to his friend Dr. Mennell. In the fulsome dedication, he makes it clear that the rather implausible medical paragon Lefevre, 'The good doctor of this story – the born surgeon and healer, the ever young and alert, the self-forgetful, the faithful friend, gifted with "that exquisite charity which can forgive all things"' is based on Menell.

A story which clearly demonstrates the complex relationship of medical professionalism to hypnotism is 'The Red Bracelet.' It is a short story which was written by L.T Meade and published in the *Strand* in 1895.[66] 'Lillie' Thomasina Meade was a highly versatile author, who quickly adapted to emerging genres and new formats. In particular, she took to the new short story form of interlinked but self-contained tales pioneered by the *Strand* magazine and exemplified by its best-known incarnation, the Sherlock Holmes stories of Arthur Conan Doyle. When Doyle took a break from writing about Holmes, it was Meade who took over.

[65] J. Maclaren Cobben, *Master of His Fate* (Edinburgh and London: Blackwood, 1890).

[66] L.T. Meade and Clifford Halifax, 'The Red Bracelet', *Strand Magazine*, 9 (May 1895), 545–61 (p. 545).

As a result of her longevity, productivity and responsiveness to prevalent trends Meade is an excellent bellwether for popular taste and attitude. Through her crime and medical mystery short stories, we get an excellent overview of evolving popular opinion in relation to many topics. Her fictions not only illustrated but also helped to mould and to fix public and medical opinion about medical hypnotism.

'The Red Bracelet' was one of 24 stand-alone stories which appeared in the *Strand*. They were published in two runs between 1893 and 1895 as 'Stories from the Diary of a Doctor' by Meade and Halifax. To highlight their medical authenticity, the book starts with the legend: 'The stories in this volume have been written with a close observance of Medical Facts and of the great advance which Surgery has made in the last decade. Several of the stories are formed on actual experience, and none of the Cures herein described will long remain impossible to the science and art of Surgery.'[67]

'The Hypnotic Patient'

Before looking at 'The Red Bracelet' in depth, it is relevant to consider the doctor sleuth Clifford Halifax's earlier encounter with hypnotism, as this is not his first medical mystery story involving the newly fashionable medical therapy. 'My Hypnotic Patient,' was Meade's first account and was her second episode for the *Strand* magazine overall.[68] Within this tale, Halifax agrees to offer locum cover to an alienist friend. He agrees to provide medical cover at a lunatic asylum over the period of his colleague's holiday. He is perplexed to find that an insane murderess, imprisoned there, could be attractive and coherent. He investigates Miss Whittaker's story and finds that she had been incarcerated for shooting a stranger in the head. He discovers that she had been previously hypnotised by Dr. Walter Anderson, her general practitioner, who had a grudge against the murder victim and decides to pay a visit to the doctor hypnotist.

During his neighbourhood inquiries, Halifax finds that Dr. Anderson lives in a poor area of Fulham and has been ostracised by his local

[67] L.T. Meade and Clifford Halifax, *Stories from the Diaries of a Doctor: Snippets of Early Medicine and Life in England* (Washington: Westphalia Press, 2015) (p. 1).

[68] L.T. Meade and Clifford Halifax, 'My Hypnotic Patient', *Strand Magazine*, 6 (August 1893) (pp. 163–77).

colleagues. The subtext is that Anderson is unprofessional. He is materially unsuccessful as he is a poor physician and unaccepted by his peers because of his fringe views in hypnotism. Halifax speaks to a local chemist who gives him this background information and simultaneously claims that Anderson has helped his wife's neuralgia but rejects hypnotism as quackery. Halifax refutes the idea that hypnotism is quackery (i.e. having no efficacy) but instead describes it as 'a dangerous remedy with small advantages to it and possibilities of much evil'.[69]

Despite his reservations, Halifax describes hypnotism as a 'science,' albeit 'little known' and 'full of dangerous capabilities'.[70] However, by 1894 it is no longer seen as the mystical, magical practice of Mesmer and Elliotson. Rather, it is a modern technique that could be investigated, understood and mastered by men of science. He visits Anderson who is professional, polite and helpful but Halifax expresses an irrational dislike of the man. He has the features of a mesmerist, olive-skinned and brown eyes with soft eyes 'that a woman would consider beautiful.' Ultimately, he is not professional as he is a hypnotist: 'He practises hypnotism, and my natural instincts as a doctor are therefore in arms against him.'

The short story concludes with the death of a hypnotised patient. When Anderson withdraws his hypnotic influence and returns her will to her, Miss Whittaker cannot cope with the stress of living in an asylum and soon expires. Dr. Anderson sees the error of his ways and vows never to dabble in hypnotism, which is shown to be beyond his expertise and competence. In the final paragraph, Halifax ruminates on the evolving relationship of the British legal system to hypnotic crime. Contemporaneously, the papers had featured several high-profile murder trials involving hypnotism, which had garnered considerable public interest in the UK. These included the Eyraud-*Bompard* case and the Dutch De Jong case. Overall, it is clear from the short story that Dr. Halifax, who is carefully depicted as an authentic, credible modern-day physician, views hypnotism as dangerous but very real and that its use is highly unprofessional.

[69] Meade, 'My Hypnotic Patient' (p. 556).

[70] Meade, 'My Hypnotic Patient' (p. 559).

'The Red Bracelet'

'The Red Bracelet' is a critical text for medical hypnotism for several reasons. It was published in January 1895 which was at the height of Trilbymania. I believe that it represents the tipping point between suggestion and medical imagination that I have previously described. It can be seen as a literary representation of the significant moment when a doctor's beneficial use of therapeutic suggestion is shown to be superior to a villain's malevolent hypnotism.

The story concerns Molly, the blind daughter of a rich country gentleman, who has been entranced by a scoundrel named Basil Winchester. He has hypnotised her to become infatuated with him so as to secure her money. This in itself is an unusual development: hypnotism had been previously portrayed and conceived as requiring a visual induction. Although the blindness is a plot device as the story hinges on Halifax later surgically curing Molly's blindness, it also suggests that Meade had already picked up on a shift in the public's perception of hypnotism. It had moved on from the primarily visual and gestural lexicon of mid-Victorian mesmerism (mesmeric passes of the hands and the fascinating gaze of the mesmerist). The active constituent of late Victorian hypnotism was essentially verbal in nature and explicable through the new science of suggestion.

Halifax is consulted by the girl's father, Stafford, and instructed to cure Molly of her hypnotically induced love-sickness by hypnotising her in 'another direction' that is re-hypnotising her to reverse the effect.[71] The hypnotic infatuation is reinforced by the titular red coral bracelet which Molly refuses to remove from her person. Halifax refuses to use hypnotism himself as he views it as unprofessional and risky but promises to go to meet Molly at her home, in Yorkshire and make up his own mind as to what can be done.

In Meade's portrayal, Halifax is the ultimate Victorian middle-class professional man: rational yet moral. He has great knowledge and power but works beneficently and crucially only within the scope of his professional code. Halifax has been described by the critic Douglas Small as the

[71] Meade, 'Red Bracelet' (p. 546).

'supreme apotheosis of middle-class values.'[72] As a result of his professional ideals, Halifax refuses to use hypnotism which he still views as 'a fearful and dangerous power'.[73] In effect, he uses his own moral authority in conjunction with his will to help Molly. He does this by reawakening her sense of filial devotion and parental obligation which has been temporarily overcome by her amorous obsession with Winchester and so helps her to return to normal behavioural conventions.

In a pivotal scene, Halifax encounters Molly for the first time. She is languishing in bed, refusing all food and deathly pale as her lover Winchester did not meet her to elope as arranged. The lethargic, disempowered woman is a common late Victorian literary trope usefully examined by the critic Elaine Showalter.[74] The link between neurasthenia and thwarted or vampiric love was common in stories like *Dracula* and Mary Elizabeth Braddon's 'Herself' (1894) and 'The Good Lady Ducayne' (1896).[75] The victim of the vampire's bite became tired and etiolated. Molly believes she is dying as she has nothing to live for. She clings to her coral bracelet for comfort.

When she becomes aware of the presence of Halifax in her bedroom, she leaps out of bed fully clothed and Halifax first notices her entirely white eyes. He learns that she is not eating due to a tightness in her throat, a clear sign of hysteria: 'Your throat is not closed, you only imagine it.'[76] He calls upon the ancient doctrine of imagination to explain her physical symptoms and then without the induction of trance or hypnosis uses his stronger will to encourage her to eat and drink: the doctrine of suggestion. She complies and he tells her that he can prevent her throat closing again (Fig. 9.3).

"But, surely, doctor, you are not going to hypnotise me?"

"I am not," I answered.

[72] Douglas Small, 'Masters of Healing: Cocaine and the Ideal of the Victorian Medical Man', *Journal of Victorian Culture*, 21 (January 2016) (pp. 3-20).

[73] Meade, 'My Hypnotic Patient' (p. 549).

[74] Elaine Showalter, 'Nervous Women—Sex Roles and Sick Roles', Ch. 5 in *The Female Malady: Women, Madness and English Culture, 1830–1980* (London: Virago, 1987) (pp. 121–44).

[75] Mary Elizabeth Braddon, 'Herself', *Sheffield Weekly Telegraph* (17 November 1894); Mary Elizabeth Braddon, 'The Good Lady Ducayne', *Strand Magazine*, 11 (February 1896) (pp. 185–99).

[76] Meade, 'My Hypnotic Patient' (p. 551).

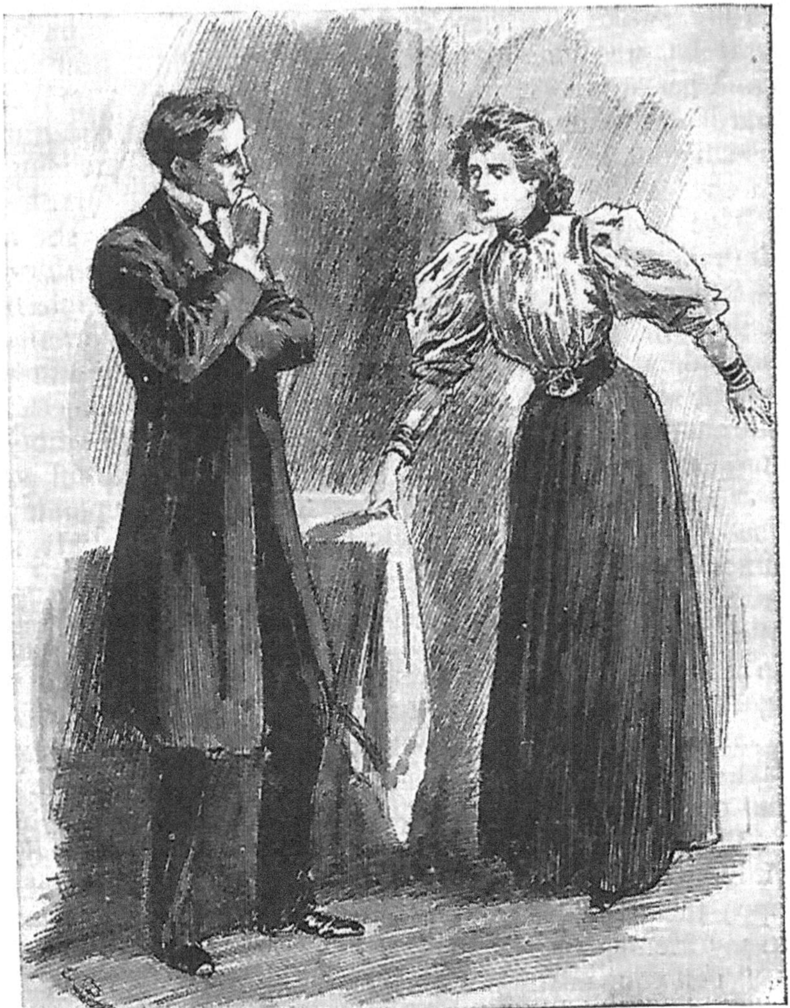

Fig. 9.3 ‘Who are you?’, illustration by Gordon Browne in the *Strand* magazine (London: George Newnes, 1895)

"Then why do you suppose that I shall obey you?"

"Because I intend to exercise my strong will over yours – yours is just now weakened by sorrow."[77]

In her fiction, Meade has clearly separated the healing power of suggestion from the mysticism of hypnotism and the trance state just as Bernheim, Tuckey and Bramwell were trying to do in their experimental and theoretical writings. In the short story, hypnotism is linked to a rupture of the social order caused by a non-medical amateur hypnotist, an immoral and sinister scoundrel. Conversely, suggestion can be used to restore order and is used by a highly ethical professional. Bernheim had already suggested that hypnotism was merely a heightened form of suggestibility and thus waking, therapeutic suggestion was possible: 'hypnotism does not really create a new condition: there is nothing in induced sleep which may not occur in the waking condition.'[78] Though these physicians were not the first to consider and attempt this separation, the logic was sound.[79] If the important therapeutic aspect of hypnosis was the suggestion, then why not dispense with the trance and all its troublesome associations altogether?

Later in the story, the supernatural and magical qualities of hypnosis are reflected in Molly's strange ability to locate her bracelet despite her blindness. The bracelet symbolises her hypnotic link to Winchester and when it is stolen, she sleepwalks to regain it. On one occasion, she is able to find it hidden in her mother's wardrobe. On another she even leaves the house to walk barefoot down the gravel drive to remove it from a gypsy baby's wrist at the lodge-keeper's house. She looks every inch the somnambule: sleepwalking in her white nightgown. Molly later describes the sensation as if a light is pointing to the bracelet that she can see and follow.

As if to further emphasise the split of suggestion from mesmerism and hypnotism which had been used historically for anaesthesia, Halifax goes on to operate on Molly using a physical medicine, the highly novel

[77] Meade, 'My Hypnotic Patient' (p. 552).

[78] Hippolyte Bernheim, *Suggestive Therapeutics* (London: G.P. Putnam, 1888) (p. 179).

[79] Braid was very much aware of the role of suggestion in hypnotic phenomena though he did not make use of this term in his early writings. One of the first to make the link explicit was the physiologist, William Carpenter. (William Carpenter, 'On the Influence of Suggestion Modifying and Directing Muscular Movement, Independently of Volition', *Proceedings, Royal Institution of Great Britain* (1852) (pp. 147–53).

agent of cocaine as a local anaesthetic despite Molly's clear suggestibility, demonstrating the triumph of the scientific as well as moral doctor. He cures her of her blindness by removing a thick membrane from the front of her eye and so breaks the hypnotic hold of Winchester. Halifax hypothesises that her blindness had exaggerated Molly's suggestibility and thus Winchester's influence. Later, Winchester returns to claim his bride but is bemused that she rejects him now that her vision is restored. Halifax receives the coral red bracelet as a gift from the grateful parents for a job well done by a superior professional and the normal moral conventions are restored.

The New Hypnotists were well aware of the need to present their use of hypnotism within a professional context. They did this in several ways. From his very first article on hypnotism, Tuckey made the case that hypnotism was a powerful agent which required safeguards. He compared the medical use of hypnotism to the medical use of toxic drugs like strychnine and aconite which were safely used by physicians but could be used to poison in the wrong hands.[80]

> Let us surround the practice of hypnotism with those precautions which the welfare of society demands, and suffer it to be employed by qualified men only, who may be trusted to use it as they use other curative agent, without any affectation of mystery or occultism.[81]

Tuckey proposed that the best safeguard would be to confine the use of hypnotism to medical men and to outlaw its use in frivolous entertainment or quackery. He and the other New Hypnotists lobbied Parliament to enact legislation to restrict the practice. This mirrored moves by the medical profession across Europe. Under pressure from their own physicians, the governments of Switzerland, Portugal and Belgium had all banned public displays of hypnotism in the late 1880s.

Tuckey made it clear that hypnotism could not be employed against someone's direct will but was keen for the UK to adopt some further safeguards to reassure and protect patients, as in continental Europe. He was aware of the reputation that mesmerism had for sexual impropriety and made the simple suggestion of the use of a chaperone to avoid this.

[80] Tuckey, 'Faith-Healing' (p. 849).

[81] Tuckey, 'Faith-Healing' (p. 850).

All of these recommendations would recur and can be found in Kingsbury's work and again in the conclusions of the committee on hypnotism set up by BMA's Section of Psychology which reported in 1893.

The hypnotic fictions of the time clearly convey the interest and anxieties which surrounded hypnosis. The themes of automatic obedience, sexual transgression and medical professionalism are seen repeatedly. By the twentieth century, the number of published fictions declines. Hypnotism is no longer interesting of itself. When hypnotism does appear, it is part of the evil powers of foreign supervillains like Guy Boothby's cosmopolitan, cultivated and unscrupulous Dr. Nikola and Sax Rohmer's inscrutable, criminal mastermind Dr. Fu Manchu.[82] It is worth noting that they are still medically trained but distanced by their foreignness. The complexities of trance are not examined and automatic obedience becomes a fixed and stable trope. I suggest that this is because the debates and anxieties are settled. The New Hypnotists had triumphed.

Bibliography

Alden, W.L. 1895. 'The Book Hunter', *Idler*, 7 (May): 567.

Arata, Stephen. 1990. 'The Occidental Tourist: "Dracula" and the Anxiety of Reverse Colonization', *Victorian Studies*, 33: 621–45.

Bagehot, Walter. 1915. 'Physics and Politics', Ch 14 in *The Works and Life of Walter Bagehot*, ed. by Mrs. Russell Barrington. London: Longman's Green.

Barlow, John. 1843. *On Man's Power Over Himself to Prevent or Control Insanity*. London: William Pickering.

Bates, Gordon. 2021. 'Arthur Conan Doyle in Mesmeric Edinburgh and Hypnotic London', *Victoriographies*, 11: 314–30.

Bates, Gordon. 2021. 'The Fascinating Fictions of Arthur Conan Doyle', in *Re-Examining Arthur Conan Doyle*, ed. by Nils Clausson. Newcastle: Cambridge Scholars. 59–74.

Bauer, Heike, ed. 2015. *Sexology and Translation: Cultural and Scientific Encounters Across the Modern World*. Philadelphia: Temple University Press.

Beer, Gillian. 1996. 'Translation or Transformation? The Relations of Science and Literature', Ch. 8 in *Open Fields, Science in Cultural Encounter*. Oxford: Oxford University Press. 173–95.

[82] Guy Boothby, *A Bid for Fortune* (New York: Appleton, 1895); Sax Rohmer, *The Mystery of Dr. Fu Manchu* (London: Methuen, 1913).

Beer, Gillian. 1983. *Darwin's Plots: Evolutionary Narrative in Darwin, George Elliot, and Nineteenth-Century Fiction*. London: Routledge and Kegan Paul. 14.

Bernheim, Hippolyte. 1889. *Suggestive Therapeutics: A Treatise on the Nature and Uses of Hypnotism*. London: G.P. Putnam.

Boothby, Guy. 1895. *A Bid for Fortune*. New York: Appleton.

Bramwell, John Milne. 1921. *Hypnotism: It's History, Practice and Theory*, 3rd ed. London: Rider.

Braddon, Mary Elizabeth. 1894. 'Herself', *Sheffield Weekly Telegraph* (17 November).

Braddon, Mary Elizabeth. 1896. 'The Good Lady Ducayne', *Strand Magazine*, 11 (February): 185–99.

Brandon, Margaret. 1891. *Hypnotized; Or a Doctor's Confession*. London: Hutchinson.

Carpenter, William. 1852. 'On the Influence of Suggestion Modifying and Directing Muscular Movement, Independently of Volition.' Proceedings, Royal Institution of Great Britain. 47–53.

Cobben, J. Maclaren. *Master of His Fate*. Edinburgh and London: Blackwood.

Corelli, Marie.2019. *A Romance of Two Worlds: Edinburgh Critical Editions of Nineteenth Century Texts*, ed. by Andrew Radford. Edinburgh: Edinburgh University Press.

Craft, Christopher. 1984. '"Kiss Me with Those Red Lips": Gender and Inversion in Dracula', *Representations*, 8: 107–33.

Cranny-Francis, Anne. 1988. 'Arthur Conan Doyle's *The Parasite*: The Case of the Anguished Author', in *Nineteenth-Century Suspense from Poe to Conan Doyle*, ed. by Clive Bloom and others. Basingstoke: Macmillan. 93–106.

Davis, Albert. 1918. *Hypnotism and Treatment by Suggestion*, 2nd ed. Liverpool: Liverpool Book Sellers.

de Roos, Hans Corneel. 2012. *Professor Abraham van Helsing: A Psychiatrist from Amsterdam? Hypnotism, Telepathy, Spiritualism and Magic in the Victorian Age*. Munich: Moonlake Editions.

de Roos, Hans Corneel. 2001. *Bram Stoker's Hidden World: A Sociogram of London's Esoteric Circles*. E-book, Munich: Moonlake Editions.

Doyle, Arthur Conan. 1884. 'John Barrington Cowles', *Cassell's Saturday Journal*, 1 (12 and 19 April).

Doyle, Arthur Conan. 1894. *The Parasite*. London: Constable.

Doyle, Arthur Conan. 1989. 'Pulling Up the Anchor', Ch. 9 in *Memories and Adventures*. Oxford: Oxford University Press. 82–93.

Doyle, Arthur Conan. 2009. 'The Parasite', in *The Parasite and The Watter's Mou*, ed. by Catherine Wynne. Kansas City: Valancourt Books: 3–47.

Doyle, Arthur Conan. 2016. 'John Barrington Cowles', in *Arthur Conan Doyle Gothic Tales*. Oxford: Oxford University Press. 91–112.

Ellis, Havelock. 1893. 'Letter to John Addington Symonds, 19 February 1893', qtd in Sean Brady. 2012. *John Addington Symonds (1840-1893) and Homosexuality: A Critical Edition of Sources.* Basingstoke: Palgrave Macmillan. 254.

Ellis, Havelock, and Symonds, John Addington. 2008. *Sexual Inversion: A Critical Edition*, ed. by Ivan Crozier. Basingstoke: Palgrave Macmillan.

Grand, Sarah. 1894. 'The New Aspect of the Woman Question', *North American Review*, 158, 448: 270–6.

Haggard, H. Rider. 1887. *Allan Quatermain.* London: Longman, Green's.

Haggard, H. Rider. 2016. *King Solomon's Mines.* Oxford: Oxford University Press.

Hamilton, Trevor. 2009. *Immortal Longings: F.W.H. Myers and the Victorian Search for Life After Death.* Exeter: Imprint Academic.

Inchbald, Elizabeth. 1788. *Animal Magnetism, A Farce of Three Acts.* Dublin: P. Byron.

Kingsbury, George. 1891. *The Practice of Hypnotic Suggestion, Being and Elementary Handbook for the Use of the Medical Profession.* Bristol: John Wright.

Krafft-Ebbing, Richard. 1965. *Psychopathia Sexualis.* London: Staples.

Maudsley, Henry. 1867. 'Hypnotism', in *Pathology of Mind.* London: Macmillan. 50–83.

Machen, Arthur. 1894. *The Great God Pan.* London: John Lane.

Maudsley, Henry. 1874. *Responsibility and Mental Disease.* London: King.

Meade, L.T., and Halifax, Clifford. 1893. 'My Hypnotic Patient', *Strand Magazine*, 6 (August): 163–77.

Meade, L.T., and Halifax, Clifford. 1895. 'The Red Bracelet', *Strand Magazine*, 9 (May): 545–61.

Meade, L.T., and Halifax, Clifford. 2015. *Stories from the Diaries of a Doctor: Snippets of Early Medicine and Life in England.* Washington: Westphalia Press.

Nordau, Max. 1895. *Degeneration.* London: William Heinemann.

Nunberg, Herman, and Federn, Ernest. 1962. 23 January 1907 *Minutes of the Vienna Psychoanalytic Society Vol. I: 1906–1908.* New York: International Universities Press. 88.

Reed, John. 1989. *Victorian Will.* Athens: Ohio University Press.

Senf, Carol. 2018. 'Dracula and Women', *The Cambridge Companion to Dracula*, ed. Roger Luckhurst. Cambridge: Cambridge University Press. 114–22.

Rohmer, Sax. 1913. *The Mystery of Dr. Fu Manchu.* London: Methuen.

Roper, Peter. 1967. 'The Effects of Hypnotherapy on Homosexuality', *Canadian Medical Association Journal*, 96: 319–27.

Von Schrenck-Notzing, Albert. 1895. *Therapeutic Suggestion in Psychopathia Sexualis*, trans. by Gilbert Chaddock. Philadelphia: F.A. Davis.

Shiel, M.P. 1898. *The Yellow Danger.* London: Grant Richards.

Showalter, Elaine. 1987. 'Nervous Women—Sex roles and Sick Roles', Ch 5 in *The Female Malady: Women, Madness and English Culture, 1830-1980*. London: Virago: 121–44.

Small, Douglas. 2016. 'Masters of Healing: Cocaine and the Ideal of the Victorian Medical Man', *Journal of Victorian Culture*, 21 (January): 3–20.

Stephen, James. 1863. *A General View of the Criminal Law of England*. London: Macmillan.

Stoker, Bram. 1910. *Famous Impostors*. London: Sidgwick & Jackson.

Stoker, Bram. 2011. *Dracula*. Oxford: Oxford University Press. 38–9.

Symonds, John Addington. 2016. *The Memoirs of John Addington Symonds: A Critical Edition*, ed. by Amber Regis. Basingstoke: Palgrave Macmillan.

T.H. 1894. 'Hypnotism in Criminal Investigation', *Sketch*, 4: 244.

Taylor, Jenny Bourne. 1988. *The Secret Theatre of Home: Wilkie Collins, Sensation Narrative, and Nineteenth-Century Psychology*. New York: Routledge. 19.

Tuckey, Charles Lloyd. 1888. 'Faith Healing as a Medical Treatment', *Nineteenth Century*, 21: 839–50.

Tuckey, Charles Lloyd. 1893. 'Letter to van Eeden, 28 December 1888', in *Van Eeden Collection*. Amsterdam: Allard Pierson, University of Amsterdam.

Tuckey, Charles Lloyd. 1891. 'The Applications of Hypnotism', *Contemporary Review*, 60: 672–86.

Tuckey, Charles Lloyd. 1891. *Psycho-Therapeutics: Treatment by Hypnotism and Suggestion*, 3rd ed. London: Baillière, Tindall and Cox.

Tuckey, Charles Lloyd. 1900. 'Case 22—Moral Breakdown', *Psycho-Therapeutics: Treatment by Hypnotism and Suggestion*, 4th ed. London: Baillière, Tindall and Cox. 308.

Tuckey, Charles Lloyd. 1905. 'Some Phases of Hypnotism', *Occult Review*, 1: 51–7.

Tuckey, Charles Lloyd. 1906. 'Perversion Sexuelle Guérie par l'Hypnotisme', *Revue de l'Hypnotisme et de la Psychologie Physiologique*, 20: 91–3.

Wells, H.G. 1896. *The Island of Doctor Moreau*. London: Heineman.

Wells, H.G. 1898. *War of the Worlds*. London: Heinemann.

CHAPTER 10

The Triumph of Medical Hypnotism

Hypnotism and suggestive therapy had first gained prominence and then started to gain acceptability and respectability in the late nineteenth century. However, their progress at the start of the twentieth century requires considerable unravelling. The previous chapters show the connections and connotations of hypnotism in the late Victorian period and how these helped to form the public perception and medical conception of hypnotism. This chapter will outline some of the evidence that this acceptance took place at the start of the twentieth century, in parallel with the transition from hypnotism to suggestive therapy in the period leading up to the First World War.

Historians of hypnotism and the psychotherapies give widely differing accounts of the status of medical hypnotism between the mid-1890s and the start of the Great War when it was used on both sides in the treatment of the psychological trauma of the soldiers. There is a surprising dearth of knowledge about the early history of the psychotherapies which has only recently been acknowledged and started to be addressed.[1] The

[1] Sarah Marks, 'Psychotherapy in Historical Perspective', *History of the Human Sciences, 30* (2017) (pp. 3–16); Sonu Shamdasani, 'Psychotherapy in Society. Historical Reflections', in *The Routledge History of Madness and Mental Health*ed. by G. Eghigian (London: Routledge, 2017) (pp. 363–78).

G. D. L. Bates, *The Uncanny Rise of Medical Hypnotism, 1888–1914*, Mental Health in Historical Perspective,
https://doi.org/10.1007/978-3-031-42725-1_10

developments in British psychotherapeutics at this time have been particularly poorly served. This had led to a privileging of the history of Freudian psychoanalytic therapy over suggestion, as the movement was far better at documenting and constructing the history of its early years.

Considering the European and more specifically the French context, the medical historian Henri Ellenberger and the French neurologist Pierre Janet both described a 'rapid decline' after Charcot's death in 1893 which was generally accepted.[2] By contrast, the North American context of the Chicago and Boston schools of psychology have been more clearly researched and the complexity of influences and developments unearthed.[3] The importance of European medicine and hypnotism (rather than German experimental psychology) to abnormal and therapeutic psychology have been revealed. The 2017 special edition of *Notes and Records*, the Royal Society's journal of the history of science, was able to discover plenty of new material about European hypnotic developments and transitions over this period but appears to have deliberately excluded the UK.[4] It seems that the editors accepted the view of the medical historian, Teri Chettiar, that in Britain hypnotism 'was decisively excluded from serious medical consideration by 1900.'[5]

By contrast, the historian Philip Kuhn, in his meticulous history of early British psychotherapeutics, states that 'The fiercely fought hypnotic

[2] Henri Ellenberger, *The Discovery of the Unconscious, the History and Evolution of Dynamic Psychiatry* (London: Allen Lane, 1970) (p. 171); Pierre Janet, *Psychological Healing: A Historical and Clinical Study*, 1 (New York: MacMillan 1925) (p. 200).

[3] George Gifford, *Psychoanalysis, Psychotherapy, and the New England Medical Scene, 1894–1944* (New York, NY: Science History Publications, 1978); Eugene Taylor, 'Psychotherapeutics and the Problematic Origins of Clinical Psychology in America', *American Psychologist*, 55 (2000) (pp. 1029–33); John Andrick, 'The "Chicago School of Psychology" and *Hypnotic Magazine*: Suggestive Therapeutics, Public Psychologies, and New Thought Pluralism, 1895–1910', *History of Psychology*, 23, 1 (2020) (pp. 1–25).

[4] Andreas-Holger Maehle and Heather Wolffram, 'Guest Editorial', *Notes and Records: The Royal Society Journal of the History of Science*, 71 (2017) Special Issue: 'History of Hypnotism in Europe', ed. by Andreas-Holger Maehle, and Heather Wolffram (pp. 119–23).

[5] Teri Chettiar, '"Looking as Little Like Patients as Persons Well Could"': Hypnotism, Medicine and the Problem of the Suggestible Subject in Late Nineteenth-Century Britain', *Medical History*, 56 (2012) (pp. 335–54).

battles of the early 1890s had…been all but won by 1898.'[6] It should be noted that Ernest Hart, hypnotism's staunchest critic, had died that year. Ironically, both Chettiar and Philip Kuhn identify Bramwell and Frederic Myers' address to the BMA annual meeting in 1898 as the pivotal moment for British medical hypnotism but come to completely different conclusions about the outcome.[7] Chettiar writes about the complexity of Myers' model of the subliminal self being unattractive or incomprehensible to British medics. Kuhn observes that even Myers' invitation demonstrates both his eminence and the increasing acceptability of hypnotism. Those who were not physicians were rarely invited to speak to the BMA. The only dissenting voice, in the absence of Hart and Kerr from the audience, was Charles Mercier who had been a regular critic in the journals and voiced the continuing fears of automatic obedience and potential criminality.[8] Bramwell directly refuted this possibility.

Kuhn's view is that hypnotism and suggestion became established medical treatments among a range of early psychotherapies. I share this opinion that hypnotism survived and made several important contributions to medical, psychological and the intellectual discourse, although it changed its name again to suggestive therapy. I will lay out the evidence for its acceptance in this chapter and the continuing role of the New Hypnotists in its establishment. I will also describe the importance of non-professional suggestive therapy and self-help books and the influx of American ideas like Christian Science and New Thought.

The Acceptance of Hypnotism and Suggestive Therapy

So, did British medical hypnotism decline or did it grow and how can we know? The absence of debate in general medical journals, does not mean that medical interest in hypnotism or its use had stopped. I have shown that Hart's successor at the *British Medical Journal*, (*BMJ*) Dawson

[6] PhilipKuhn, 'The Medical Society for the Study of Suggestive Therapeutics', Ch. 7 in *Psychoanalysis in Britain, 1893–191, Histories and Historiography* (Lanham: Lexington, 2017) (pp. 159–180) (p. 174).

[7] Kuhn, 'The 1898 BMA Hypnotism Debates', Ch. 3 in *Psychoanalysis* (pp. 31–45) (p. 35).

[8] Charles Mercier, 'Suggestion and Crime', *British Medical Journal* (10 September 1898) (p. 678).

Williams was more favourably inclined to hypnotism and the non-material aspects of the doctor-patient relationship. However, the *BMJ* did publish fewer papers and editorials about hypnotism after Hart. Chettiar suggests that this shows the rejection of the technique but another interpretation would be that the debate had been settled favourably.

In any case, Chettiar's observation about the absence of hypnotism from the medical journals, as a whole, is not true. Adopting a more objective measure, historian Alan Gauld has charted that the number of publications on the topic of hypnotism (as identified by the medical cataloguing system the *Index Medicus*) over the time. While falling in Europe, the coverage in British medical journals actually rises between 1895 and 1914.[9]

Charles Lloyd Tuckey and John Milne Bramwell continued to write for medical and lay journals as well as publish new editions of their books which continued to sell and seemed oblivious to any decline, particularly one on the scale indicated by Janet. In 1897, Bramwell gave a public lecture in Charing Cross, London in which he stated that hypnotism had a bright future: 'While those who study and practise hypnotism differ widely in their theoretical explanations of its phenomena, what is common to all [...] is the belief in its future—the profound conviction that this science, so ridiculed, constitutes one of the greatest advances of the human mind and one of its most precious possessions.'[10] Tuckey contributed an article on hypnotism and suggestion to the *Medical Annual* of 1898, a book widely read by doctors as it doubled as a directory of all UK medical practitioners: 'During the last few years hypnotism has met with increasing favour at the hands of the medical profession. Prejudice against it has largely died out and it has come to be regarded as a possible remedy in many cases without ordinary treatment.'[11]

Gauld's overall view is that 'while the interest in and practice of hypnotism continued to grow for several years [after the early 1890s] but it never wholly, or even largely, overcame the strong conservatism of the British medical profession' and notes that interest rose in the UK while

[9] Alan Gauld, *A History of Hypnotism* (Cambridge: Cambridge University Press, 1992) (p. 561).

[10] John Milne Bramwell, *Suggestion: Its place in Medicine and Scientific Research* (N.P., 1897).

[11] Charles Lloyd Tuckey, 'Hypnotism and Suggestion', *The Medical Annual and Practitioners Index* (Bristol: John Wright, 1898) (pp. 77–85) (p. 77).

falling in most other countries over the same period.[12] It may be true that hypnotism did not conquer the traditionalists of British medicine but I will show how the tenets of suggestive therapy did find their way into orthodox medical practice in the UK.

It should not be surprising that the majority of British doctors failed to adopt hypnotism in their work. There are several reasons for this. None of its British exponents claimed hypnotism to be a panacea. They had demonstrated it to be efficacious in pain reduction and sleep problems in physical health, functional illness and in the treatment of mental disorders like neurasthenia, addiction and hysteria. These were the sort of problems that usually presented to general practitioners and psychiatrists not to general hospital doctors. Consequently, the practice of hypnotism would have been most useful for general practitioners and those psychiatrists managing community-based neurotic conditions and this seems to have been the case. Uptake was therefore much greater in these specialties. Of course, even among these two groups there were varying professional beliefs about efficacy and legitimacy. The medical historian, Rhodri Hayward has acknowledged the enduring influence of hypnotism and suggestive therapy on the psychological aspects of primary care.[13]

Specialisation was a relatively recent innovation at this time. Medicine had split from surgery but had not yet fully subdivided itself before the First world war. Psychological medicine and general practice also had a history of separation from medicine.[14] However, even within psychological medicine, work outside of large asylums was a relatively new development as 'anxiety, neurasthenia and other forms of neurosis (as they were increasingly called) seemed more common.'[15] For example, the medical psychologist L. Forbes Winslow had opened one of the first outpatient mental hospitals in London in 1890, allowing treatment of the poor who could not afford the lodging fees.[16] A figure of considerable controversy and a medical maverick, Winslow had been an exposer

[12] Gauld, *Hypnotism* (p. 350).

[13] Rhodri Hayward, 'The Emergence of the Unconscious', Ch. 1 in *The Transformation of the Psyche in British Primary Care, 1889–1970* (London: Bloomsbury, 2015) (pp. 1–30).

[14] William Bynum, *Science and the Practice of Medicine in the Nineteenth Century* (Cambridge: Cambridge University Press, 1994) (pp. 191–6).

[15] Bynum, *Science* (p. 196).

[16] L. Forbes Winslow, *Recollections of Forty Years* (London: John Ouseley, 1910) (p. 374).

of séance fraud and a vocal critic of American spiritualism, claiming that it was a cause of insanity and responsible for the high number of residents in American asylums.[17] However, by the start of the twentieth century, he recanted his previous materialist views in a lecture to a spiritualist society in Merthyr Tydfil.[18] He too, had started to use hypnotism in his medical practice and had joined the lay group, the London Psycho-Therapeutic Society (LPS), serving as its vice-president from 1910. While Winslow's personal Damascene conversion is not indicative of all physicians' views, it does suggest that the suspicion with which hypnotism was viewed was shifting.

The London Psycho-Therapeutic Society

The PTS had been founded by the journalist and part-time hypnotist Arthur Hallam (1878–1948) and the spiritualist and 'clairvoyant healer,' George Spriggs (1850–1912) in 1901. Its aims were the advocacy of health reform, medical hypnotism, suggestive therapeutics, curative human radiations, specialist diet and general drugless healing. Spriggs became the principal therapist and Hallam administered the organisation and ran the journal, the *Health Record and Psycho-Therapeutic Journal* later just the *Health Record (HR)* and the regular lecture series. They achieved a remarkable reach, seeing 2500 patients and providing 200,000 treatments without charge, in their first ten years. In 1910, their fundraising had been so fruitful that they were able to move the organisation and their treatment centre to Bloomsbury Square in upmarket north London.

Despite attracting the derision of the medical press because of their fringe beliefs and non-medical backgrounds, they did initially attract at least a dozen medical practitioners, both to lecture and attend their events. In the early years of the society, they attracted some older 'free-thinking' physicians including the homoeopath, theosophist and mesmerist George Wyld and the maverick, publicity-hungry L. Forbes Winslow. As a lay organisation, there was no imperative to stick to a materialist scientific schema and they were a broad church. Their membership

[17] L. Forbes Winslow, *Spiritualistic Madness* (London: Baillère, 1877).

[18] Anon, 'Lyttleton Forbes Winslow's Obituary', *Light,* 33, 1692 (14 June 1913) (p. 288).

included Theosophists, mesmerists, spiritual healers and Swedenborgians, followers of the scientist and mystic Emanuel Swedenborg (1688–1772).

The lectures and journal articles demonstrate a wide range of ideas and beliefs about the trance state and the power of the mind to heal the body. The majority of those which concerned hypnotism refer to it as magnetism and rely on older mystical mesmeric dogma of fluid, aura, higher mental functioning and rapport. Nevertheless, the number of interested physicians in the audience and as lecturers continued to increase. A sign of the progress of the organisation and hypnotism as a whole, was the coverage in the *Lancet* of a 1906 lecture by Dr. Edwin Ash, a Manchester-trained doctor who was one of the most active and highest profile of the second wave of medical hypnotists who emerged in the early 1900s.[19] The *Lancet*, which had previously published only a handful of scientific papers on hypnotism, had published two of Ash's hypnotism papers earlier in the year.[20] The article not only publicised the *PTS* but mentioned the presence of the physicians in the audience. Only ten years before, there would have been talk of quackery and the loss of professionalism as a result of sharing healing practices and education with non-professionals.

Around 1910, an *HR* editorial clearly reflected the optimistic mood of the editor and the members.[21] Hallam described the rapid growth of the society and claimed credit for the journal's role in changing the public mood towards mind cure which I have shown was mostly suggestive therapy. However, by 1913 the PTS was in serious financial and existential trouble. The rent on the Bloomsbury Square building jumped significantly and the journal *HR* was a major drain on their resources. Perhaps most seriously they had lost their principal therapist the charismatic, George Spriggs the previous year.[22] They were forced to abandon the journal and the building. Ultimately, Hallam himself disappeared

[19] Edwin Ash, 'Modern Hypnotism. A lecture delivered before the PTS', *Lancet*, 168, 4341 (10 November 1906) (p. 1308).

[20] Edwin Ash, 'Some Experiments in Hypnotism', *Lancet*, 167, 4300 (27 January 1906) (pp. 216–20); Edwin Ash, 'The Induction of Hypnosis', *Lancet*, 168, 4330 (25 August 1906) (pp. 501–4).

[21] Arthur Hallam, 'Editorial', *Health Record* (July 1911) (p. 74).

[22] Kuhn, 'The London Psycho-Therapeutic Society (1900–1915)' Ch. 4 in *Psychoanalysis* (pp. 49–95).

mysteriously in 1915 and this spelled the end for this version of the PTS and the *Health Record* journal.

The PTS played an important part in the democratisation of therapeutic hypnotism. Such was its scale that its free treatments did much to popularise hypnotism in London as an early mind cure and reassure many about its safety. Despite threatening the medical monopoly, the response of the medical institutions mellowed over time. Perhaps as a result of his previous experience of the early fear of hypnotism and public resistance, Tuckey held stronger views about medical professionalism and the need for a medical psychotherapeutic cartel and wished to ban medical members of the PTS from the MSSST.

The Medical Society for the Study of Suggestive Therapy

The roots of the MSSST can be traced back to one of the new specialist journals, the *General Practitioner (GP).* It was a key publication for the propagation of the principles and practice of hypnotism and suggestive therapy to physicians in community practice. Like the *Journal of Mental Science* for psychiatrists and asylum superintendents, it continued to regularly publish articles on hypnotism and suggestion in the late 1890s and first decade of the new century.

In 1903, Percy Allan (1869–1927) had joined George Brown at the *GP* as an editorial assistant. Allan was a general practitioner in Croydon who had met Tuckey quite early in his career. After introducing Allan and three other Guy's hospital students to hypnotism at his Green Street home, Tuckey and Allan had enjoyed 'a long and intimate friendship.'[23] Allan would become a medical member of the Society for Psychical Research and later contributed to Tuckey's obituary for its journal. Allan was very receptive to any work on hypnotism and encouraged Tuckey to write for the *GP.* Between June 1903 and April 1907, Tuckey wrote six papers for the journal on hypnotic topics from pain management to treatment of homosexuality and obsessions.[24] He encouraged others to share

[23] Anon. 'Obituary—C. Lloyd Tuckey', *Journal of the Society for Psychical Research*, 22 (1925) (pp. 115–7) (p. 116).

[24] Charles Lloyd Tuckey, 'Some Notes on Hypnotic Suggestion', *General Practitioner* (6 June 1904) (pp. 350–1); Charles Lloyd Tuckey, ' Some Notes on Hypnotic Suggestion', *General Practitioner* (13 June 1904) (pp. 367–8); Charles Lloyd Tuckey, 'Some

their experiences in the *GP* as Allan and Brown were sufficiently 'open-minded' to print them. This was an important contribution. The historian Philip Kuhn claims that 'there is little doubt that Tuckey's writings, especially in the *GP*, were to be a significant factor in its [hypnotism as a therapeutic approach] growing popularity during the first long decade of the new century.'[25]

The growing enthusiasm for hypnotism among general practitioners had an unexpected result. Two GPs from outside of London, decided that it would be useful to establish a national society to support and educate doctors who wished to practice this way and to promote the wider use of suggestion by doctors. They were Alfred Betts Taplin (1856–1939) and Douglas Bryan (1879–1955). Betts Taplin had been qualified for over 20 years but in 1900, decided to practice solely in mental health primarily using hypnotism. Without a post at a local Liverpool hospital or asylum this was a brave move but he successfully built up his practice by word of mouth.[26] He presented one of his cases treated by hypnotic suggestion at the Liverpool Medical Institute which was written up in the *BMJ*.[27] Bryan was Leicester GP who had also tried his hand at hypnotism and was surprised by his success. He wrote up some of his case reports in the *GP* journals. It is not clear how Bryan and Betts Taplin came into contact with each other although Kuhn has suggested that it might have been the result of these scientific journal contributions.[28]

Over the summer of 1906, the pair sounded out the 52 year old Tuckey, about becoming president of their new organisation. His initial response was negative. Seventeen years before, he had gloomily written to

Notes on Hypnotic Suggestion', *General Practitioner* (20 June 1904) (pp. 382–4); Charles Lloyd Tuckey, 'Notes on Some Cases of Obsession', *General Practitioner* (26 September 1903) (pp. 607–8); Charles Lloyd Tuckey, 'Notes on Sexual Perversion', *General Practitioner* (7 November 1903) (pp. 703–4); Charles Lloyd Tuckey, 'The Utility of the Study of Suggestion to the Student and Practitioner', *General Practitioner* (6 April 1907) (pp. 210–3).

[25] Kuhn, 'Medical Society for the Study of Suggestive Therapeutics', Ch. 7 in *Psychoanalysis* (p. 162).

[26] C.M. Vaillant, 'An Historical Sketch of the Emergence of Liverpool Psychiatry', *Journal of the Liverpool Psychiatric Club*, 1 (1963). http://www.priory.com/homol/livpsy/19th.htm [accessed 6 May 2020].

[27] Anon. 'Treatment by Hypnotic Suggestion', *British Medical Journal* (28 April 1906) (pp. 979–80).

[28] Kuhn, *Psychoanalysis* (pp. 164–6).

the *Lancet* suggesting that a medical hypnotic society could never flourish in the UK.[29] However they must have persuaded him of the changed cultural environment and he eventually agreed, another indicator of the improving profile of hypnotism. The newly formed group publicised itself in the *GP* and *Journal of the Society for Psychical Research* and first met at Tuckey's Park Lane home on November 8th.[30] Far from rejection or critical voices, the response was overwhelmingly positive from the medical and lay press: 'We wish the best success to the Medical Society for the study of Suggestive Therapeutics of which Charles Lloyd Tuckey is the president. Psychology in this country has an unparalleled record, it should no longer be behind in the modern age.'[31]

The MSSST, the eventual choice of name for the new society was proposed by Milne Bramwell. The terminology used is highly significant. When people decide to rename things, they can be striving for more technically precise terminology or they can be attempting to distance an object or idea from previous unhelpful associations and sometimes both at once. In their attempts to rid animal magnetism of its disproven mechanism, adherents renamed it mesmerism after its most famous proponent. Then to separate it from the theatrical, magical and Romantic associations it became hypnotism. Stage entertainers and mediums were quite happy to re-appropriate the newer concept and word and as a result tarnished it for the medics and scientists. Suggestive therapy was the latest attempt to separate the induction of the trance state from its previous iterations. Additionally, Bramwell like many of the medical hypnotists, found sleep unnecessary and did not always use hypnotic induction at all but continued to use suggestion and wanted this conveyed in the name of the society.

One of the founding principles of the society was that hypnotism and suggestion were powerful therapeutic tools that should be restricted to medical professionals. They went so far as to exclude membership to any medics that might work with lay-people who either used hypnotism or attempted to cure disease. They had no wish to lose the hard-won monopoly of doctors in treating the sick or the potential loss of status

[29] Charles Lloyd Tuckey, 'Correspondence', *Lancet* (12 October 1889) (p. 776).

[30] Percy Allan, 'M.S.S.S.T.', *General Practitioner* (24 November 1906) (p. 748); Anon. 'The M.S.S.S.T', *Journal of the Society for Psychical Research*, 13 (1906) (pp. 14–5).

[31] Anon. 'The M.S.S.S.T.', *Morning Post* (4 July 1907) (p. 3).

if others were competent to do their work. Presumably, they had in mind the PTS, though they permitted Edwin Ash to join despite his connections to the PTS.

In 1910, they decided to change the name to the Psycho-Medical society (PMS). This may have been to better reflect and accommodate the range of psychotherapies that the members followed. Suggestive therapy had separated into three forms of treatment: hypnotism, hypnotism with suggestion and pure suggestion. There was also a growing interest in using hypnotism to uncover supressed traumatic memories as part of a hybrid of suggestion and Freudian catharsis.[32] In his book on hypnotism, L. Forbes Winslow characterised the British context which has been called the early British Eclectic: 'there are schools in Psychotherapeutics on the continent. In England we have none.'[33] With the enthusiasm of the recent convert, he concludes, 'It is the bounden duty of the physician to be properly instructed in every possible subject which bears directly or indirectly on his profession.'

The mixed form of hypnotism and cathartic therapy was prevalent enough to find its way into popular fiction. Algernon Blackwood's short story 'The Man who Found Out (A Nightmare)' written in 1912, features a physician, Laidlaw who is permanently relieved of a terrible traumatic memory which is destroying him, by medical hypnotism.[34] Blackwood had not only been taught hypnotism by medical student friends at Edinburgh University but was also a member of the SPR. In addition, the hybrid therapy was a feature of Rebecca West's novel *The Return of the Soldier* (1918) in which hypnotism is considered as part of the early mind cure of Chris, a soldier with severe amnesia and regression, damaged by the First World War. His physician glibly suggests: 'Oh, hypnotism is a silly trick. It releases the memory of a dissociated personality which can't be related [...] to the waking personality. I'll do it by talking to him. Getting him to tell his dreams.'[35] West was a suffragette and her sister

[32] The story of the interconnections between suggestion and psychoanalysis and their subsequent representations are beyond the scope of this book but are well covered by Ellenberger and Borsch-Jacobsen. Ellenberger, *Discovery*; Mikkel Borch-Jacobsen, 'Hypnosis in Psychoanalysis', *Representations* 27 (1989) (pp. 92–110).

[33] L. Forbes Winslow, *Suggestive Power of Hypnotism* (London: Rebman, 1910) (p. 20).

[34] Algernon Blackwood, 'The Man who Found Out', in *Ancient Sorceries and Other Weird Stories* (London: Penguin, 2002) (pp. 131–46).

[35] Rebecca West, *The Return of the Soldier* (London: Virago, 2010) (p.126).

was one of the early female British qualified doctors. It is likely that she had links to Jessie Murray and May Sinclair of the Medico-Psychological Clinic, an important early centre for psychotherapeutics.

In the pre-war period those doctors with an interest in forms of mind cure would join medical societies like the MSSST to learn more to help their work. Part of the reason for the growth and prosperity of the MSSST was the quality of the presenters in its lecture series. Since so many of its early members were also members of the SPR, they had access to some of the best scholars and most up-to-date information on British and Continental ideas about the mind.

In addition to the highly experienced, Bramwell and Tuckey there were lectures from other medical members and suggestion enthusiasts of the SPR: Hugh Wingfield, previously a Cambridge physiologist and early psychologist; T.W Mitchell, who joined the SPR in 1906 and became its president after Bramwell in 1910; and William McDougall, the professor of psychology at Oxford and a major figure in early twentieth-century psychology. The links between the MSSST and SPR were even closer than shared members and overlapping interests. From its inception, the MSSST had access to the SPR's journal, as well as the use of its library and offices at 20 Hanover Square. This existing infrastructure would have been really useful to the MSSST in its early years.[36]

In conclusion, the MSSST/PMS was an important early medical institution not only for the promotion of hypnotism but as a site of knowledge for early psychotherapeutics and medical psychology. Its existence demonstrates the persistence of medical hypnotism into the twentieth century. Although the membership numbers were relatively small compared with the number of practising physicians, its members were highly influential and the ideas of suggestion and dual consciousness can be traced into many if not all of the psychotherapies which followed. Twenty years after their arrival, the New Hypnotists were continuing to play a leading role in the promotion of hypnotism through the MSSST organisation and its teaching programme. Its records and lectures illustrate the transition that was occurring in mind cure. Pre-war British psychotherapeutics was diverse and eclectic with a variety of therapeutic approaches. Hypnotism and the trance were becoming less critical to the effectiveness of suggestion while suggestion remained. Additionally, the medical hypnotists were

[36] Kuhn, *Psychoanalysis* (p. 167).

quite open to the psychoanalytic ideas of Freud, particularly the idea of catharsis of traumatic memories, even if Freud himself had rejected hypnotism as part of the therapeutic process, for practical as well as theoretical reasons.[37]

The Medical Mainstream

One of the ways that suggestion came to be accommodated within British medical orthodoxy was an expansion in the idea of which aspects of the therapeutic encounter could promote therapeutic suggestion. While hypnotism was being decoupled from suggestive therapy, suggestion was being reinvented as a part of the 'bedside manner' or healing persona of the best physicians. The prolific English writer, devout Christian and physician, Alfred Schofield did much to promote the idea of 'unconscious therapeutics' or the way that the personality of a doctor could impact positively on their patient.[38] He did not claim ownership of this idea but claimed that it he was expounding from his reading and that this was accepted wisdom in North America. In his book *Unconscious Therapeutics: or, the Personality of the Physician,* his main US sources for the importance of medical character, manners and appearance appears to be the Bostonian physician and author Oliver Wendell Holmes (1809–1894) and the Philadelphian physician, S. Weir Mitchell.[39] It appears that Weir Mitchell (1829–1914) had little time for psychotherapeutics but the efficacy of his famous 'rest cure' was attributed to his personality by his colleagues.[40]

To ensure that a physician is unconsciously therapeutic, Schofield suggests he should be clean and smartly-dressed, calm, unrushed, sympathetic and of 'helpful, buoyant spirit'.[41] He summarises its importance: 'It

[37] Borch-Jacobsen convincingly argues that although Freud removed hypnotism from his mind cure it was impossible to completely remove suggestion from the therapeutic encounter. Mikkel Borch-Jacobsen, 'Hypnosis in Psychoanalysis', *Representations* 27 (1989) (pp. 92–110).

[38] Alfred Schofield, *Unconscious Therapeutics: or, the Personality of the Physician* (Philadelphia: Blakiston, 1904).

[39] S. Weir Mitchell, *Doctors and Patients* (Philadelphia and London: Lippincot, 1888).

[40] Richard Cabot, 'The Use and Abuse of Rest in the Treatment of Disease', *Psychotherapy: A Course of Instruction in Sound Psychology, Sound Medicine, and Sound Religion*, 2 (1909) (pp. 23–38) (p. 28).

[41] Schofield, *Unconscious Therapeutics* (p. 100).

is not too much to say that inferior medical skill with a good and assuring manner, is more likely to effect cure than a superior skill with a different, depressing personality.'[42]

An exemplar of the increasing prominence of these values was the stellar career of the Canadian physician William Osler, who personified a more sympathetic professionalism. Osler made his name at Johns Hopkins hospital in Baltimore before being appointed the Oxford Regius professor of Medicine in 1905 and made a baronet by King George V in 1911. He was famous for his clinical skills, teaching, medical knowledge but particularly his engaging bedside manner. His colleagues agreed on the force of his personality and the potency of what he called his 'general cheer-up prescription'.[43] He was probably the most prominent and influential doctor of his time, certainly in the English-speaking world. He was described by his peers as sociable, charming, cultured and well read.

Osler strongly believed in the importance of the non-material aspects of the doctor-patient encounter. He described himself as 'an unconscious faith-healer'.[44] Resonating with Schofield's description of the role of faith and the character of the physician in projecting confidence to effect cure, Osler recommended a certain attitude: 'A man must have faith in himself to be of any use in the world [...] Confidence once won, the rest follows naturally; and with a strong faith in himself a man becomes a strong centre for its local radiation.'[45]

In Osler's speech to a group of medical students he opined that 'it is hard to maintain good spirits amid the trials and tribulations of the day, but it is an unpardonable mistake to go about among patients with a long face.'[46] This not dissimilar to an extract from Tuckey's *Psycho-Therapeutics*: 'No physician adopting a psychical method of treatment can

[42] Schofield, *Unconscious Therapeutics* (p. 100).

[43] Michael Bliss, *William Osler, A Life in Medicine* (New York: Oxford University Press, 1999) (p. 264).

[44] William Osler, 'The Faith that Heals', *British Medical Journal* (18 June 1910) (pp. 1470–2) (p. 1470).

[45] Osler, 'Faith' (p. 1471).

[46] William Osler, 'The Student Life' in *Aequinamitas* (Philadelphia: Blakiston, 1910) (pp. 413–44) (p. 424).

afford to ignore any legitimate means of influencing the patient's imagination. The best way to attain that end is the assumption and maintenance of a firm yet sympathetic demeanour.'[47]

There is further evidence in the journals of increasing orthodox acceptance and enthusiasm for psychological treatments in general before the war. In 1904, the Hunterian Society oration, an annual speech hosted by one of the more prestigious and longstanding London medical societies was awarded to a medical hypnotist and future member of the MSSST, John Woods. He spoke on his speciality, 'On the Psychic Side of Therapeutics,' 'There are however, signs that the opposition which treatment by suggestion has met with is growing daily less and less and that this potent therapeutic method bids fair soon to be taught in our schools as a matter of routine.'[48] The speech was generally well-received by all the medical journals.

Five years later, another MSSST member Dr Claye Shaw gave the annual speech for another medical club the Harveian society. Titled 'The Influence of Mind as a Therapeutic Agent,' it was printed in full in the *BMJ* with an editorial introduction suggesting that the medical profession needed to be 'aware of this trend of public opinion and to ascertain how far suggestion may operate in the treatment of morbid conditions.'[49]

Under Dawson Williams, the *BMJ* had become less materialistic than under Hart. Consider this modern-sounding formulation from an educational supplement of 1897: 'Disease of the body is so much influenced by the mind that in each case we have to understand the patients quite as much as the malady. This is not learnt in hospitals.'[50] The culmination of this interest combined in part with the rise of Christian Science movement led to a *BMJ* special edition on the subject of Faith-Healing in June 1910.[51]

[47] Charles Lloyd Tuckey, *Psycho-Therapeutics*, 4th ed (London: Baillière, Tindall and Cox, 1900) (p. 157).

[48] John Woods, 'Abstract of an Address on the Psychic Side of Therapeutics', *Lancet* (20 February 1904) (pp. 489–92) (p. 492).

[49] Thomas Claye Shaw, 'The Influence of Mind as a Therapeutic Agent', *Lancet* (6 November 1909) (pp. 1369–73); Thomas Claye Shaw, 'The Influence of Mind as a Therapeutic Agent', *British Medical Journal* (6 November 1909) (pp. 1352–6) (p. 1352).

[50] Anon, 'Educational Number: The Training of the Medical Profession', *British Medical Journal* (28 August 1897), (p. 509).

[51] Anon, Special Edition, *British Medical Journal* (18 June 1910).

The BMA as a monolithic institution came around to hypnotism and the psychological treatments eventually. At the BMA national meeting of 1910, Dr. Gardner's presidential address is remarkable for not only the acknowledgement of the importance of the science of psychology but also its recognition of the early pioneers at the SPR. He specifically mentions its lay members Frederic Myers, Henry Sidgwick, William Crookes and Oliver Lodge but highlights the importance of the British medical hypnotists, Bramwell and Tuckey and their European colleagues: 'These are names that will go down to posterity as the pioneers of a movement to study these phenomena from a scientific standpoint and rescue the wheat of psychological therapeutics from the chaff and humbug of Christian Science and spiritual knavery.'[52]

The Spiritual Healing Commission

Dr. Gardner's reference to the 'humbug of Christian Science' in his speech to the BMA, indicates not only the contemporaneous rise of the Church of Christian Science but also the scale of the threat that it was felt to pose to the medical profession. The unorthodox Christian Scientists were an American church founded upon spiritual healing which came to prominence in the UK in the early 1900s. However, there were other orthodox church branches like the Emmanuel movement from Boston, USA and individual faith-healers like James Hickson and Edward Montagu, Earl of Sandwich who also emerged and flourished at this time.[53] A *BMJ* editorial from August 1910 commented that spiritual healing was 'one of the most notable features of the present day.'[54]

Christian Science itself was established by Mary Baker Eddy in 1866 after she had experienced the complete and spontaneous cure of all her injuries, sustained in a fall, by reading the Gospel and discovering the 'healing truth.' Her beliefs are contained in *Science and Health* published in 1875, which became the handbook of the church. The main precept of

[52] T. Frederic Gardner, 'President's Address', *British Medical Journal (Supplement)* (11 June 1910) (pp. 362–6) (p. 363).

[53] Louis Rose, *Faith Healing* (Harmondsworth: Penguin Books, 1970).

[54] Anon, 'Modern Miracles of Healing', *British Medical Journal* (20 August 1910) (p. 479).

the Christian Scientists was the illusory nature of the physical world.[55] It followed that sickness and pain were also illusions and that to be healthy only required the acceptance of man's wholly spiritual form. There was therefore no need for science or medicine or any conceivable reason to consult a doctor.

Christian Science was first mentioned in the *BMJ* in 1898. It was reported that Major Cecil Lester had died after dismissing his military physicians and seeking Christian Science treatment for his tuberculous peritonitis. The healer charged him a guinea per week for absent healing through prayer and 'right thought.' The case was described as 'a depressing exhibition of folly and cruelty'.[56] The Christian Scientists were the most extreme faith-healing group in their wholesale disavowal of medical intervention; most faith-healers viewed doctors as 'a relatively junior or flawed part of God's ordained healing process.'[57] The Emmanuel movement was unusual in adopting hypnotism as their means of religious healing.

The physicians were not the only professional group feeling threatened by the rise of Christian Science and the new faiths. The number of followers of the religion had increased rapidly in the United States in the 1890s and spread further with the first Christian Science lecturer's arrival in the UK in 1897. The number of churches had risen from 28 in 1892 to a staggering 1500 congregations by 1915.[58] The majority, but not all, members would have been defections from the Church of England. The American Episcopalian bishops who were so concerned about the new religion that they requested a coordinated response from the Anglican Church at the 1908 Lambeth conference.[59] There was a growing interest among the public and the clergy about, 'the power of the subconscious mind and the possibilities of using psychological suggestion allied to faith

[55] Mary Baker Eddy, *Science and Health with Key to the Scriptures* (Boston: Christian Science Publishing Society, 1934) (pp. 112–3).

[56] Anon, 'Faith-Healing', *British Medical Journal* (15 October 1898) (p. 1187).

[57] Sheryl Root, *The Healing Touch: Spiritual Healing in England c.1870–1955* (Unpublished PhD thesis, University of Warwick, 2005) (p. 76).

[58] Charles Herman Lea, *A Plea for the Thorough and Unbiased Investigation of Christian Science and a Challenge to its Critics*, 2nd ed. (London: Dent, 1915) (p. 7).

[59] Stuart Mews, 'The Revival of Spiritual Healing in the Church of England', *Studies in Church History*, 19 (1982) (pp. 299–332) (p. 312).

for the alleviation of functional disorders' which appeared in several articles late Edwardian religious journals.[60] Additionally, there were still a few Anglican clergy who wished to reclaim religious healing as an integral part of their work and prevent the monopoly of their rivals.

All these factors culminated in a Lambeth conference resolution to set up a meeting with representatives of the British medical establishment to consider a way forward. The joint conference met in October 1910 and established a joint 'committee of inquiry,' whose purpose was to define the scope and meaning of faith, religious and mental healing; examine the safety of medically unqualified healers and to promote cooperation between the two professions.[61] The historian Sheryl Root has argued that the Anglican Church itself was an important factor in helping to engage medical interest and raise awareness of spiritual healing during this period. She suggested that doctors were more willing to debate with 'respectable clergymen' than respond to 'the demands and criticisms of vocal but radical individuals.'[62]

Both Tuckey and Bramwell were invited to give evidence to the committee which met 19 times and interviewed nine expert witnesses before publishing in 1914. Hypnotism and suggestion had by now entered the mainstream and they were considered professional experts in this form of healing. Their testimony appears along with that of the other witnesses called, the faith healer Edward Montagu, the Earl of Sandwich and five Anglican clerics. The Christian Scientists were notable by their absence and the report makes no mention of the church despite being one of the main triggers for the unusual cooperative venture.

In his evidence, Tuckey gave a summary of his views of the time. There is a strong suggestion that he held an Anglican faith and had not completely relinquished some of his non-materialist views, maintaining the needy agnosticism of the SPR. He was cautious in separating spiritual healing from mental and faith healing. He said that spiritual healing was

[60] Mews, 'Spiritual Healing' (p. 313); Samuel McComb, 'The Christian Religion as Healing Power', *Hibernian Journal* (October 1909) (pp. 10–27); Harrington Sainsbury, 'Christianity, Science and "Christian Science"', *Church Quarterly Review* (April 1910) (pp. 63–8).

[61] Anon, *Spiritual Healing: Report of a Clerical and Medical Committee of Inquiry into Spiritual Faith, and Mental Healing* (London: Macmillan, 1914) (p. 8).

[62] Root, *Healing Touch* (p. 246).

'miraculous, Divine help from outside, non-physical and outside the ordinary laws of nature.' He should like to think that it existed but had no personal experience.'[63] Bramwell, who had always been more of a sceptic, was unable to distinguish between the three forms of healing, seeing them as equivalent.

Both explained their view that suggestion was the basis of all mental healing. They described its mechanism using a mix of models from the subliminal consciousness and hypnotism to the imagination, though the brief format of the report may not do justice to the complexity of their views. These ideas can be clearly traced back to those outlined by SPR members Frederic and Arthur Myers in 'Mind-cure, Faith-cure and the Miracle of Lourdes'.[64] The historian Ruth Harris has observed the way that the spiritual healing phenomena at Lourdes a couple of decades earlier could not be adequately explained by the existing positivism of medical science and the importance of suggestion and Myers' work in a new formulation.[65]

Paradoxically, it was the threat of Christian science and religious healing to the medical profession which forced the medical profession to accept the non-material and relationship aspect of their work. Suggestion became the 'catch-all' theory to make sense of the phenomenon. The joint religious and medical commission demonstrates the seriousness of the perceived threat and the invitations to Tuckey and Bramwell from Lambeth Palace show how far the New Hypnotists had come from the fringes to the mainstream of medicine and public discourse.

Popular Psychology

In any history of psychology and psychological ideas, there is a risk of looking at institutional or professional histories exclusively. The focus of the book has been upon the New Hypnotists, who were medical and therefore institutional if not initially orthodox. In this chapter, there has been coverage of medical and public acceptance and evidence for hypnotism and suggestion in the medical literature and formation of medical

[63] Anon, *Spiritual Healing* (pp. 52–3).

[64] Arthur Myers and Frederic Myers, 'Mind Cure, Faith-Cure and the Miracles of Lourdes', *Proceedings of the Society for Psychical Research*, 9 (1893) (pp. 160–209).

[65] Ruth Harris, *Lourdes: Body and Spirit in a Secular Age* (London: Allen Lane, 1999) (p. 351).

societies like the MSSST. However, I have also discussed noninstitutional histories, like the pre-war story of the MPS and the rise of the Church of Christian Science. There was one final important influence that helped to secure acceptability and credibility which should be considered and it is noninstitutional. The last section of this chapter looks at the rise of what historian of psychology Lesley Hearnshaw called popular or 'practical' psychology between the 1890s and 1914.[66]

This area of psychological history has been generally neglected, partly because it was not previously considered to be important and partly because it is harder to research. There are several threads of practical psychology to consider. Key to all strands was the belief that an understanding of basic psychological ideas was beneficial to the individual and the use of psychological techniques could improve mental functioning. Many of the techniques did not require a doctor or therapist and fitted naturally with the Victorian ethos of self-improvement and later the Edwardian English drive for National Efficiency.

The story of Pelmanism is quite representative and has been recovered by the historian Mathew Thomson.[67] Pelmanism was a form of mind-training offered as a correspondence course by Londoner William Joseph Ennever. He established the business in 1899, working with early psychologists and naming it after one of his colleagues Christopher Pelman, who had died soon after the business was launched. Initially at least, Pelmanism used memory drills to improve overall mental functioning. One of the early products that grew out of the course was the card game also called Pelmanism, a pair-matching game which is known today as 'patience.' The course was advertised in the *Times* as early as 1903 which gave it the apparent approval of the establishment.[68] The Pelman Institute claimed to have taken on 200,000 students by 1915.

After 1900, there was a general outpouring of new psychological publications aimed at the public: self-help books, journals and mail-order course pamphlets. The book titles provide a pretty clear idea of the subject matter. Some of the Edwardian best-sellers included *The New Psychology,*

[66] Lesley Hearnshaw, *A Short History of British Psychology 1840–1940* (London: Routledge, 1986).

[67] Mathew Thomson, 'Practical Psychology', Ch. 1 in *Psychological Subjects: Identity, Culture and Health in Twentieth-Century Britain* (Oxford: Oxford University Press, 2006) (pp. 23–6).

[68] Anon, 'Memory Means Money', *Times* (21 February 1903).

or the Secret of Happiness, being Practical Instructions as to How to Develop and Employ Thought Power (1903) which was based on Theosophist and journalist Richard Harte's fascination with mesmerism and hypnotism; the US naturalist philosopher Stanton Kirkham wrote *The Philosophy of Self-Help: An Application of Practical Psychology to Daily Life* (1909) and the English novelist Arnold Bennett wrote several self-help books including *Mental Efficiency and other Hints to Men and Women* (1912).[69]

Reading through the general, occult, Theosophy and spiritualist journals of the time, one cannot help but be struck by the sheer number of advertisements for such mind-developing material published in the spaces around the articles. The majority were placed by American companies, where advertising standards, business and publishing was much less regulated. Many of the books and mail-order self-help courses were based (sometimes very loosely) upon the principles of suggestion and hypnosis. Some were just reprints of the books of the European medical hypnotists printed out of copyright.

Of course, not all of these courses or books were reputable or legal. The advertisements would focus on what the reader lacked (friends, money or influence) and offer mechanisms for success (personal magnetism, spiritual attraction or suggestive therapeutics). The most notorious mail-order swindler of the time was the American Elmer Sidney Prather (1872–1939) an ex-stage hypnotist who went into the mail-order occultism business. He styled himself 'Professor Elmer Ellsworth Knowles' and offered his 'Complete System of Personal Influence and Healing' from 1899. This course came in six modules which could be purchased separately. Four of the modules included aspects of mesmerism, hypnotism or suggestive therapy. The fourth one for example was entitled 'Magnetic Healing, Distance Healing, Treatment by Suggestion.'

Prather initially charged between $1 and $10 for his correspondence course but became more grandiose, running the Metropolitan Institute of Science from his New York Office in 1905. The Institute offered doctorates in suggestive therapeutics taught and assessed by post. In 1909, after two fraudulent payments and assault charges, Prather and his

[69] Richard Harte, *The New Psychology or the Secret of Happiness, Being Practical Instructions as to How to Develop and Employ Thought Power* (London: Fowler, 1903); Stanton Kirkham, *The Philosophy of Self-Help: An Application of Practical Psychology to Daily Life* (London: Puttnams, 1909); Arnold Bennet, *Mental Efficiency* (London: Hodder and Stoughton 1912).

wife emigrated to England. They set up a mail-order business supplying astrology books, magnetism lessons, hypnotic devices, cosmetics and dietary supplements. This provided them with a staggering income of over $100,000 a year while their previously established US companies continued to operate. In 1911, a former English employee tried to blackmail the couple and the coverage of the resulting court case revealed that the Prathers had over a hundred employees and that the German correspondence alone involved 5000 letters a week.[70] When he died in 1939, Prather's American heirs shared $530,000 in 1943, the equivalent in 2017, of $7.5 million.[71] His business model and focus on hypnotism and suggestion was highly lucrative but also clearly illustrates the level of interest in practical psychology and hypnotism and suggestion, in particular.

All of the events described in the chapter contradict the popular misconception that Britain was either unaware or rejecting of wider developments in psychological thinking before the First World War. Instead it is clear that there were an array of new psychological ideas and therapies which reached had from the institutions of medicine and academe to the general public through magazines, papers and a new genre of psychological self-help literature. Recent research has helped to revise the previous view, which was part of the founding myth of Freudian psychoanalysis promulgated by Ernest Jones, a pioneer psychoanalyst. He effectively controlled the development of classic Freudian analytic practice through the London Psycho-Analytical Society and wrote an influential history of early psychoanalysis. This depicted the early Freudian analysts battling against British conservativism, sexual repression and ignorance.

Bibliography

Allan, Percy. 1906. 'M.S.S.S.T.', *General Practitioner* (24 November): 748.

[70] Bernard Petitdant, 'Professor Elmer Ellsworth Knowles and its [sic] Radio Hypnotic Crystal' *Kinésithérapie Revue,* 20 (2020) (pp. 41–4).

[71] Marc Demarest, 'Latent Powers, Latent Demand. A Look at the Mail-Order Occult in Anglo-American Culture 1895–1920' (The International Association for the Preservation of Spiritualist and Occult Periodicals: Forest, OR, 2017). http://www.ehbritten.org/docs/demarest_popular_occulture_july_2017.pdf [accessed 14 July 2017].

Andrick, John. 2020. 'The "Chicago School of Psychology" and *Hypnotic Magazine*: Suggestive Therapeutics, Public Psychologies, and New Thought Pluralism, 1895–1910', *History of Psychology*, 23, 1: 1–25.

Anon. 1897. 'Educational Number: The Training of the Medical Profession', *British Medical Journal* (28 August): 509.

Anon. 1898. 'Faith-Healing', *British Medical Journal* (15 October): 1187.

Anon. 1903. 'Memory Means Money', *Times* (21 February).

Anon. 1906. 'Treatment by Hypnotic Suggestion', *British Medical Journal* (28 April): 979–80.

Anon. 1906. 'The M.S.S.S.T', *Journal of the Society for Psychical Research* 13: 14–5.

Anon. 1907. 'The M.S.S.S.T', *Morning Post* (4 July): 3.

Anon. 1910. 'Special Edition', *British Medical Journal* (June 18).

Anon. 1910. 'Modern Miracles of Healing', *British Medical Journal* (20 August): 479.

Anon. 1910. *Spiritual Healing: Report of a Clerical and Medical Committee of Inquiry into Spiritual Faith, and Mental Healing.* London: Macmillan.

Anon. 1913. 'Lyttleton Forbes Winslow's Obituary' *Light*, 33, 1692: 288.

Anon. 1925. 'Obituary—C. Lloyd Tuckey', *Journal of the Society for Psychical Research*, 22: 115–7.

Ash, Edwin. 1906. 'Some Experiments in Hypnotism', *Lancet*, 167 (27 January): 216–20.

Ash, Edwin. 1906. 'Modern Hypnotism. A Lecture Delivered Before the PTS', *Lancet*, 168 (10 November): 1308.

Ash, Edwin. 1906. 'The Induction of Hypnosis', *Lancet*, 168 (25 August): 501–504.

Bennet, Arnold. 1912. *Mental Efficiency.* London: Hodder and Stoughton.

Blackwood, Algernon. 2002. 'The Man Who Found Out', in *Ancient Sorceries and Other Weird Stories.* London: Penguin. 131–46.

Bliss, Michael. 1999. *William Osler, A Life in Medicine.* New York: Oxford University Press. 264.

Borch-Jacobsen, Mikkel. 1989. 'Hypnosis in Psychoanalysis', *Representations*, 27: 92–110.

Bramwell, John Milne. 1897. *Suggestion: Its Place in Medicine and Scientific Research.* N.P.

Bynum, William. 1994. *Science and the Practice of Medicine in the Nineteenth Century.* Cambridge: Cambridge University Press. 191–6.

Cabot, Richard. 1909. 'The Use and Abuse of Rest in the Treatment of Disease', *Psychotherapy: A Course of Instruction in Sound Psychology, Sound Medicine, and Sound Religion*, 2: 23–38.

Chettiar, Teri. 2012. '"Looking as Little Like Patients as Persons Well Could": Hypnotism, Medicine and the Problem of the Suggestible Subject in Late Nineteenth-Century Britain', *Medical History*, 56: 335–54.

Demarest, Marc. 2017. 'Latent Powers, Latent Demand. A Look at the Mail-Order Occult in Anglo-American Culture 1895–1920'. The International Association for the Preservation of Spiritualist and Occult Periodicals: Forest, OR, 2017. http://www.ehbritten.org/docs/demarest_popular_occulture_july_2017.pdf [accessed 14 August 2017].

Eddy, Mary Baker. 1934. *Science and Health with Key to the Scriptures*. Boston: Christian Science Publishing Society.

Ellenberger, Henri. 1970. *The Discovery of the Unconscious, the History and Evolution of Dynamic Psychiatry*. London: Allen Lane.

Gardner, T. Frederic. 1910. 'President's Address', *British Medical Journal* (Supplement) (11 June): 362–6.

Gauld, Alan. 1992. *A History of Hypnotism*. Cambridge: Cambridge University Press.

Gifford, George. 1978. *Psychoanalysis, Psychotherapy, and the New England Medical Scene, 1894–1944*. New York: Science History Publications.

Hallam, Arthur. 1911. 'Editorial', *Health Record* (July): 74.

Harris, Ruth. 1999. *Lourdes: Body and Spirit in a Secular Age*. London: Allen Lane.

Harte, Richard. 1903. *The New Psychology, or the Secret of Happiness, Being Practical Instructions as to How to Develop and Employ Thought Power*. London: Fowler.

Hayward, Rhodri. 2015. 'The Emergence of the Unconscious', Ch. 1 in *The Transformation of the Psyche in British Primary Care, 1889–1970*. London: Bloomsbury. 1–30.

Hearnshaw, Lesley. 1986. *A Short History of British Psychology 1840–1940*. London: Routledge.

Janet, Pierre. 1925. *Psychological Healing: A Historical and Clinical Study*, vol 1. New York: MacMillan. 200.

Kirkham, Stanton.1909. *The Philosophy of Self-Help: An Application of Practical Psychology to Daily Life*. London: Puttnams.

Kuhn, Philip. 2017. *Psychoanalysis in Britain, 1893-1913, Histories and Historiography*. Lanham: Lexington.

Lea, Charles Herman. 1915. *A Plea for the Thorough and Unbiased Investigation of Christian Science and a Challenge to its Critics*, 2nd ed. London: Dent.

Maehle, Andreas-Holger and Wolffram, Heather. 2017. 'Guest Editorial', in *Notes and Records: The Royal Society Journal of the History of Science*, 71, Special Issue: 'History of Hypnotism in Europe', ed. by Andreas-Holger Maehle, and Heather Wolffram. 119–23.

Marks, Sarah. 2017. 'Psychotherapy in Historical Perspective', *History of the Human Sciences*, 30: 3–16

McComb, Samuel. 1909. 'The Christian Religion as Healing Power', *Hibernian Journal* (October): 10–27.

Mercier, Charles. 1898. 'Suggestion and Crime', *British Medical Journal* (10 September): 678.

Mews, Stuart. 1982. 'The Revival of Spiritual Healing in the Church of England', *Studies in Church History*, 19: 299–332.

Mitchell, S. Weir. 1888. *Doctors and Patients*. Philadelphia and London: Lippincot.

Myers, Arthur and Myers, Frederic. 1893. 'Mind Cure, Faith-Cure and the Miracles of Lourdes', *Proceedings of the Society for Psychical Research*, 9: 160–209.

Osler, William. 1910. 'The Student Life', in *Aequinamitas*. Philadelphia: Blakiston. 413–44.

Osler, William. 1910. 'The Faith that Heals', *British Medical Journal*, (June 18): 1470–2.

Petitdant, Bernard.2020. 'Professor Elmer Ellsworth Knowles and its [sic] Radio Hypnotic Crystal' *Kinésithérapie Revue* 20: 41–4.

Root, Sheryl. 2005. *The Healing Touch: Spiritual Healing in England c. 1870–1955*. Unpublished PhD thesis, University of Warwick.

Rose, Louis. 1970. *Faith Healing*. Harmondsworth: Penguin Books.

Sainsbury, Harrington. 1910. 'Christianity, Science and "Christian Science"', *Church Quarterly Review* (April): 63–8.

Schofield, Alfred. 1904. *Unconscious Therapeutics: Or, the Personality of the Physician*. Philadelphia: Blakiston.

Shamdasani, Sonu. 2017. 'Psychotherapy in Society: Historical Reflections' ,in *The Routledge History of Madness and Mental Health*, ed. by G. Eghigian. London: Routledge. 363–378.

Shaw, Thomas Claye. 1909. 'The Influence of Mind as a Therapeutic Agent', *Lancet* (6 November): 1369–73.

Shaw, Thomas Claye. 1909. 'The Influence of Mind as a Therapeutic Agent', *British Medical Journal* (6 November): 1352–6.

Taylor, Eugene. 2000. 'Psychotherapeutics and the Problematic Origins of Clinical Psychology in America', *American Psychologist*, 55: 1029–33.

Thomson, Mathew. 2006. 'Practical Psychology', Ch. 1 in *Psychological Subjects: Identity, Culture, and Health in Twentieth-Century Britain*. Oxford: Oxford University Press. 23–6.

Tuckey, Charles Lloyd. 1889. 'Correspondence', *Lancet* (12 October): 776.

Tuckey, Charles Lloyd. 1898. 'Hypnotism and Suggestion', *Medical Annual and Practitioners Index*. Bristol: John Wright. 77–85.

Tuckey, Charles Lloyd. 1904. 'Some Notes on Hypnotic Suggestion', *General Practitioner* (6 June): 350–1.
Tuckey, Charles Lloyd. 1904. 'Some Notes on Hypnotic Suggestion', *General Practitioner* (13 June): 367–8.
Tuckey, Charles Lloyd. 1904. 'Some Notes on Hypnotic Suggestion', *General Practitioner* (20 June): 382–4.
Tuckey, Charles Lloyd. 1903. 'Notes on Some Cases of Obsession', *General Practitioner* (26 September): 607–8.
Tuckey, Charles Lloyd. 1903. 'Notes on Sexual Perversion', *General Practitioner* (7 November): 703–4.
Tuckey, Charles Lloyd. 1907. 'The Utility of the Study of Suggestion to the Student and Practitioner', *General Practitioner* (6 April): 210–3.
Tuckey, Charles Lloyd. 1900. *Psycho-Therapeutics: Treatment by Hypnotism and Suggestion*, 4th ed. London: Baillière, Tindall and Cox.
Vaillant, C.M. 1963. 'An Historical Sketch of the Emergence of Liverpool Psychiatry', *Journal of the Liverpool Psychiatric Club*, 1. http://www.priory.com/homol/livpsy/19th.htm [accessed 6 May 2020].
West, Rebecca. 2010. *The Return of the Soldier*. London: Virago. 126.
Winslow, L. Forbes. 1877. *Spiritualistic Madness*. London: Baillère.
Winslow, L. Forbes. 1910. *Recollections of Forty Years*. London: John Ouseley.
Winslow, L. Forbes. 1910. *Suggestive Power of Hypnotism*. London: Rebman.
Woods, John. 1904. 'Abstract of an Address on the Psychic Side of Therapeutics', *Lancet* (20 February): 489–92.

CHAPTER 11

Post-Hypnotic Suggestion: WWI and Beyond

With the coming of the First World War, the New Hypnotists saw the final realisation of their lives' work: the acceptance of hypnotism and the therapeutic use of suggestion on a massive scale. None of them would have wanted it to have seen it happen that way. The industrial scale of the slaughter and destruction caused by the mechanisation of warfare led to the armies of all countries experiencing large numbers of both physical and psychological casualties. The term 'shell-shock' was used for their mental symptoms, popularised by the medical psychologist Charles Myers in a *Lancet* article.[1] It originally matched his belief in a physical cause like concussion for the symptoms ranging from dulling of the senses, loss of hearing and speech to dazedness, neurasthenia and full unconsciousness. Myers soon realised the term to be inaccurate because for the majority the causation was psychic and trauma-related not physical but the name stuck.

Myers and his junior colleague William Brown, a reader in psychology at London University had been co-opted by the army to treat those

[1] Charles Myers, 'A Contribution to the Study of Shell Shock'. *Lancet*, 1 (13 February 1915) (pp. 316–20).

G. D. L. Bates, *The Uncanny Rise of Medical Hypnotism, 1888–1914*, Mental Health in Historical Perspective,
https://doi.org/10.1007/978-3-031-42725-1_11

affected and return them to the fighting as quickly as possible.[2] They introduced a combination of suggestion and hypnotism to treat the private infantrymen at field hospitals close to the frontline.[3] Brown was an experienced hypnotist and member of the SPR and MSSST. He claimed a remarkably high success rate of returning 70% of soldiers to the front after two weeks of rest and treatment. The poet Wilfred Owen described him as 'a kind of wizard, who mesmerises when he likes.'[4]

It was only the severely affected officers who were allowed to leave the fighting to return to the UK, so their numbers were very few. The two most famous centres for the treatment of shellshock in Britain were at Seale Hayne College in Devon and Craiglockhart, near Edinburgh. The former was run by Dr. Arthur Hurst, whose work has been immortalised by the silent black and white films of his patients before and after treatment.[5] Hurst used a combination of suggestion under hypnosis and persuasion with electrotherapy (applying currents to the tongue or to limbs to cause them to move involuntarily). Some of the physical 'assistance' to the patients shown in the films looks painful but any cries and the content of his persuasion is lost without the sound. Although Hurst was an excellent self-publicist, his colleagues questioned his superficial approach and suggested that the patients quickly relapsed away from the centre.

Craiglockhart became famous for another reason. The hospital became closely associated with the treatment of one of its most famous patients, the war poet Siegfried Sassoon. The treatment at Craiglockhart was eclectic including hypnotism, suggestion and Freudian analysis but as a result of Siegfried Sassoon's therapy there, the Freudian aspect has been mythologised. Both Sassoon's autobiography *Sherston's Progress* and Pat Barker's *Regeneration* trilogy have romanticised Sassoon's recovery under Freudian therapy by psychologist William Rivers. There are two problems

[2] William Brown, 'The Treatment of Cases of Shell Shock in an Advanced Neurological Centre', *Lancet*, 2 (1918), 2 (p. 197).

[3] Ben Shepherd, *A War of Nerves: Soldiers and Psychiatrists 1914–1994* (London: Pimlico, 2002) (pp. 60–62).

[4] Harold Owen and John Bell, *Wilfred Owen: The Collected Letters* (Oxford: Oxford University Press, 1967) (p. 455).

[5] Edgar Jones, 'War Neuroses and Arthur Hurst: A Pioneering Medical Film about the Treatment of Psychiatric Battle Casualties', *Journal of the History of Medicine and Allied Sciences*, 67 3 (2012) (pp. 345–73).

with this. Firstly, a closer study of Rivers technique and psychological framework reveals that despite his familiarity with Freudian ideas he was no purist. Indeed, he was aware that he relied heavily on the 'personality of the healer' and his relationship with the patient, which had been a later development in suggestion theory. Second, the accounts have led to the impression that the main treatment for shellshock was early Freudian therapy which would have been practically impossible given the number affected and the hours of treatment required.

There were other less well-known centres of treatment. Early in the war, Lord Knutsford, the fund-raising chairman of the London Hospital, had put forward an appeal for charitable donations in order to buy or rent a large and quiet house in London for 'the men suffering from very severe mental and nervous shock, due to exposure strain and tension'.[6] Lord Northcliffe's brother had offered one of his London residences for the purpose. Charles Lloyd Tuckey was one of the 23 doctors who volunteered to give their services for free to help the psychological casualties of the First World War.[7]

It is not clear how much work Tuckey was able to perform for the war effort or privately, as by this time his health was not good. His long-standing valvular heart disease was likely to have caused worsening heart failure. Earlier in the year, he had turned down a senior position at the new Medico-Psychological Clinic, also known as the Brunswick Square clinic, one of the early centres of psycho-therapeutics in London. Ostensibly, this was because they were using therapists who were not medically qualified and their main fundraiser was Edward Montagu Lord Sandwich, an eccentric aristocratic faith healer. Even the resignation of Lord Sandwich did not mollify him.

At the age of 61, Tuckey married Beatrice Wood Marsland, a woman 13 years his junior. As a lifelong bachelor, it seems likely that the marriage was one of convenience as his deteriorating health meant that he needed a carer. Percy Allan suggested in his obituary that despite Tuckey's good looks and healthy demeanour he 'never enjoyed robust health.'[8] The

[6] Myers, 'Shell Shock'.

[7] Anon. 'Lord Knutsford's Appeal', *Times* (4 November 1914), (p. 5); Anon. 'Psycho-Therapy and the War', *Journal of the Society for Psychical Research*, 16 (1914) (pp. 310–6) (p. 311).

[8] Anon, 'Obituary: Charles Lloyd Tuckey', *Journal of the Society for Psychical Research*, 22, Oct 1925 (pp. 115–7) (p. 116).

references in his work to his foreign trips to Spain, the Canary Islands, the United States and Australia all support this. Only the year before he had written positively about marriage but from the vantage point of a bachelor and physician of mature age.[9] He gave no hint in the article for a gentleman's journal that he planned to marry soon. The wedding ceremony took place in Eastbourne in December 1915.[10] Beatrice was the only daughter of a London solicitor and a friend of his sister, Deborah.[11] They lived for a couple of years at his Mayfair residence on Upper Brook Street until his final retirement. They then moved to her family home, *Ingarsby* in Eastbourne on the South Coast.

Despite his poor health, he published the seventh and final edition of *Psycho-Therapeutics* in 1921, with the help of his friend, Percy Allan. Tuckey and Allan chose to omit a prior chapter on Psychoanalysis from the sixth edition 'as we felt it is now a recognised and separate treatment with its own literature' not because they had 'ceased to sympathise with this form of therapy.'[12] Tuckey like the other early British psychotherapists was eclectic and pragmatic in outlook. It was Freud and his disciples who were the purists, rejecting all other psychological approaches to enhance the homogeneity of treatment and to emphasise their own unique contributions. In the seventh edition, Tuckey included a couple of chapters written by Allan which outlined in short case histories, his positive experience of using hypnotism and suggestion during the Great War.[13]

Tuckey remained on the council of the SPR until a stroke meant that he was unable to travel to London to attend the meetings. He lived longer than expected and struggled to support himself financially. He was prophetic when he told his friend van Eeden in 1893, that he would

[9] Charles Lloyd Tuckey, 'Some Thoughts on Marriage', *Contemporary Review*, 96 (1914) (pp. 366–75).

[10] Anon. 'Marriages', *Lancet*, (18 December 1915) (p. 1381).

[11] On census day 1901, Deborah Tuckey was Staying with Robert Wood Marsland and His Family. Sally Davis 'Charles Tuckey', *Work on the Hermetic Order of the Golden Dawn*. http://www.wrightanddavis.co.uk/GD/TUCKEYCHARLESL.htm [accessed 9 May 2020].

[12] Charles Lloyd Tuckey, 'Preface to the Seventh Edition', in *Treatment by Hypnotism and Suggestion or, Psycho-Therapeutics*, 7th ed. (London: Baillière, Tindall and Cox, 1921) (p. vii).

[13] Percy Allan, 'Treatment by Suggestion During the War', Ch. 11 in CLT, *Psycho-Therapeutics*, 7th ed. (pp. 347–55).

'never be a rich man.'[14] However, he remained a popular figure and his friends and colleagues were concerned by his impecunious state. One of his friends from the MSSST, Thomas (T.W.) Mitchell petitioned the Home Secretary for a pension for him from the public purse.[15]

The impressive letter now resides at the National Archive in Twickenham and sets out the reasons for the Home Secretary to provide Tuckey with a Civil list pension. The letter is signed by nineteen 'memorialists' as they described themselves. The names of the signatories are an indication of the networks of influential and prominent people that Tuckey had cultivated throughout his life. Perhaps unsurprisingly, thirteen of them were physicians, including William Osler and the eminent medical psychologists Charles Myers and William MacDougall. Five were Fellows of the Royal Society, the pinnacle of British scientific esteem, including the physicists and spiritualists Oliver Lodge and William Barrett with whom Tuckey had worked on the council of the SPR. Other distinguished SPR members like the philosopher F.C.S. Schiller, the public intellectual Gilbert Murray and the member of parliament for Hampstead, George Balfour also contributed. As a sign of the increasing contribution of women to medicine and public life, six of the cosignatories were female. These include Eleanor Sidgwick, former president of the Society for Psychical Research and principal of Newnham College and Constance Long, a protégé of Tuckey's who was the president of the Women's Medical Association and an important member of the Psycho-Medical Society (the renamed MSSST) .[16]
The letter sets out Tuckey's achievements:

> Our present day knowledge of the principles and practice of Psychotherapeutics in all its forms would have been impossible but for the hypnotists. Lloyd Tuckey was the pioneer in this country of the revival of Hypnotism and Suggestion as therapeutic agents in medical practice, which

[14] Charles Lloyd Tuckey to van Eeden Correspondence (24 October 1893). *Van Eeden Collection*. Amsterdam, Allard Pierson, University of Amsterdam, Hs. XXIV C 81.

[15] Thomas (T.W.) Mitchell, 'Memorial on Behalf of Charles Lloyd Tuckey,' National Archive, PROT1/12460 C677293.

[16] Long was a doctor and psychoanalyst who eventually gave up hypnotic suggestion for Jungian influenced psychoanalysis. She translated Jung and wrote *The Psychology of Phantasy*. Anon, 'Obituary—Constance Long', *British Medical Journal*, (3 March 1923) (p. 399).

took place about thirty years ago. Forty years earlier, James Braid had shown that hypnotic phenomena were identical with those of so-called animal-magnetism, and when Tuckey began his psychotherapeutic work the prejudices which had arisen in connexion [sic] with Mesmerism or Animal-Magnetism were still very prevalent. Consequently great courage and singleness of purpose were required by any man who advocated the use of Hypnotism in medical practice. Tuckey had these virtues in an eminent degree. In 1889 he published his work on "Treatment by Hypnotism and Suggestion" [sic] which has been a standard treatise on the subject up to the present time and has gone through many editions; the then president of the Royal College of Physicians in Dublin, the late Sir Francis Cruise M.D. having written the preface to the fifth edition.

Dr. Tuckey's work has prepared the way for the recent great increase of the practice of psycho-therapeutics, a branch of medicine which, after long neglect in this country, is generally recognised as one of the first importance and destined to undergo great further development in the future.

Tuckey was provided with a pension of £200 a year which came from the secret Bounty Fund.[17] This was an unaccountable trust that only the Prime Minister could use without public scrutiny. The pension came from this source as the civil service advice was that hypnotism was 'not scientific enough' for a civil list pension, according to the supporting documentation in the archive.[18] Hypnotism had not lost its non-scientific mesmeric undertones for everyone. Tuckey survived for another six years, dying of valvular heart disease and the complications of an arterial clot in his left leg on 12th August 1925.[19]

The other New Hypnotists also retreated from public life after the war. John Milne Bramwell had published a third edition of *Hypnotism: Its History, Practice and Theory* in 1913 but there were few changes to the text.[20] As Tuckey had foreseen, Bramwell did become prosperous as a

[17] Gordon Bates, 'Charles Lloyd Tuckey and the "New Hypnotism"—Psychiatry in History' *British Journal of Psychiatry*, 214, 1 (2019) (p. 19). 10.1192/bjp.2018.168.

[18] Mitchell, 'Memorial'.

[19] Certificate of Death, *Charles William Lloyd Tuckey* (12 August 1925), Eastbourne District Registrar's Office, File no 298. Informant: Beatrice Mary Lloyd Tuckey [wife of deceased], Eastbourne, Sussex.

[20] John Milne Bramwell, *Hypnotism: Its History, Practice and Theory,* 3rd ed. (London: William Rider, 1913).

result of his hypnotic therapy. After the war, Bramwell indulged his interests in fishing and yachting but died earlier the same year as Tuckey at the Miramare Palace Grand Hotel in Ospedaletti, Italy. Felkin had tried to serve during the war but illness prevented him and prompted his move to New Zealand. He died in Havelock North in 1926 where he had set up his new temple Whare Ra. He was buried in the local cemetery, wearing the full regalia of the Knight of the Ordo Tabulae Rotundae, his neo-Arthurian mystical and chivalric order.

George Kingsbury had moved from Blackpool to London, two years after his unsuccessful campaign to become an MP. His obituary records that he was a 'brilliant speaker and debater' and was called to the Bar at the Middle Temple.[21] He continued to practise both medically and as a barrister specialising in medicolegal cases until the war and beyond. He took a special interest in prosecutions and inquests of Christian Scientists, helping to defend those prosecuted for their own or their relative's rejection of orthodox medicine.[22] In 1935, at the age of 75, he was still taking cases. He died nine years after his wife at home in London in 1936.

Hypnotism refers to a physiological state of consciousness as well as to a relationship between the hypnotist and hypnotised. By investigating the state, Charcot's eminence in the late nineteenth century gave hypnotism legitimacy once more. However, the Nancy school under Bernheim and Liébeault were more interested in the hypnotic relationship and it was this aspect that had the greatest cultural impact and through the concept of suggestion became the most productive.

The end of the century was an inflection point in Europe and Britain. Hypnotism, like mesmerism before it, had become a magical word with powerful positive and negative associations and as much wide-eyed enthusiasm as reactionary scientific backlash. At this opportune time, Lloyd Tuckey and the New Hypnotists adopted the ideas of the Nancy school and combined them with the emerging theories of the Society for Psychical Research. In so doing, they succeeded in conferring legitimacy to medical hypnotism and suggestion in Britain.

The stories of these remarkable Victorian medical men have been neglected and deserve recovery. Their lives and contributions to early

[21] Anon, 'Death of Dr. G. C. Kingsbury', *West Lancashire Evening Gazette* (17 March 1938) (p. 12).

[22] Anon, 'Death of Christian Scientist', *Liverpool Echo* (11 October 1930) (p. 14).

psycho-therapeutics reveal important insights into the construction of medical history and the public and professional internal struggles to achieve legitimacy and credibility. It is striking that their contributions to psychosomatic medicine and early psychological therapies have been overlooked by both medical and psychological institutions. The transitions from imagination and hypnotism to suggestion may have been necessary for reasons of acceptability but this removed the unique aspects of the trance state. Perhaps one reason for the collective amnesia regarding these events is that the 'power of suggestion' appeared too close to common sense, but that may be a measure of its widespread acceptance today.[23]

Bibliography

Anon. 1914. 'Lord Knutsford's Appeal', *Times* (4 November): 5.

Anon. 1914. 'Psycho-Therapy and the War', *Journal of the Society for Psychical Research* 16: 310–6.

Anon. 1915. 'Marriages', *Lancet* (18 December): 1381.

Anon. 1923. 'Obituary—Constance Long', *British Medical Journal* (3 March): 399.

Anon. 1925. 'Obituary: Charles Lloyd Tuckey', *Journal of the Society for Psychical Research*, 22 (October): 115–7.

Anon. 1930. 'Death of Christian Scientist', *Liverpool Echo* (11 October): 14.

Anon. 1938. 'Death of Dr. G. C. Kingsbury', *West Lancashire Evening Gazette* (17 March): 12.

Bates, Gordon. 2019. 'Charles Lloyd Tuckey and the "New Hypnotism"—Psychiatry in History' *British Journal of Psychiatry*, 214 1: 19.

Bramwell, John Milne. 1913. *Hypnotism: Its History, Practice and Theory*, 3rd ed. London: William Rider.

Brown, William. 1918. 'The Treatment of Cases of Shell Shock in an Advanced Neurological Centre', *Lancet* 2 (1918): 197.

Davis, Sally. 'Charles Tuckey', *Work on the Hermetic Order of the Golden Dawn*. http://www.wrightanddavis.co.uk/GD/TUCKEYCHARLESL.htm [accessed 9 May 2020].

Ewart, C. Theodore. 1890. *The Power of Suggestion*. London: Kegan Paul, Trench.

Jones, Edgar. 2012. 'War Neuroses and Arthur Hurst: A Pioneering Medical Film about the Treatment of Psychiatric Battle Casualties', *Journal of the History of Medicine and Allied Sciences*, 67, 3: 345–73.

[23] The first time that this ubiquitous phrase was used in a title was in 1890. C. Theodore Ewart, *The Power of Suggestion* (London: Kegan Paul, Trench, 1890).

Long, Constance. 1920. *Psychology of Phantasy*. London: Baillière, Tindall and Cox.

Mitchell, T. W. et al. 1919. 'Memorial on Behalf of Charles Lloyd Tuckey'. Bounty Fund. London, National Archive. PROT1/12460.

Myers, Charles. 1915. 'A Contribution to the Study of Shell Shock', *Lancet*, 1 (13 February): 316–320.

Office, E.D.R. 1925. Death Certificate: Charles William Lloyd Tuckey. Eastbourne.

Owen, Harold, and Bell, John. 1967. *Wilfred Owen: The Collected Letters*. Oxford: Oxford University Press.

Shepherd, Ben. 2002. *A War of Nerves: Soldiers and Psychiatrists 1914–1994*. London: Pimlico.

Tuckey, Charles Lloyd. 1893. Letter to van Eeden, October 24th, 1893. In *Van Eeden Collection*. Hs. XXIV C 81. Amsterdam, Allard Pierson, University of Amsterdam.

Tuckey, Charles Lloyd. 1914. 'Some Thoughts on Marriage', *Contemporary Review* 96: 366–75.

Tuckey, Charles Lloyd. 1921. *Treatment by Hypnotism and Suggestion or, Psycho-Therapeutics*, 7th ed. London: Baillière, Tindall and Cox.

Index

G. D. L. Bates, *The Uncanny Rise of Medical Hypnotism, 1888–1914*, Mental Health in Historical Perspective,
https://doi.org/10.1007/978-3-031-42725-1

The manufacturer's authorised representative in the EU is Springer
Nature Customer Service Centre GmbH, Europaplatz 3, 69115 Heidelberg,
Germany. If you have any concerns regarding our products, please
contact ProductSafety@springernature.com

Printed and bound by CPI Group (UK) Ltd, Croydon, CR0 4YY
05/10/2026
02228122-0002